Endocrine Diseases

Guest Editor

RAMIRO E. TORIBIO, DVM, MS, PhD

VETERINARY CLINICS OF NORTH AMERICA: EQUINE PRACTICE

www.vetequine.theclinics.com

Consulting Editor
ANTHONY SIMON TURNER, BVSc, MS

April 2011 • Volume 27 • Number 1

SAUNDERS an imprint of ELSEVIER, Inc.

W.B. SAUNDERS COMPANY
A Division of Elsevier Inc.

1600 John F. Kennedy Boulevard • Suite 1800 • Philadelphia, Pennsylvania 19103

http://www.vetequine.theclinics.com

VETERINARY CLINICS OF NORTH AMERICA: EQUINE PRACTICE Volume 27, Number 1

April 2011 ISSN 0749-0739, ISBN-13: 978-1-4557-0518-4

Editor: John Vassallo; j.vassallo@elsevier.com
Developmental Editor: Donald Mumford

Veterinary Clinics of North America: Equine Practice (ISSN 0749-0739) is published in April, August, and December by Elsevier Inc., 360 Park Avenue South, New York, NY 10010-1710. Business and Editorial Offices: 1600 John F. Kennedy Blvd., Suite 1800, Philadelphia, PA 19103-2899. Subscription prices are $238.00 per year (domestic individuals), $373.00 per year (domestic institutions), $117.00 per year (domestic students/residents), $277.00 per year (Canadian individuals), $466.00 per year (Canadian institutions), $320.00 per year (international individuals), $466.00 per year (international institutions), and $159.00 per year (international and Canadian students/residents). To receive student/resident rate, orders must be accompanied by name of affiliated institution, date of term, and the signature of program/residency coordinator on institution letterhead. Orders will be billed at individual rate until proof of status is received. Foreign air speed delivery is included in all *Clinics* subscription prices. All prices are subject to change without notice. **POSTMASTER:** Send address changes to *Veterinary Clinics of North America: Equine Practice*, 3251 Riverport Lane, Maryland Heights, MO 63043. Customer Service (orders, claims, online, change of address): Elsevier Health Sciences Division, Subscription Customer Service, 3251 Riverport Lane, Maryland Heights, MO 63043. Tel: 1-800-654-2452 (U.S. and Canada); 314-447-8871 (outside U.S. and Canada). Fax: 314-447-8029. E-mail: journalscustomer service-usa@elsevier.com (for print support); E-mail: journalsonlinesupport-usa@elsevier (for online support).

Reprints. For copies of 100 or more of articles in this publication, please contact the Commercial Reprints Department, Elsevier Inc., 360 Park Avenue South, New York, NY 10010-1710. Tel.: 212-633-3812; Fax: 212-462-1935; E-mail: reprints@elsevier.com.

Veterinary Clinics of North America: Equine Practice is covered in *MEDLINE/PubMed (Index Medicus), Excerpta Medica, Current Contents/Agriculture, Biology and Environmental Sciences, and ISI.*

Printed and bound by CPI Group (UK) Ltd, Croydon, CR0 4YY

Transferred to Digital Print 2011

Contributors

CONSULTING EDITOR

ANTHONY SIMON TURNER, BVSc, MS
Diplomate, American College of Veterinary Surgeons; Professor, Department of Clinical Sciences, College of Veterinary Medicine and Biomedical Sciences, Colorado State University, Fort Collins, Colorado

GUEST EDITOR

RAMIRO E. TORIBIO, DVM, MS, PhD
Diplomate, American College of Veterinary Internal Medicine; Associate Professor, Department of Veterinary Clinical Sciences, College of Veterinary Medicine, The Ohio State University, Columbus, Ohio

AUTHORS

ROSA J. BARSNICK, Dr. med vet, MS
Diplomate, American College of Veterinary Internal Medicine; Pferdeklinik in Kirchheim (Kirchheim Equine Hospital), Kirchheim/Teck, Germany

MICHELLE H. BARTON, DVM, PhD
Diplomate, American College of Veterinary Internal Medicine; Fuller E. Callaway Endowed Chair and Professor of Large Animal Internal Medicine, Department of Large Animal Medicine, University of Georgia College of Veterinary Medicine, Athens, Georgia

BABETTA A. BREUHAUS, DVM, PhD
Diplomate, American College of Veterinary Internal Medicine; Associate Professor of Equine Medicine, Department of Clinical Sciences, North Carolina State University, Raleigh, North Carolina

TIM J. EVANS, DVM, MS, PhD
Diplomate, American College of Theriogenology; Diplomate, American Board of Veterinary Toxicology; Associate Professor, Department of Veterinary Pathobiology; Toxicology Section Leader, Veterinary Medical Diagnostic Laboratory, College of Veterinary Medicine, Columbia, Missouri

NICHOLAS FRANK, DVM, PhD
Diplomate, American College of Veterinary Internal Medicine; Associate Professor and Section Chief of Large Animal Medicine, Department of Large Animal Clinical Sciences, University of Tennessee College of Veterinary Medicine, Knoxville, Tennessee; Associate Professor of Large Animal Medicine, Division of Medicine, School of Veterinary Medicine and Science, University of Nottingham, Leicestershire, United Kingdom

KELSEY A. HART, DVM, PhD
Diplomate, American College of Veterinary Internal Medicine; Assistant Professor of Large Animal Internal Medicine, Department of Large Animal Medicine, University of Georgia College of Veterinary Medicine, Athens, Georgia

SAMUEL D.A. HURCOMBE, BVMS, MS
Diplomate, American College of Veterinary Internal Medicine; Diplomate, American College of Veterinary Emergency and Critical Care; Clinical Assistant Professor in Equine Emergency and Critical Care, Department of Veterinary Clinical Sciences, Galbreath Equine Center, The Ohio State University, Columbus, Ohio

DIANNE MCFARLANE, DVM, PhD
Diplomate, American College of Veterinary Internal Medicine (Large Animal); Department of Physiological Sciences, Oklahoma State University, Stillwater, Oklahoma

KENNETH HARRINGTON MCKEEVER, PhD, FACSM
Professor of Equine Exercise Physiology; Associate Director for Research, Equine Science Center, Department of Animal Science, School of Environmental and Biological Sciences, Rutgers, The State University of New Jersey, New Brunswick, New Jersey

HAROLD C. MCKENZIE III, DVM, MS
Diplomate, American College of Veterinary Internal Medicine; Associate Professor of Equine Medicine, Marion duPont Scott Equine Medical Center, Virginia/Maryland Regional College of Veterinary Medicine, Virginia Polytechnic and State University, Leesburg, Virginia

HAROLD C. SCHOTT II, DVM, PhD
Diplomate, American College of Veterinary Internal Medicine; Professor and Equine Division Head, Department of Large Animal Clinical Sciences, College of Veterinary Medicine, Veterinary Medical Center, Michigan State University, East Lansing, Michigan

ALLISON J. STEWART, BVSc (Hons), MS
Diplomate, American College of Veterinary Internal Medicine; Diplomate, American College of Veterinary Emergency and Critical Care; Associate Professor of Equine Internal Medicine, Department of Clinical Sciences, John Thomas Vaughan Large Animal Teaching Hospital, College of Veterinary Medicine, Auburn University, Auburn, Alabama

RAMIRO E. TORIBIO, DVM, MS, PhD
Diplomate, American College of Veterinary Internal Medicine; Associate Professor, Department of Veterinary Clinical Sciences, College of Veterinary Medicine, The Ohio State University, Columbus, Ohio

Contents

Preface: Endocrine Diseases xi

Ramiro E. Toribio

Hypothalamic-Pituitary Gland Axis Function and Dysfunction in Horses 1

Samuel D.A. Hurcombe

Hypothalamic-pituitary (HP) dysfunction has been documented in a limited capacity in horses and foals associated with critical illness, stress, and pain. This article reviews species-specific details of anatomy, function, hormones, receptors, and testing of the HP axis in the horse. A discussion of critical care medicine relevant to HP dysfunction in the horse with some reference to current understanding in human medicine is made, focusing primarily on current and relevant literature. A brief mention of other conditions described in human and veterinary medicine is also provided for reference only, such as syndrome of inappropriate antidiuretic hormone secretion and other conditions.

Adrenocortical Insufficiency in Horses and Foals 19

Kelsey A. Hart and Michelle H. Barton

The adrenal cortices produce various steroid hormones that play vital roles in several physiologic processes. Although permanent adrenocortical insufficiency is rare in all species, emerging evidence in both human and equine medicine suggests that transient reversible adrenocortical dysfunction resulting in cortisol insufficiency frequently develops during critical illness. This syndrome is termed relative adrenal insufficiency (RAI) or critical illness–related corticosteroid insufficiency (CIRCI) and can contribute substantially to morbidity and mortality associated with the primary disease. This review discusses the mechanisms, diagnosis, and clinical consequences of adrenocortical insufficiency, with particular focus on the current understanding of RAI/CIRCI in horses and foals.

Endocrine Dysregulation in Critically Ill Foals and Horses 35

Ramiro E. Toribio

Critical illness challenges many endocrine homeostatic systems to overcome diseases, stress, and hostile conditions that threaten survival. Coordinated and consecutive responses by the autonomic nervous system, endocrine metabolic adaptations to mobilize and conserve energy and electrolytes, cardiovascular adjustments to maintain organ perfusion, and immunomodulation to overcome infections and inflammation are required. Because most admissions to equine intensive care units are related to horses with gastrointestinal disease and septic foals, most endocrine information during critical disease are generated from these populations. This article presents an overview on endocrine responses to critical illness in horses and foals and also some comparative information.

Endocrinology of the Equine Neonate Energy Metabolism in Health and Critical Illness 49

Rosa J. Barsnick and Ramiro E. Toribio

Hormonal control of energy metabolism plays an important role in the peripartum development and health of the equine neonate. The endocrine system is generally functional at birth, but the maturation of the endocrine system and the associated energy metabolism is delayed and continues during the postnatal period. The energy metabolism is susceptible to disturbances, especially when illness occurs. Hormones involved in energy metabolism have recently been studied in healthy and critically ill neonatal foals. Understanding these hormones in the equine neonate will support appropriate therapeutic interventions as well as prognostic assessment of the sick foal.

Equine Hyperlipidemias 59

Harold C. McKenzie III

Hyperlipidemia is the presence of elevated lipid concentrations in the blood and is associated with periods of negative energy balance and physiologic stress. In increased concentrations, circulating lipids typically occur in the triglyceride form, which may interfere with numerous normal physiologic functions, particularly by reducing insulin sensitivity. Although the hyperlipidemia risk is greatest in ponies, miniature horses, and donkeys, all equids are at risk if they are in a situation involving negative energy balance. The sedentary lifestyle of many modern horses and the frequent feeding of high-carbohydrate diets contribute substantially to the risk of excessive fat mobilization and the development of hyperlipidemias.

Equine Metabolic Syndrome 73

Nicholas Frank

The concept of an equine metabolic syndrome (EMS) was first proposed in 2002. This concept has developed over time, and EMS was recently described in a consensus statement released by the American College of Veterinary Internal Medicine. In human medicine, metabolic syndrome (MetS) refers to a set of risk factors that predict the risk of cardiovascular disease, including obesity, glucose intolerance and insulin resistance (IR), dyslipidemia, microalbuminuria, and hypertension. EMS shares some of the features of MetS, including increased adiposity, hyperinsulinemia, IR, but differs in that laminitis is the primary disease of interest.

Equine Pituitary Pars Intermedia Dysfunction 93

Dianne McFarlane

Equine pituitary pars intermedia dysfunction (PPID), also known as equine Cushing's syndrome, is a widely recognized disease of aged horses. Over the past two decades, the aged horse population has expanded significantly and in addition, client awareness of PPID has increased. As a result, there has been an increase in both diagnostic testing and treatment of the disease. This review focuses on the pathophysiology and clinical syndrome, as well as advances in diagnostic testing and treatment of PPID, with an emphasis on those findings that are new since the excellent comprehensive review by Schott in 2002.

Disorders of the Equine Thyroid Gland **115**

Babetta A. Breuhaus

Regulatory control of the thyroid gland in horses is similar to other species. Clinical signs of hypothyroidism in adult horses are minimal. Several drugs and physiologic and pathophysiological states can cause circulating thyroid hormone concentrations to be low without actual pathology of the thyroid gland. Thus, nonthyroidal factors must be ruled out before a diagnosis of hypothyroidism can be made. Thyroid hormone supplementation seems to be well tolerated, even in euthyroid horses. Neonatal foals have very high circulating thyroid hormone concentrations, and deficiencies result in significant clinical signs. Unlike in adults, two syndromes of hypothyroidism are well described in foals.

Disorders of Calcium and Phosphate Metabolism in Horses **129**

Ramiro E. Toribio

Calcium and phosphate have structural and nonstructural functions, and their concentrations in the extracellular compartment are affected by the physiologic status of the animal as well as diseases. Important progress in understanding calcium and phosphorus metabolism in healthy and diseased horses and foals has been made in recent years. For example, several studies have confirmed that hypocalcemia is frequent in horses with gastrointestinal disease and that calcium endocrine dysregulation is associated with survival in foals. One critical point in the homeostasis of these minerals is their interaction and interdependence with other ions, including potassium and magnesium. In this review, the author provides a clinical overview on disorders of calcium and phosphate in the horse.

Magnesium Disorders in Horses **149**

Allison J. Stewart

Magnesium (Mg) is an essential macroelement that is required for cellular energy-dependent reactions involving adenosine triphosphate and for the regulation of calcium channel function. Subclinical hypomagnesemia is common in critically ill humans and animals and increases the severity of the systemic inflammatory response syndrome; worsens the systemic response to endotoxins; and can lead to ileus, cardiac arrhythmias, refractory hypokalemia, and hypocalcemia. This article discusses the clinical signs, consequences, and treatment of hypomagnesemia in horses and describes the association of Mg and endotoxemia, insulin resistance, and brain injury.

The Endocrine Disruptive Effects of Ergopeptine Alkaloids on Pregnant Mares **165**

Tim J. Evans

During equine gestation, ergopeptine alkaloid exposure is not uncommon, and pregnant mares are particularly sensitive to the endocrine disruptive effects of these compounds on lactogenesis and steroidogenesis.

Agalactia, prolonged gestation, abortion, dystocia, and placental and fetal abnormalities are all clinical manifestations of changes in the endocrine milieu induced by the ingestion of ergopeptine alkaloid-contaminated feedstuffs by mares during late gestation. An understanding of the endocrine disruptive effects of gestational exposure to ergopeptine alkaloids is necessary for the diagnosis of potential exposures to these compounds and for effective prophylaxis and therapy.

Water Homeostasis and Diabetes Insipidus in Horses **175**

Harold C. Schott II

Diabetes insipidus (DI) is a rare disorder of horses characterized by profound polyuria and polydipsia (PU/PD), which can be caused by loss of production of arginine vasopressin (AVP). This condition is termed neurogenic or central DI. DI may also develop with absence or loss of AVP receptors or activity on the basolateral membrane of collecting-duct epithelial cells. This condition is termed nephrogenic DI. Equine clinicians may differentiate true DI from more common causes of PU/PD by a systematic diagnostic approach. DI may not be a correctable disorder, and supportive care of affected horses requires an adequate water source.

Endocrine Alterations in the Equine Athlete: An Update **197**

Kenneth Harrington McKeever

Horses spend most of their day eating, standing, and occasionally exercising. Exercise can range from running in a pasture to athletic training. Under resting conditions, horses easily maintain the internal environment. The performance of work or exercise is a major physiologic challenge, a disturbance to homeostasis that invokes an integrative response from multiple organ systems. The response to exercise involves endocrine and neuroendocrine signaling associated with the short-term and adaptive control of many systems. The coordinated control of multiple physiologic variables is essential for achieving regulation to maintain the integrity of the internal environment of the body.

Index **219**

FORTHCOMING ISSUES

August 2011

Regenerative Medicine

Matthew C. Stewart, BVSc, PhD,
and Allison A. Stewart, DVM, MS,
Guest Editors

December 2011

Clinical Neurology

Thomas J. Divers, DVM,
and Amy L. Johnson, DVM,
Guest Editors

April 2012

Therapeutic Farriery

Stephen E. O'Grady, DVM, MRCVS, and
Andrew Parks, VetMB, MS, MRCVS,
Guest Editors

RECENT ISSUES

December 2010

Pain in Horses: Physiology, Pathophysiology and Therapeutic Implications

William W. Muir, DVM, PhD, *Guest Editor*

August 2010

Advances in Laminitis, Part II

Christopher C. Pollitt, BVSc, PhD,
Guest Editor

April 2010

Advances in Laminitis, Part I

Christopher C. Pollitt, BVSc, PhD,
Guest Editor

RELATED INTEREST

Veterinary Clinics of North America: Small Animal Practice
March 2010 (Vol. 40, No. 2)
Obesity, Diabetes, and Adrenal Disorders
Thomas K. Graves, DVM, PhD, *Guest Editor*

Preface
Endocrine Diseases

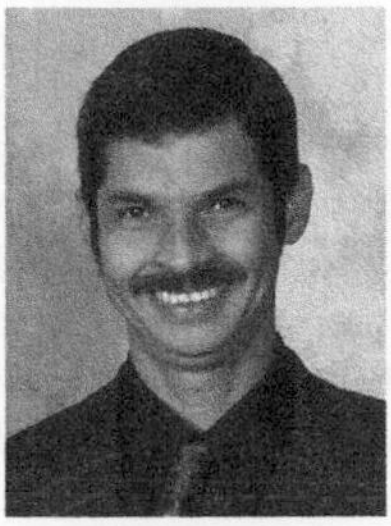

Ramiro E. Toribio, DVM, MS, PhD
Guest Editor

I feel honored to have the opportunity to share with the readers of the *Veterinary Clinics of North America: Equine Practice* this issue dedicated to endocrine diseases of horses and foals. It is my hope that we meet your expectations in content and applicable information.

For decades, most interest in equine endocrinology has been focused on reproductive function, while insight to other hormonal systems has remained limited. As our understanding of equine endocrine diseases expands, there is more recognition that a number of hormonal disorders are interlinked to the function of most body systems. It is also evident that acute or chronic equine diseases can disturb endocrine homeostasis, leading to additional complications. This knowledge has clinical relevance as interventional decisions are largely based on how well we comprehend equine pathophysiology, from inflammation to acid-base and electrolyte disorders, but also pharmacology and clinical endocrinology. This becomes clear, for example, when treating mares with fescue toxicosis, horses with pituitary pars intermedia dysfunction and metabolic syndrome, or foals with sepsis and hypotension, where all this information needs to be integrated.

In the previous issue dedicated to equine endocrine diseases, edited by Drs Nat Messer and Philip Johnson (August 2002), the contributors did a comprehensive review on endocrine pathologies. Since then, our understanding of specific equine endocrinopathies has improved considerably. It is worth mentioning that collaborations between academic institutions and the private sector deserve some of the credit for advancing this field.

Endocrine disorders can be primary in nature as those affecting the pituitary and thyroid glands, or secondary as those the result of systemic inflammation, chronic disease, abnormal mineral metabolism, organ dysfunction (eg, renal failure), or poor management (obesity). Conditions such as pituitary pars intermedia dysfunction, hypothyroidism, equine metabolic syndrome, endocrine dysregulation in critically ill

Vet Clin Equine 27 (2011) xi–xii
doi:10.1016/j.cveq.2011.01.003 vetequine.theclinics.com
0749-0739/11/$ – see front matter

foals, disorders of mineral homeostasis, and the effect of exercise on various hormones are presented in detail.

It is apparent by the quality of the articles included in this issue that the field of equine clinical endocrinology has taken major strides. As discussed by Nick Frank, weight loss and diet management are practical measures to treat horses with metabolic syndrome, a condition that greatly results from excessive caloric intake, leading to a deregulated energy metabolism and a pro-inflammatory state. The discovery that there are seasonal variations on pro-opiomelanocortin-derived peptides in horses, and that testing in the wrong time of the year (eg, autumn) could result in misdiagnosis of pituitary pars intermedia dysfunction, was an important contribution by Dianne McFarlane. The overviews by Sam Hurcombe on hypothalamic and pituitary function, and by Kelsey Hart on adrenocortical function, give clinical relevance to the hypothalamic-pituitary-adrenal gland axis in critical illness. Integration between hypothalamic and renal physiology, in particular in the context of water conservation and diabetes insipidus, is eloquently described by Hal Schott. Rosa Barsnick and Harold McKenzie provide great reviews on energy metabolism in neonates and adult horses. Clinical aspects of magnesium, calcium, and phosphorus dysregulation in different pathological conditions are presented by Allison Stewart and Ramiro Toribio.

To the contributors of this issue, your time and effort to share your expertise with the readers are deeply appreciated. To John Vassallo and Simon Turner, many thanks for considering me for this task. To those that, in one way or another, have supported my professional endeavors, from Panama to Argentina, Costa Rica, and the United States, I am indebted to you.

Ramiro E. Toribio, DVM, MS, PhD
Department of Veterinary Clinical Sciences
College of Veterinary Medicine
The Ohio State University
601 Vernon Tharp Street
Columbus, OH 43210, USA

E-mail address:
Toribio.1@osu.edu

Hypothalamic-Pituitary Gland Axis Function and Dysfunction in Horses

Samuel D.A. Hurcombe, BVMS, MS

KEYWORDS

• Horse • Vasopressin • ACTH • Hypothalamus • Pituitary

The importance of hypothalamic-pituitary (HP) interactions in mammals is well recognized. In health, this highly regulated and integrated system is involved in the homeostasis of intermediary metabolism, immune responses, body temperature, hunger, thirst, growth, reproduction, and cardiovascular function, to name a few functions. The hypothalamus coordinates many hormonal and behavioral circadian rhythms and complex neuroendocrine inputs/outputs and behaviors, including level/content of consciousness, mood, instinctive behaviors (eg, maternal), and feeding.

The HP axis is critical for evoking the biologic responses to internal and external stressors, where activation of both the HP axis and sympathetic nervous systems results in adrenocortical and adrenomedullary secretion of corticosteroids and catecholamines, respectively. These biologically active messengers modulate important responses, such as heightened alertness, glucose mobilization/use, vasomotor tone, cardiac output to improve delivery of metabolic fuel (notably glucose and oxygen), and removal of metabolic waste (lactic acid and carbon dioxide) during times of physiologic and pathologic stress. Like many biologic systems, there is a limit and capacity for these responses to work and when they are reached or exceeded, HP axis dysfunction results in serious compromises that can lead to increased morbidity and mortality.

Dysfunctions of any of the multiple HP axes can modify many physiologic functions and, if severe, can be life threatening. Individual and species differences exist regarding HP activation, stimulation, hormonal secretion, and effector organ responses. Disorders of the hypothalamic-pituitary-adrenal axis (HPAA) are better described in the human and comparative literature, with a paucity of available information in the horse. In humans, HPAA dysregulation related to sepsis/septic shock, traumatic central diabetes insipidus, and syndrome of inappropriate antidiuretic hormone secretion (SIADH) are examples of diseases that affect one or more components of the HP system. Although the HPAA has been the most studied HP axis in the horse, when compared with other species, available information is lacking.

Department of Veterinary Clinical Sciences, Galbreath Equine Center, The Ohio State University, 601 Vernon L Tharp Street, Columbus, OH 43210, USA

E-mail address: Samuel.Hurcombe@cvm.osu.edu

Vet Clin Equine 27 (2011) 1–17
doi:10.1016/j.cveq.2010.12.006 vetequine.theclinics.com

The focus of this article is primarily on the anatomy, physiology, and pathophysiology of the HPAA in horses with emphasis on arginine vasopressin (AVP), corticotropin-releasing hormone (CRH) (or corticoliberin), and their downstream response by the pituitary and adrenal glands. A discussion of the HP response to critical illness of humans and animals, from experimental and clinical research, is provided. Other HP axes include the hypothalamic-pituitary-thyroid (HPT) axis with thyrotropin-releasing hormone (TRH) and thyroid-stimulating hormone (TSH) and the hypothalamic-pituitary growth hormone (GH) axis with growth hormone–releasing hormone (GHRH) and GH. HP axes involved in reproduction are not discussed. Pathologic conditions associated with HPT and GH axes relevant to energy metabolism and skeletal development are discussed by Barsnick elsewhere in this issue. A complete discussion of the adrenal gland and its interactions with the hypothalamus and pituitary gland in health and disease can be found in the article by Hart and Barton elsewhere in this issue. Similarly, the article by McFarlane includes a thorough discussion of pituitary pars intermedia dysfunction (PPID).

ANATOMY

The hypothalamus, located in the ventral diencephalon, is a complex anatomic and organizational structure, with many nuclei (preoptic, supraoptic, paraventricular, anterior, suprachiasmatic, dorsomedial, ventromedial, and arcuate nuclei) and areas involved with control of body temperature, energy metabolism, blood pressure regulation (water and sodium), stress response, reproduction, and environment integration. The hypothalamus is highly connected to other higher structures of the central nervous system (eg, limbic system) and with the pituitary gland downstream. Because of its unconscious and regulatory functions, the hypothalamus is a major component of the autonomic nervous system.

In vertebrates, the pituitary gland is divided into 3 distinct lobes: pars nervosa (neurohypophysis or posterior pituitary), pars intermedia (intermediate lobe), and pars distalis (adenohypophysis or anterior pituitary), each having a unique role in endocrine homeostasis. In the equine species, the adenohypophysis surrounds the other pituitary lobes.

Hypothalamic neuroendocrine neurons control pituitary gland function. Magnocellular neurons in the paraventricular and supraoptic nuclei synthesize AVP and oxytocin, which are transported (hypothalamic-hypophyseal tract) by unmyelinated axons and stored in secretory vesicles in the nerve terminals (Herring bodies) in the neurohypophysis. Parvocellular neurons in various hypothalamic nuclei make direct connection to blood vessels in the median eminence (hypothalamic-hypophyseal portal system) to release factors that control the synthesis and secretion of hormones by the adenohypophysis.[1] These hypothalamic factors include CRH, TRH, and AVP. Although the median eminence is part of the central nervous system, it is strategically located outside the blood-brain barrier to mediate a rapid pituitary response to factors present in portal and systemic circulation.

Neurons from other hypothalamic nuclei and areas (arcuate nucleus and preoptic area) also connect to the portal system to regulate hormones involved with somatic, metabolic, and reproductive functions, including GHRH to release GH, TRH to increase TSH and prolactin release, gonadotropin-releasing hormone to increase follicle-stimulating hormone and luteinizing hormone secretion, somatostatin to inhibit GH secretion, and dopamine (DA) to inhibit prolactin and TSH release. Reproductive hormones are not discussed in this review. The cells of the pars intermedia are primarily controlled by hypothalamic TRH stimulation and dopaminergic inhibition (see the article by McFarlane elsewhere in this issue).

HPAA DYNAMICS

The HPAA responses are essential for life and have been investigated in the equine fetus,[2–4] preterm foal, and neonatal foal.[5] In healthy, term foals, increases in AVP; adrenocorticotropic hormone (ACTH), also known as corticotropin or adrenocorticotropin; and cortisol concentrations occur as a physiologic adaptation to hypovolemia and hypotension,[6] indicating that at birth foals have a functional HPAA.

The secretion of inhibitory or stimulatory endocrine factors by a higher endocrine center (hypothalamus) controls the response of its target organ (pituitary gland), which releases hormones with various critical functions. In addition, these hormones inhibit (negative feedback) or stimulate (positive feedback) the higher controlling center to create an endocrine homeostatic system.

Stimulation of the HP axis starts with excitation of the hypothalamus by different inputs. CRH and AVP are released into the pituitary portal system to increase ACTH secretion by the pituitary corticotrophs. AVP is considered the main secretagogue for ACTH in adult horses,[1,7–11] late-term equine fetuses, and foals.[2–4] AVP is also responsible for the short-term fluctuations in ACTH concentrations.[12] This has been confirmed in exercising horses where CRH seemed to play a minor regulatory role on ACTH secretion. ACTH in turn controls the secretion of cortisol by the adrenal cortex (zona fasciculata). Cortisol has direct and indirect pathways to negatively feedback on the hypothalamus, limbic system, and pituitary gland. This attenuates or decreases the release of CRH, AVP, and ACTH. It seems that the glucocorticoid negative feedback effect on AVP secretion is less robust than that for CRH because AVP secreting neurons are less sensitive to glucocorticoids.[1] Therefore, the reciprocal interactions among CRH, AVP, ACTH, and cortisol, rather than one signaling hormone, modulate HPAA dynamics.[13]

Recently, Keenan and colleagues[13] described the complex feedback and feedforward interactions between AVP, CRH, ACTH, and cortisol in healthy horses. Simply stated, they showed that hypocortisolemia amplifies CRH and AVP secretion when mean cortisol feedback concentrations decrease 0% to 25% and both CRH and AVP synergize in evoking ACTH secretion. There was also an autostimulation/autoinhibition mechanism for the hypothalamic peptides independent of cortisol concentration, where reduced feedback by CRH of 0% to 25% and AVP by 50% augments both CRH and AVP secretion.[13]

ACTH binds receptors in the adrenal gland cortex to stimulate sterold synthesis and secretion via the adenylate cyclase second messenger system. In the mitochondria, cholesterol is converted to pregnenolone. Through the action of 3β-hydroxysteroid dehydrogenase and 17α-hydroxylase, pregnenolone is biotransformed to progesterone and 17α-hydroxyprogesterone, the precursors of aldosterone and cortisol, respectively.[14] The principle function of ACTH is to stimulate cortisol release and, to a lesser extent, also aldosterone.

In addition to its function in the adenohypophysis, AVP is transported through the hypothalamic-neurohypophyseal tract to the neurohypophysis to be released in systemic circulation to act on the renal collecting ducts to retain water and on smooth muscle cells of the vasculature to induce constriction.

HORMONES

Corticotropin-Releasing Hormone

In horses, CRH is a 41-amino acid peptide derived from a 195-amino acid preprohormone (196 amino acids in humans and dogs). CRH is synthesized by parvocellular neurons in the paraventricular nucleus of the hypothalamus and released by neurosecretory terminals into the primary capillary plexus of the HP portal system to stimulate ACTH secretion.[15] Factors that affect CRH release include stress and cortisol concentrations. CRH is also produced by the placenta in late gestation where it seems to determine pregnancy length and parturition.

Arginine Vasopressin

AVP is a 9-amino acid peptide synthesized by the magnocellular neurons of the paraventricular and supraoptic nuclei of the hypothalamus. Because AVP has a short half-life in humans (5–15 minutes), blood concentrations reflect recent hormonal release.[16] AVP has several physiologic functions, including water reabsorption by renal collecting tubules and vasoconstriction. Major stimuli for AVP secretion are controlled by osmotic and nonosmotic factors. Plasma hypertonicity stimulates hypothalamic osmoreceptors to release AVP. This system is very sensitive and increases in plasma tonicity of 1% to 2% can induce AVP release. Volume depletion (hypotension) is sensed by baroreceptors in the left atrium, aortic sinus, and carotid sinus. A decrease in blood volume of 5% to 10% results in rapid AVP release.[17]

Growth Hormone–Releasing Hormone and Somatostatin

GHRH is a neurosecretory hormone of the hypothalamic arcuate nucleus that is transported to the adenohypophysis to stimulate release of GH. GHRH stimulates GH release through interaction with the GHRH receptor on somatotrophs via G_s-protein/cyclic adenosine monophosphate and inositol triphosphate/diacylglycerol signal transduction. GHRH is secreted in a pulsatile manner and of critical importance for postnatal growth, bone growth, and intermediary metabolism.

Somatostatin, or GH inhibitory hormone, is a peptide produced by hypothalamic neurons as well as cells in the stomach, intestine, and pancreas. Similar to GHRH, somatostatin is released into the HP portal system and its main function is to inhibit the secretion of GH and TSH. Somatostatin and insulinlike growth factor 1 are the main components of the negative feedback system for GH release.

Thyrotropin-Releasing Hormone

TRH is synthesized by neurons of the paraventricular nucleus from a polypeptide precursor that is cleaved by proteases to the active tripeptide hormone. TRH stimulates the secretion TSH (thyrotropin) by the pituitary thyrotrophs. In turn, TSH increases thyroid hormone release from the thyroid gland. Increased metabolic demand and metabolic rate activate the HPT axis, leading to increases in TRH, TSH, and thyroid hormones. TRH also acts in other pituitary cell types. For example, TRH stimulates the secretion of prolactin by the lactotrophs, ACTH by the corticotrophs, and GH by the somatrotrophs. In the melanotrophs of the pars intermedia, TRH promotes the synthesis and secretion of proopiomelanocortin (POMC) peptide, in particular ACTH. These effects seem to be primarily mediated by the TRH's ability to decrease DA secretion. DA is a cell inhibitory factor in the pituitary pars distalis and pars intermedia. TRH release is suppressed by TSH, thyroid hormones (endogenous and exogenous) and glucocorticoid (endogenous and exogenous) through a negative feedback system.

Dopamine

The functions of DA in the pituitary gland are by far inhibitory. Dopaminergic neurons, also known as tuberoinfundibular DA neurons, are primarily located in the arcuate nucleus of the hypothalamus. Axons from tuberoinfundibular DA neurons project into the HP portal system to inhibit prolactin, GH, and TSH secretion. These neurons also make contact with melanotrophs in the pars intermedia to inhibit the synthesis and secretion of POMC peptides, including ACTH and α-melanocyte–stimulating hormone (α-MSH). Basic knowledge of the dopaminergic system is important to understand the pathogenesis of equine PPID, tall fescue toxicosis, and their treatment.

Proopiomelanocortin

POMC is a precursor polypeptide with 267 amino acid residues. The *POMC* gene encodes a polypeptide hormone precursor that undergoes extensive, tissue-specific, post-translational processing via cleavage by subtilisin-like enzymes (prohormone convertases). There are 8 potential cleavage sites within the polypeptide precursor, and, depending on tissue type and the available convertase, processing may yield as many as 10 biologically active peptides involved in diverse cellular functions. POMC is primarily expressed in the corticotrophs of the pars distalis and melanotrophs of the pars intermedia. POMC processing differs between the pars distalis and pars intermedia of horses. ACTH, beta-lipotropic hormone (β-LPH), gamma-lipotropic hormone (γ-LPH), and β-endorphin (β-END) are the main peptides in the pars distalis, whereas ACTH, β-LPH, and α-MSH are primarily produced in the pars intermedia. ACTH undergoes further cleavage to yield additional active hormones (see discussion of ACTH later).

Adrenocorticotropic Hormone

ACTH is a 39-amino acid peptide produced in the pituitary pars distalis from post-translational processing of POMC. ACTH main function is to stimulate glucocorticoid production by the adrenal cortex. ACTH is metabolized to $ACTH_{1\text{-}13}$, which is identical to α-MSH. Corticotropin-like peptide is another major ACTH metabolite, which represents $ACTH_{18\text{-}39}$. α-MSH, β-LPH, and corticotropin-like peptide are the main fragments in the pars intermedia, with ACTH production being minimal. DA has inhibitory effects on the synthesis and secretion of POMC peptides, including ACTH. DA agonists are used to decrease ACTH production in horses with PPID.

β-Endorphin

β-END is a 31-amino acid peptide generated from cell-specific cleavage of POMC. It is an agonist of various endogenous opioid receptors ($\mu_{1,2,3}$; $\delta_{1,2}$; and $\kappa_{1,2,3}$), but μ_1 is considered the main receptor by which β-END (and morphine) mediates analgesia, sedation, and narcosis.

α-Melanocyte–Stimulating Hormone

α-MSH is a post-translational product of POMC cleavage in the pars intermedia. It has important roles in the regulation of appetite and sexual behavior, and it is a prime regulator for melanin production by melanocytes in skin and hair. Plasma α-MSH has been measured in horses in the context of diagnosing pars intermedia dysfunction (Cushing disease) and, like ACTH, its concentrations are affected by season.[18]

RECEPTORS

AVP exerts its effects through 5 potential receptors, named V_1, V_2, V_3, oxytocin-receptor, and a purinergic (P_2) receptor. These are G-protein transmembrane receptors found in specific tissues. In horses, the 3 AVP receptors are the likely mediators of the responses to endogenous and exogenous AVP and analogs.

V_1

These receptors mediate the pressor actions of AVP on vascular smooth muscle. V_1 receptors are also located in the liver, testis, brain, and renal medulla. V_1 receptor agonism activates $G_{q/11}$ protein signaling, leading to the release of second messengers (inositol triphosphate and diacylglycerol), which in turn activate protein kinase C to increase intracellular calcium flux.[19] This sequence of events increases vasomotor tone and vasoconstriction.

V_2

These receptors are located in the renal collecting ducts. Through cyclic adenosine monophosphate signaling, V_2 receptor activation increases the translocation of aquaporin-2 channels from intracellular vesicles into the cell membrane of the tubular epithelial cells. Without the effect of AVP, urinary osmolality can be as low as 50 mOsm/L by continued sodium reabsorption without water reabsorption.[20] Other effects include increasing von Willebrand factor production and release from endothelial stores.

V_3

V_3 receptors (also termed V_1b receptors) are primarily located in the corticotrophs of the adenohypophysis and upon AVP stimulation there is a rapid release of ACTH into systemic circulation.

CRH Receptors

Two types of CRH receptors have been identified, namely CRH-1 and CRH-2. CRH-1 is the main receptor in s populating the pituitary corticotrophs and its activation increases POMC expression and ACTH production.

TRH Receptors

TRH receptors are present in the thyrotrophs and lactotrophs of the pars distails and melanotrophs in the pars intermedia.

TSH Receptors

Receptors for TSH are primarily located in the follicular cells of the thyroid gland where, on activation, lead to increased synthesis of triiodothyronine and thyroxine.

TESTING THE HYPOTHALAMIC-PITUITARY AXIS

Testing of HP function can be done by measuring hormonal concentrations or by performing dynamic tests. Hormone concentrations can be measured in systemic venous blood, pituitary venous blood, saliva, and urine.[21] Determination of systemic blood hormone concentrations is the most commonly used method. Many hormones are released in small amounts (eg, pg/dL to ng/dL), have similar amino acid sequences (eg, AVP and oxytocin), or are different between species. Therefore, to determine their blood concentrations, sensitive and specific methods, such as radioimmunoassays, immunoradiometric assays, immunochemiluminometric assays, and ELISAs, are used. Be aware that there are species differences between hormones and that assay validation is necessary before making any interpretation of the data.

Measurement of AVP and other small peptides requires appropriate sample handling and expedient analysis because plasma proteases may result in hormone degradation in vitro. Several studies advocate the use of protease inhibitors, such as aprotinin, to preserve sample integrity especially when processing may be delayed.

Assessing HP or HPAA function generally requires stimulation or suppression of the axis via the administration of a specific hormone. For example, ACTH administration stimulates the zona fasciculata to secrete cortisol, where ACTH is the administered stimulator and cortisol is the target organ measured response. This indicates an actual response to provocation, which is superior to single random sample hormone concentration determinations in the assessment of axis functionality. A thorough discussion of the methodology, utility, and pitfalls of the ACTH and TRH stimulation tests is covered in the articles by Breuhaus and McFarlane elsewhere in this issue.

A well-accepted test for assessing the HPAA in humans is the CRF (corticorelin) challenging test. In addition, this test is for differentiating whether or not high blood ACTH concentrations are from the pituitary gland or an ectopic source. A recent study in horses evaluated the effect of ovine CRH on plasma and salivary total cortisol responses and found that for the same challenge dose of ovine CRH, salivary cortisol concentrations peaked 5 times higher compared with baseline whereas plasma cortisol concentrations increased up to 1.5 times higher compared with baseline.[21] The CRH stimulation test has been used in calves with chronic activation of the HPAA as a result of external stressors.[22]

Some investigators believe that salivary cortisol concentrations are more reflective of biologically active systemic cortisol concentrations because only unbound (free) cortisol can diffuse into saliva and may have utility in HPAA function testing in horses.[21,23]

Another test of pituitary function is the TRH stimulation test where exogenous TRH is administered and the expected response should be an increase in TSH from the thyrotrophs of the pars distalis. Exogenous TRH also stimulates ACTH secretion by the melanotrophs of the pars intermedia and this finding has been used to aid in the diagnosis of PPID.[24,25] More recently, the TRH stimulation test was assessed in horses with anhidrosis where anhidrotic horses had different TSH responses to TRH stimulation than normal horses. There was no difference in thyroid hormone concentrations between horses and, as such, the biologic significance of an altered pituitary (TSH) response is unknown.[26]

HYPOTHALAMIC-PITUITARY DYSFUNCTION IN CRITICAL ILLNESS

Human Perspective

Disorders of HP axes with emphasis on hypothalamic dysfunction are better described in humans than in veterinary patients. Endocrinopathies of critical illness, including those related to critical illness related corticosteroid insufficiency (CIRCI), also known as relative adrenal insufficiency [RAI]); diabetes insipidus (DI) (central and nephrogenic); SIADH; and many heritable conditions are examples that are described. Conversely, although the body of evidence is being gathered in equine patients, in particular those afflicted with critical illness, many of these clinical conditions are by and large poorly understood, poorly defined, and/or poorly recognized if they exist. Dysfunction of the HPAA is better understood in septic and critically ill foals, largely through prospective multicenter research endeavors,[27–30] and further investigation is ongoing.

In people, HPAA dysfunction is becoming increasingly recognized. For specific patient populations, hormonal/peptide supplementation, including AVP and cortisol (and their analogs), is used as therapy. Notable are patients with septic shock, defined as patients with severe sepsis and refractory hypotension despite fluid resuscitation. The 2008 Surviving Sepsis Campaign guidelines illustrate the usefulness of these treatments in providing hemodynamic support, among many other therapeutics, to improve survival in septic human patients.[31]

Changes in AVP and ACTH have been well documented in humans,[32] including children[33] and adults with early sepsis.[34] Alterations seemingly follow a pattern of having an increase in AVP, ACTH, and cortisol during the acute early stages of sepsis and with prolonged stimulation, followed by decreases of these same hormones occurring proportionally to the magnitude of disease severity and/or duration of disease. Increases in plasma AVP concentrations have been found in baboons, dogs,[35] rats,[9] and foals.[28] In children with acute septic shock, nonsurvivors are reported to have increased AVP concentrations.[33] Proposed mechanisms for the increased AVP concentration during sepsis include a physiologic response to stress,[6] changes in blood pressure[6,33,36] and blood volume in relation to blood pressure,[6,33] changes in serum osmolality,[16,19,33] and response to circulating endotoxin and proinflammatory mediators, including IL-1β, IL-6, and tumor necrosis factor (TNF)-α.[8,33,37,38] Moreover, in fulminant septic shock, AVP concentrations have been shown to be lower than anticipated for the degree of critical illness.[39] As the shock state progresses, the early increased AVP concentrations decrease to normal or subnormal values despite a lack of resolution or even worsening of a patient's clinical condition. This has been called relative vasopressin deficiency because in the presence of hypotension, vasopressin is expected to be elevated.[34] The author and coworkers have evidence that a similar phenomenon may occur in septic foals (discussed later).

In light of these observations in humans, AVP is administered as an adjunctive pressor agent after volume resuscitation, inotropes (eg, dobutamine), and first-line pressors, such as norepinephrine. Primary use of AVP for refractory hypotension alone or in high doses is not recommended due to concerns of coronary and splanchnic ischemia and conflicting efficacy findings.[40,41] To date, large protocol driven trials investigating the use of AVP or cortisol administration in critically ill veterinary patients are lacking. Infrequent and sparse case reports/case series have been reported.[42–44] Given the surfeit of research, investigation, and success in the human critical care field, however, the therapeutic utility of AVP and/or cortisol supplementation deserves more investigation in critically ill foals and adult horses.

Information on other endocrine axes in critical illness is provided in the article by Toribio elsewhere in this issue.

Animal Studies

There are few studies that have investigated the clinical utility of AVP or AVP analogs for the treatment of hypotension, either as single therapy or in combination with other inotrope or vasopressor agents. One of the significant negative effects of AVP use in septic patients is its ability to shunt blood flow from the skin and splanchnic circulation to other vital organs. Splanchnic perfusion is vital to maintain intestinal integrity, and when significant hypoperfusion occurs, this is permissive for bacterial translocation, bacteremia, systemic inflammatory response syndrome (SIRS), and sepsis. In a study of isoflurane-induced hypotension in foals, AVP administration decreased splanchnic perfusion in excess of that caused by systemic hypotension and to a greater extent than other vasoactive substances, including dobutamine and norepinephrine.[45]

Similarly, in a porcine model of endotoxemia, cutaneous and splanchnic microcirculation measured by microsphere flow was depressed after the administration of AVP and was not improved when dobutamine was coadministered.[46]

Vasopressin Use in Horses

The use of vasopressin as a therapeutic in horses is poorly documented in clinical practice. Some clinicians use vasopressin (0.25–8 mU/kg/min) as a continuous rate of infusion to treat catecholamine-refractory hypotension in endotoxemia/sepsis of adult horses and foals with variable results. Given the lack of evidence for its use in septic foals, it is prudent to consider AVP when other pressors and intropes have failed. Also, for similar reasons, starting at a low dose and gradually titrating up is a recommended safe practice when using vasoactive substances.

AVP is used in people for cardiopulmonary cerebral resuscitation (0.2–0.8 U/kg) as a first-line treatment or when epinephrine has failed to yield return of spontaneous circulation.[17] This treatment recommendation might also have utility in resuscitation of critically ill foals. AVP was approximately a 5 times more potent vasopressor in rats and human subjects with septic shock/endotoxemia than in normal subjects.[47,48] Reasons for this effect may be due in part to the ability of AVP to reset ATP-sensitive potassium channels, potentiate endogenous catecholamines, and inhibit inducible nitric oxide synthase.[49]

Equine Perspective

There are few reports investigating the pathophysiology or treatment of HP dysfunction in horses. Most studies are observational and physiologic in nature, assessing the normal HP axis (and HPAA) response or interaction.[1,6,28,50,51] Recently, Wong and colleagues[51] published normal values for AVP in foals during the first 3 months of life, with minimal changes over time (6.2 $\pm$ 2.5 pg/mL). These values were similar to those previously reported in healthy foals.[28]

Critical Illness (Endotoxemia and Sepsis)

Endotoxemia and sepsis are frequent findings in adult horses and foals, respectively. Studies have shown that bacterial toxins (exotoxins and endotoxin) can induce activation of the mononuclear phagocyte system and the production of proinflammatory cytokines in septic foals,[52,53] notably TNF-α, interleukin (IL)-1β, and IL-6, which are thought to be responsible, in part, for the development of systemic inflammation and the progression to SIRS. Endotoxin and proinflammatory cytokines themselves also are AVP secretagogues in humans[16,37] and horses[8] by activating AVP magnocellular neurons. TNF-α is an early mediator in endotoxemia and is correlated with the severity of clinical signs.[52–54] Similarly, detectable endotoxin concentrations in plasma of septic foals are correlated with nonsurvival.[52]

In a prospective study of 111 neonatal foals (septic n = 51, sick nonseptic n = 29, and healthy n = 31), septic foals, determined by clinical findings, blood culture status, and/or sepsis score greater than or equal to 14, had increases in plasma AVP, ACTH, and cortisol concentrations. The median age was 24 hours, confirming that hormone determinations occurred early during the course of disease. In that same study, foals with negative blood culture and sepsis score[55] less than or equal to 10 hospitalized for conditions other than sepsis, for example, neonatal isoerythrolysis or neonatal encephalopathy (also known as perinatal asphyxia syndrome and dummy foal), also had elevations in HPAA hormones, to a lesser magnitude, however, than septic foals. AVP concentration was also found significantly associated with survival; foals with high AVP concentrations were more likely to die.[28]

Systemic hypotension is reported commonly in septic foals[49,56–59] and is also associated with increased AVP concentration in the acute stage of sepsis in humans.[34] In a study by Hurcombe and colleagues,[28] a normal calculated serum osmolality was found in foals with high AVP concentrations, suggesting that nonosmotic stimuli were responsible for AVP release (ie, hypotension or hypoperfusion [baroreceptor-mediated release] and systemic inflammation [stress-mediated release]). In further assessment of HP axis activation in septic foals, ACTH concentrations were measured in conjunction with AVP. Septic foals and sick nonseptic foals had proportionally higher plasma ACTH concentrations compared with healthy foals. Median plasma ACTH concentrations were significantly higher in septic than in sick nonseptic foals, which, in turn, were significantly higher than in healthy foals. In addition to CRH,[10,60] AVP is a major pituitary ACTH secretagogue,[7–11] which may explain why foals with increased AVP also had increases in ACTH, as seen in a previous study in foals.[61]

Again, proposed mechanisms for increased ACTH concentrations are likely similar to those described for increased AVP release. Other mechanisms may include RAI or CIRCI, where adrenocortical exhaustion and lack of cortisol production provide a positive stimulus for ACTH release in times of extreme stress. This phenomena has been described in critically ill people[34,62–64] and more recently in septic foals.[29,30] RAI is diagnosed in foals by a decreased baseline cortisol concentration and/or subnormal response in cortisol release after administration of low- and/or high-dose exogenous ACTH[29,65] (see article elsewhere in this issue by Hart and Barton). In human critical care, an increase in cortisol by at least 9 μg/dL is useful to rule out RAI (delta-9 rule); however, this cutoff is both controversial and species specific.

These results are consistent with limited published data in septic foals[27] but differ from some results of sepsis studies in humans, where ACTH and cortisol concentrations often were low. Differences may be explained by species variation, age of subject, duration of illness, and severity of illness.[62–64]

The utility of determining hormone ratios can also provide a rough estimation of function. This is not a substitute but a surrogate for more accurate measure of assessing HPAA function, such as cosyntropin (exogenous ACTH) stimulation testing.

AVP:ACTH and ACTH:cortisol ratios were determined and significantly higher in septic foals compared with sick nonseptic foals and healthy foals in two studies.[27,28] In those critically ill foals where a marked increase in AVP and concomitant normal or low ACTH concentration were found, this finding would be supportive of pituitary dysregulation or relative pituitary insufficiency. CRH:ACTH ratios may also indicate dysfunction at the level of the pituitary gland. To test this theory, a CRH stimulation test might be useful to determine appropriate pituitary responsiveness.

An increase in AVP and ACTH may indicate an appropriate HPAA response to critical illness. Despite increases in these hormones, affected foals were likely to have systemic perfusion impairment. This observation may indicate an inappropriate target organ response, such as adrenocortical unresponsiveness or exhaustion (CIRCI), or inappropriate vascular endothelium responsiveness, where physiologic increases in AVP concentration were insufficient to mediate vasoconstriction, through unknown mechanisms. One could postulate that potential V_1 receptor refractoriness or exhaustion was a possible cause. Increases in AVP and ACTH were in agreement with previous studies assessing HPAA maturity in newborn foals[3] and suggest that HPAA stimulation occurs as a result of acute critical illness in young foals and that the magnitude of stimulation is proportional to the severity of disease and outcome and not necessarily changes in serum osmolality.[28] In light of these findings, further evaluation of hormone dynamics over time would be required to assess if AVP depletion or relative vasopressin deficiency occurs in septic foals, as has been described in people; however, this information is currently lacking.

To date, much of the available information regarding endocrinopathies of critical illness center on the adrenal as the target organ; however, HPA dysfunction likely occurs at multiple levels and further identification and definition of these abnormalities may yield therapeutic targets.

Colic (Abdominal Pain)

Acute abdominal pain represents a major stress to activate the HPAA in horses. Blood cortisol and catecholamine concentrations have been associated with survival in horses with colic. The mean cortisol concentration was 7.1 μg/dL in survivors and 15.4 μg/dL in nonsurvivors, and nonsurvivors were 1.28 times more likely to die than survivors (crude, unadjusted odds ratio; $P = .037$).[66] These results are consistent with a more recent study evaluating baseline (admission) β-END, heat shock protein 72, cortisol, and ACTH concentrations in horses with colic. β-END, ACTH, and cortisol were related to the severity of colic and likelihood of survival.[67] More recently, Ludders and colleagues[50] showed that horses with colic had an 8-fold preanesthesia AVP elevation than horses with elective arthroscopy, and AVP concentrations remained elevated longer during anesthesia ($P<.001$).

Hypothalamic-Pituitary Dysfunction, Stress, and the Performance Horse

Stress has been defined as any event that results in increased activity of the HPAA and a subsequent increase in plasma corticosteroid concentrations.[68] In times of stress, stimulation of the HPAA to yield an increase in cortisol has several life-preserving functions, including permissive effects on intermediary metabolism, such as catecholamine-mediated lipolysis and free fatty acid synthesis. Glucocorticoids also promote energy production through glycolysis, lipolysis, and protein catabolism. Another important action of cortisol is to enhance the vascular responsiveness to endogenous catecholamines, which facilitates vascular integrity and blood flow to vital organs during stress.[1,14]

A neuroendocrine disorder at the level of the HP axis has been suggested as the cause of the overtraining syndrome, defined as a homeostatic disturbance at the cellular level resulting in longer recovery post-training times in horses. Clinical findings in these horses include poor performance, poor appetite, weight loss, mental instability/irritability, lack of competitive drive, reproductive cycling abnormalities, increased susceptibility to illness, and persistent tachycardia after exercise, to name a few.[69] Chronic stress in horses has also been found to result in poor fractional change in pituitary venous concentrations of ACTH after administration of human CRH (2 μg). Of importance, there is 100% amino acid homology between human and equine CRH,[1] which has clinical value for testing the pituitary and adrenal components of the axis. Similarly, Alexander and Irvine looked at social stress and found that horses showed decreased in corticosteroid-binding globulin) concentrations, resulting in increased free cortisol concentrations in plasma.[70]

The stress endocrine response to transport has also been evaluated in horses submitted to different lengths of transportation. One study measured β-END, ACTH, and cortisol responses in healthy stallions transported 300 km with jugular venous blood sampling every 100 km. Increases in all 3 hormones were observed with cortisol concentrations remaining elevated over the entire distance, indicating persistent activation and/or a longer half life.[71] The HPAA responses to transportation can result in altered pulmonary macrophage function, which is permissive for the development of (pleuro)pneumonia.

VASOPRESSIN AND THE KIDNEY

Relative and absolute AVP deficiency can result in DI. The hallmark feature of this uncommon condition of horses is polyuria without renal failure and hyposthenuric specific gravity (<1.008). Serum osmolality is increased due to loss of water in the urine. This alone should be a potent stimulus for AVP release; however, either the target organ is unresponsive to the circulating AVP (nephrogenic DI) or no AVP is released in response to hyperosmolality (central or pituitary-dependent DI). Nephrogenic DI results from a lack of AVP signaling in the collecting ducts to assemble and mobilize aquaporin-2 channels and reclaim water despite adequate AVP response stimulation (eg, hypertonicity, hypovolemia). Central DI results from a lack of synthesis and release of AVP. Without AVP, water reabsorption does not occur, resulting in voiding of large volumes of hyposthenuric urine. In both forms, the ability of the nephron to concentrate tubular fluid is lacking. Horses with central DI should respond to exogenous AVP administration (water reabsorption) by increasing their urine-specific gravity (adequately >1.015) and osmolality and decreasing their urine volume and serum osmolality. A thorough review of DI can be found elsewhere in this issue in the article by Schott.

Finally, another disorder of AVP control is the SIADH, where there is an inappropriate release of AVP. This can be due to structural central nervous system disease or drugs or can be idiopathic. SIADH is recognized in humans and dogs[72] and characterized by hyponatremia, increased urine osmolality, and possible circulatory overload, although most patients are euvolemic. Currently, this has not been reported in horses but may be possible.

HYPOTHALAMIC-PITUITARY DYSFUNCTION AND DOPAMINE

As discussed previously, dopamine is an inhibitory neurotransmitter to several cell types of the pars distalis and pars intermedia. Increased dopaminergic input to the pituitary gland results in a reduction in the synthesis and secretion of prolactin, GH, TSH, and POMC peptides. A decrease in dopaminergic input to the pituitary pars intermedia can result in melanotroph hyperplasia and is the pathogenic basis for the development of equine PPID. Under the premise that dopamine is an inhibitory factor for melanotroph function, dopamine agonists are used to treat PPID (see the article by MacFarlane elsewhere in this issue).

Exogenous dopaminergic alkaloids can lead to reproductive and perinatal abnormalities in the mare and foal. Tall fescue (*Festuca arundinacea*) infested with the endophyte, *Neotyphodium coenophialum*, has toxic amounts of dopaminergic ergopeptine alkaloids (derivatives of lysergic acid).[73] This dopaminergic dominance over the pituitary gland inhibits prolactin secretion, causing agalactia and poor/absent mammary gland development.[74] Many other manifestations, including thickened placenta, abortion, prolonged gestation, dystocia, and weak or dead foals can occur in late-term pregnant mares. Foals born to mares exposed to *Neotyphodium*-infested fescue have altered HPA and HPT axis dysfunction, where ACTH, thyroxine, triiodothyronine, progestagen, and cortisol concentrations are lower than healthy foals.[75] These fetal endocrine abnormalities are associated with prolonged gestation. For detailed information on dopaminergic alkaloids, see the article by Evans elsewhere in this issue.

Exogenous DA receptor antagonists (domperidone and metoclopramine [DA2 receptor antagonists], sulpiride [DA2 and DA3 receptor antagonist], and phenothiazines [DA receptor antagonists]) can reverse the inhibitory effects of DA, increasing prolactin secretion. Removal of pregnant mares from infested pastures by day 300 of gestation results in a rapid decline in alkaloid exposure, increasing progestagen and prolactin concentrations. Thus, mares should be off tall fescue pastures 30 to 60 days before the expected foaling date.

SUMMARY

The HP axis (and HPAA) is a tightly regulated endocrine feedback and feed-forward system essential to cellular and organ function as well as physiologic adaptation in horses. Although an understanding of the normal responses to stress is fairly well understood, the responses to critical illness are limited. The body of evidence that HP axis dysfunction in the horse truly exists is mounting. Further investigation as to complete endocrine dynamics in response to critical illness (eg, endotoxemia/sepsis, SIRS, multiple-organ dysfunction syndrome, and trauma), methods to diagnose HP dysfunction, and specific therapies (eg, fluid therapy, antiendotoxic therapies, anti-inflammatory drugs, and hormone replacement therapy) is ongoing. Specifically, the rationale for glucocorticoid administration in septic patients with CIRCI/RAI is evident. The benefit, however, is yet to be determined. This important adaptive axis deserves more attention and investigation because therapies targeting different levels of the HPAA may yield favorable outcomes and increase survival in critically ill horses/foals, as seen in other species.

REFERENCES

1. Alexander SL, Irvine CH, Donald RA. Dynamics of the regulation of the hypothalamo-pituitary-adrenal (HPA) axis determined using a nonsurgical method for collecting pituitary venous blood from horses. Front Neuroendocrinol 1996;17:1–50.
2. Giussani DA, Forhead AJ, Fowden AL. Development of cardiovascular function in the horse fetus. J Physiol 2005;565(part 3):1019–30.
3. Wood CE, Cudd TA. Development of the hypothalamus-pituitary-adrenal axis of the equine fetus: a comparative review. Equine Vet J Suppl 1997;24:74–82.
4. Challis JR, Bassett N, Berdusco ET, et al. Foetal endocrine maturation. Equine Vet J Suppl 1993;14:35–40.
5. Rossdale PD, Silver M, Ellis L, et al. Response of the adrenal cortex to tetracosactrin (ACTH1-24) in premature and full-term foals. J Reprod Fertil Suppl 1982;32: 545–53.
6. Hada T, Onaka T, Takahashi T, et al. Effects of novelty stress on neuroendocrine activities and running performance in thoroughbred horses. J Neuroendocrinol 2003;15:638–48.
7. Evans MJ, Marshall AG, Kitson NE, et al. Factors affecting ACTH release from perifused equine anterior pituitary cells. J Endocrinol 1993;137:391–401.
8. Alexander SL, Irvine CHG. The effect of endotoxin administration on the secretory dynamics of oxytocin in follicular phase mares: relationship to stress axis hormones. J Neuroendocrinol 2002;14:540–8.
9. Brackett DJ, Schaefer CF, Tompkins P, et al. Evaluation of cardiac output, total peripheral vascular resistance, and plasma concentrations of vasopressin in the conscious, unrestrained rat during endotoxemia. Circ Shock 1985;17:273–84.
10. Minton JE. Function of the hypothalamic-pituitary-adrenal axis and the sympathetic nervous system in models of acute stress in domestic farm animals. J Anim Sci 1994;72:1891–8.
11. Delmas A, Leone M, Rousseau S, et al. Clinical review: vasopressin and terlipressin in septic shock patients. Crit Care 2005;9:212–22.
12. Alexander SL, Irvine CH, Ellis MJ, et al. The effect of acute exercise on the secretion of corticotropin-releasing factor, arginine vasopressin, and

adrenocorticotropin as measured in pituitary venous blood from the horse. Endocrinology 1991;128:65–72.
13. Keenan DM, Alexander S, Irvine C, et al. Quantifying nonlinear interactions within the hypothalamo-pituitary-adrenal axis in the conscious horse. Endocrinology 2009;150:1941–51.
14. Ganong WF. Adrenal cortex in review of medical physiology. 22nd edition. New York: McGraw-Hill Company Inc; 2005. p. 361–5.
15. Evans MJ, Mulligan RS, Livesey JH, et al. The integrative control of adrenocorticotrophin secretion: a critical role of corticotrophin-releasing hormone. J Endocrinol 1996;148:475–83.
16. Barrett LK, Singer M, Clapp LH. Vasopressin: mechanisms of action on the vasculature in health and in septic shock. Crit Care Med 2007;35:33–40.
17. Scroggin RD, Quandt J. The use of vasopressin for treating vasodilatory shock and cardiopulmonary resuscitation. J Vet Emerg Crit Care (San Antonio) 2009; 19:145–57.
18. McFarlane D, Donaldson MT, Mc Donnell SM, et al. Effects of season and sample handling on measurement of plasma alpha-melanocyte-stimulating hormone concentrations in horses and ponies. Am J Vet Res 2004;65:1463–8.
19. Holmes CL, Landry DW, Granton JT, et al. Science review: vasopressin and the cardiovascular system part 1- receptor physiology. Crit Care 2003;7:427–34.
20. DiBartola SP. Disorders of sodium and water: hypernatremia and hyponatremia. In: DiBartola SP, editor. Fluid, electrolyte, and acid-base disorders in small animal practice. St. Louis (MO): Saunders Elsevier; 2006. p. 47–79.
21. Reijerkerk EPR, Visser EK, van Reenen CG, et al. Effects of various doses of ovine corticotrophin-releasing hormone on plasma and saliva cortisol concentrations in horses. Am J Vet Res 2009;70:361–4.
22. Veissier I, van Reenen CG, Andanson S, et al. Adrenocorticotropic hormone and cortisol in calves after corticotropin-releasing hormone. J Anim Sci 1999;77: 2047–53.
23. Lebelt D, Shonreiter S, Zanella A. Salivary cortisol in stallions: relationships with plasma levels, daytime profile and changes in response to semen collection. Pferdeheilkunde 1996;12:411–4.
24. Frank N, Andrews FM, Sommardahl CS, et al. Evaluation of the combined dexamethasone suppression/thyrotropin-releasing hormone stimulation test for detection of pars intermedia pituitary adenomas in horses. J Vet Intern Med 2006;20:987–93.
25. Beech J, Boston R, Lindborg S, et al. Adrenocorticotropin concentration following administration of thyrotropin-releasing hormone in healthy horses and those with pituitary pars intermedia dysfunction and pituitary gland hyperplasia. J Am Vet Med Assoc 2007;231:417–26.
26. Breuhaus BA. Thyroid function in anhidrotic horses. J Vet Intern Med 2009;23: 168–73.
27. Gold JR, Divers TJ, Barton MH, et al. Plasma adrenocorticotropin, cortisol, and adrenocorticotropin/cortisol ratios in septic and normal-term foals. J Vet Intern Med 2007;21:791–6.
28. Hurcombe SDA, Toribio RE, Slovis N, et al. Blood arginine vasopressin, adrenocorticotropin hormone and cortisol concentrations at admission in septic and critically ill foals and their association with survival. J Vet Intern Med 2008; 22:639–47.
29. Hart KA, Slovis NM, Barton MH. Hypothalamic-pituitary-adrenal axis dysfunction in hospitalized neonatal foals. J Vet Intern Med 2009;23:901–12.

30. Wong DM, Vo DT, Alcott CJ, et al. Baseline plasma cortisol and ACTH concentrations and response to low-dose ACTH stimulation testing in ill foals. J Am Vet Med Assoc 2009;234:126–32.
31. Dellinger RP, Levy MM, Carlet JM, et al. Surviving sepsis campaign: international guidelines for management of severe sepsis and septic shock: 2008. Crit Care Med 2008;36:296–327.
32. Jochberger S, Mayr VD, Luckner G, et al. Serum vasopressin concentrations in critically ill patients. Crit Care Med 2006;34:293–9.
33. Lodha R, Vivekanandham S, Sarthi M, et al. Serial circulating vasopressin levels in children with septic shock. Pediatr Crit Care Med 2006;7:220–4.
34. Sharshar T, Blanchard A, Paillard M, et al. Circulating vasopressin levels in septic shock. Crit Care Med 2003;31:1752–8.
35. Wilson MF, Brackett DJ, Hinshaw LB, et al. Vasopressin release during sepsis and septic shock in baboons and dogs. Surg Gynecol Obstet 1981;153:869–72.
36. Holmes CL, Patel BM, Russel JA, et al. Physiology of vasopressin relevant to the management of septic shock. Chest 2001;120:989–1002.
37. Kasting NW, Mazurek MF, Martin JB. Endotoxin increases vasopressin release independently of known physiologic stimuli. Am J Physiol 1985;248:E420–4.
38. Beishuizen A, Thijs LG. Endotoxin and the hypothalamo-pituitary-adrenal (HPA) axis. J Endotoxin Res 2003;9:3–24.
39. Landry DW, Levin HR, Gallant EM, et al. Vasopressin deficiency contributes to the vasodilation of septic shock. Circulation 1997;95:1122–5.
40. Russell JA, Walley KR, Singer J, et al. Vasopressin versus norepinephrine infusion in patients with septic shock (VASST Investigation). N Engl J Med 2008;358:877–87.
41. Torgersen C, Dunser MW, Wenzel V, et al. Comparing two different arginine vasopressin doses in advanced vasodilatory shock: a randomized, controlled, open-label trial. Intensive Care Med 2010;36:57–65.
42. Silverstein DC, Waddell LS, Drobatz KJ, et al. Vasopressin therapy in dogs with dopamine-resistant hypotension and vasodilatory shock. J Vet Emerg Crit Care 2007;17(4):399–408.
43. Yoo JH, Kim MS, Park HM. Vasopressor therapy using vasopressin prior to crystalloid resuscitation in irreversible hemorrhagic shock under isoflurane anesthesia in dogs. J Vet Med Sci 2007;69:459–64.
44. Peyton JL, Burkitt JM. Critical illness-related corticosteroid insufficiency in a dog with septic shock. J Vet Emerg Crit Care (San Antonio) 2009;19:262–8.
45. Valverde A, Giguere S, Sanchez LC, et al. Effects of dobutamine, norepinephrine, and vasopressin on cardiovascular function in anesthetized neonatal foals with induced hypotension. Am J Vet Res 2006;67:1730–7.
46. Holt DB, Delaney RR, Uyehara CF. Effects of combination dobutamine and vasopressin therapy on microcirculatory blood flow in a porcine model of severe endotoxic shock. J Surg Res 2010. [Epub ahead of print].
47. Baker CH, Sutton ET, Zhou Z, et al. Microvascular vasopressin effects during endotoxin shock in the rat. Circ Shock 1990;30:81–95.
48. Landry DW, Levin HR, Gallant EM, et al. Vasopressin pressor hypersensitivity in vasodilatory septic shock. Crit Care Med 1997;25:1279–82.
49. Corley KTT. Inotropes and vasopressors in adults and foals. Vet Clin North Am Equine Pract 2004;20:77–106.
50. Ludders JW, Palos H-M, Erb HN, et al. Plasma arginine vasopressin concentration in horses undergoing surgery for colic. J Vet Emerg Crit Care (San Antonio) 2009;19:528–35.

51. Wong DM, Vo DT, Alcott CJ, et al. Plasma vasopressin concentrations in healthy foals from birth to 3 months of age. J Vet Intern Med 2008;22:1259–61.
52. Barton MH, Morris DD, Norton N, et al. Hemostatic and fibrinolytic indices in neonatal foals with presumed septicemia. J Vet Intern Med 1998;12:26–35.
53. Allen GK, Green EM, Robinson JA, et al. Serum tumor necrosis factor alpha concentrations and clinical abnormalities in colostrum-fed and colostrum-deprived neonatal foals given endotoxin. Am J Vet Res 1993;54:1404–10.
54. Bentley A, Barton M, Lee M, et al. Antimicrobial-induced endotoxin and cytokine activity in an in vitro model of septicemia in foals. Am J Vet Res 2002;63:660–8.
55. Brewer BD, Koterba AM. Development of a scoring system for the early diagnosis of equine neonatal sepsis. Equine Vet J 1988;20:18–22.
56. Roy MF. Sepsis in adults and foals. Vet Clin North Am Equine Pract 2004;20: 41–61.
57. Furr MO. Systemic inflammatory response syndrome, sepsis and antimicrobial therapy. Clin Tech Equine Pract 2003;2:3–8.
58. Corley KTT. Monitoring and treating the cardiovascular system in neonatal foals. Clin Tech Equine Pract 2003;2:42–55 [2].
59. Nout YS, Corley KTT, Donaldson LL. Indirect oscillometric and direct blood pressure measurements in anesthetized and conscious neonatal foals. J Vet Emerg Crit Care 2002;12:75–80.
60. Livesey JH, Donald RA, Irvine CH, et al. The effects of cortisol, vasopressin (AVP), and corticotropin releasing factor administration on pulsatile adrenocorticotrophin, alpha-melanocyte-stimulating hormone, and AVP secretion in the pituitary venous effluent of the horse. Endocrinology 1988;123:713–20.
61. Gold JR, Divers TJ, Barton MH, et al. ACTH, cortisol and vasopressin levels of septic (survivors and non-survivors) in comparison to normal foals [abstract]. J Vet Intern Med 2006;20:720.
62. Fernandez E, Schrader R, Watterberg K. Relevance of low cortisol values in term and near-term infants with vasopressor resistant hypotension. J Perinatol 2005; 25:114–8.
63. Johnson KL. The hypothalamic-pituitary-adrenal axis in critical illness. AACN Clin Issues 2006;17:39–49.
64. Soliman AT, Taman KH, Rizk MM, et al. Circulating adrenocorticotrophic hormone (ACTH) and cortisol concentrations in normal, appropriate-for-gestational-age newborns versus those with sepsis and respiratory distress: cortisol response to low dose and standard dose ACTH tests. Metabolism 2004;53: 209–14.
65. Hart KA, Huesner GL, Norton NA, et al. Hypothalamic-pituitary-adrenal axis assessment in healthy term neonatal foals utilizing a paired low dose/high dose ACTH stimulation test. J Vet Intern Med 2009;23:344–51.
66. Hinchcliff KW, Rush BR, Farris JW. Evaluation of plasma catecholamine and serum cortisol concentrations in horses with colic. J Am Vet Med Assoc 2005; 227:276–80.
67. Niinisto KE, Korolainen RV, Raekallio MR, et al. Plasma levels of heat shock protein 72 (HSP72) and beta-endorphin as indicators of stress, pain and prognosis in horses with colic. Vet J 2010;184:100–4.
68. Harbuz MS, Lightman SL. Stress and the hypothalamo-pituitary-adrenal axis: acute, chronic and immunological activation. J Endocrinol 1992;134:327–39.
69. de Graaf-Roelfsema E, Keizer HA, van Breda E, et al. Hormonal responses to acute exercise, training and overtraining. A review with emphasis on the horse. Vet Q 2007;29:82–101.

70. Alexander SL, Irvine CH. The effect of social stress on adrenal axis activity in horses: the importance of monitoring corticosteroid-binding globulin capacity. J Endocrinol 1998;157:425–32.
71. Fazio E, Medica P, Aronica V, et al. Circulating beta-endorphin, adrenocorticotrophic hormone and cortisol levels of stallions before and after short road transportation: stress effect of different distances. Acta Vet Scand 2008;50:6.
72. Shiel RE, Pinilla M, Mooney CT. Syndrome of inappropriate antidiuretic hormone secretion associated with congenital hydrocephalus in a dog. J Am Anim Hosp Assoc 2009;45:249–52.
73. Putnam MR, Bransby DI, Schumacher J, et al. Effects of the fungal endophyte acremonium coenophialum in fescue on pregnant mares and foal viability. Am J Vet Res 1991;52:2071–4.
74. Brendemeuhl JP. Fescue and agalactia: pathophysiology, diagnosis and management. Periparturient mare and neonate. San Antonio (TX): Society of Theriogenology; 2000. p. 25–32.
75. Brendemeuhl JP, Williams MA, Boosinger TR, et al. Plasma progestagen, tri-iodothyronine, and cortisol concentrations in postdate gestation foals exposed in utero to the tall fescue endophyte Acremonium coenophialum. Biol Reprod 1995;1:53–9.

Adrenocortical Insufficiency in Horses and Foals

Kelsey A. Hart, DVM, PhD*, Michelle H. Barton, DVM, PhD

KEYWORDS

- Adrenal gland • Adrenal insufficiency • CIRCI • Cortisol
- Hypoadrenocorticism

The adrenal cortices produce a variety of steroid hormones (corticosteroids), including mineralocorticoids (eg, aldosterone), glucocorticoids (eg, cortisol), and adrenal androgens (eg, dehydroepiandrosterone [DHEA]). These corticosteroids play vital roles in several physiologic processes, including electrolyte and fluid balance; cardiovascular homeostasis; carbohydrate, protein, and lipid metabolism; immune and inflammatory responses; and sexual development and reproductive function. Like other endocrine organs, adrenocortical dysfunction may manifest as either abnormal increases or abnormal decreases in activity. Increased adrenocortical activity (hyperadrenocorticism) may occur in horses with pituitary pars intermedia dysfunction, but primary hyperadrenocorticism and permanent adrenocortical insufficiency (hypoadrenocorticism, Addison's Disease) are rare in horses. However, emerging evidence in both human and equine medicine suggests that transient reversible adrenocortical dysfunction resulting in cortisol insufficiency frequently develops during critical illness. This syndrome is termed relative adrenal insufficiency (RAI) or critical illness–related corticosteroid insufficiency (CIRCI) and can contribute substantially to morbidity and mortality associated with the primary disease. Thus, this review discusses the mechanisms, diagnosis, and clinical consequences of adrenocortical insufficiency, with particular focus on our current understanding of RAI/CIRCI in horses and foals.

ADRENOCORTICAL ANATOMY AND PHYSIOLOGY

The adrenal glands are located at the craniomedial aspect of each kidney, and each gland is divided into an outer cortex that secretes corticosteroids and an inner medulla that secretes catecholamines. The adrenal cortices are divided into 3

The authors have no disclosures.
Department of Large Animal Medicine, University of Georgia College of Veterinary Medicine, 501 DW Brooks Drive, Athens, GA 30602, USA
* Corresponding author.
E-mail address: khart4@uga.edu

Vet Clin Equine 27 (2011) 19–34
doi:10.1016/j.cveq.2010.12.005 vetequine.theclinics.com

cellular zones: (1) the outer zona glomerulosa; (2) the middle zona fasciculata, which is the largest zone and comprises 75% of the weight of the entire adrenal gland; and (3) the narrow inner zona reticularis.[1] Cells in the zona glomerulosa are primarily responsible for the secretion of mineralocorticoids (eg, aldosterone), whereas zona fasciculata cells synthesize and secrete glucocorticoids (eg, cortisol). Cells in the zona reticularis also secrete small amounts of glucocorticoids but predominantly produce adrenal androgens such as DHEA and androstenedione.[2]

All corticosteroid hormones are structurally similar and share a common synthetic pathway (**Fig. 1**). All steroid hormones are synthesized from cholesterol and contain a common sterol backbone with three 6-carbon and one 5-carbon rings. Steroid hormone synthesis occurs in the mitochondria and endoplasmic reticulum and begins with mitochondrial uptake of cytoplasmic cholesterol via the steroidogenic acute regulatory (StAR) transporter protein.[3] Binding of a regulatory hormone to adrenocortical cell surface receptors stimulates cyclic AMP-mediated uptake of circulating plasma lipoproteins and liberation of cholesterol via lysosomal lipases to provide the major source of such cholesterol for steroid hormone synthesis.[1] De novo cholesterol synthesis also occurs in the adrenal cortex and can serve as an alternative source of cytoplasmic cholesterol for corticosteroid synthesis.[1]

Once cholesterol is taken up into the mitochondrion via StAR, it is converted to pregnenolone via side chain cleavage enzyme (p450SCC, SCC, or cholesterol desmolase). Both cholesterol deliveries to the mitochondria via StAR and p450SCC-catalyzed pregnenolone synthesis have been proposed as the rate-limiting step in corticosteroid biosynthesis.[4,5] All other steroid hormones are derivatives of pregnenolone; the specific steroids that are produced by a particular adrenocortical cell depend on the biosynthetic enzymes that are expressed in that cell (see **Fig. 1**).[1,6]

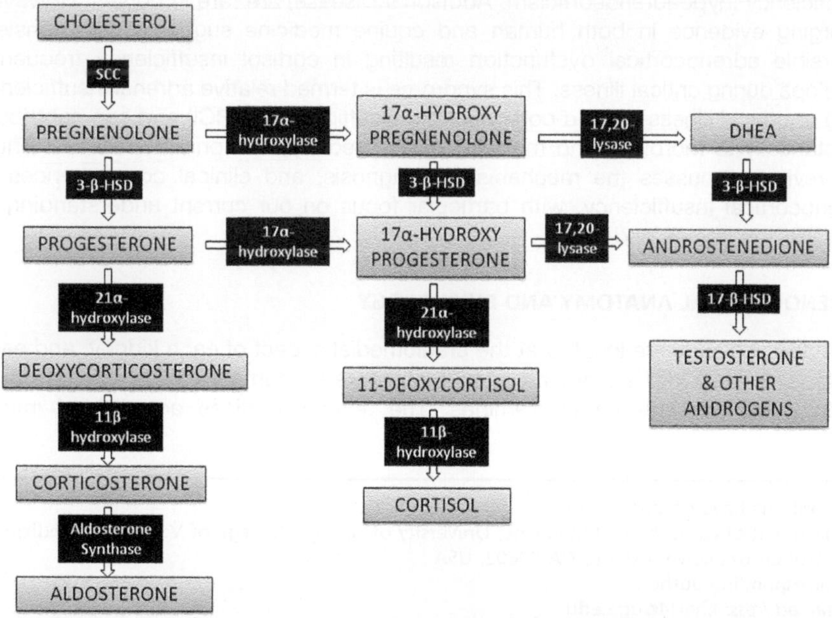

Fig. 1. Biosynthetic pathway for adrenal corticosteroids. The enzymes responsible for catalyzing each biotransformation are shown in the black boxes over the arrows. 3β-HSD, 3β-hydroxysteroid dehydrogenase; SCC, side chain cleavage enzyme.

Glucocorticoids: Synthesis, Secretion, and Systemic Effects

Glucocorticoids are the predominant adrenal corticosteroids and the most prevalent circulating steroid hormones. The synthesis of glucocorticoids is regulated by the hypothalamic-pituitary-adrenal (HPA) axis (**Fig. 2**), and these corticosteroids play an integral role in the endocrine response to stress. The HPA axis is activated when physiologic, pathophysiologic, or environmental stressors activate the peripheral and central nervous system components whose signals are then interpreted and integrated in the hypothalamus. Activation of the hypothalamic paraventricular nuclei culminates in the release of the peptide hormone corticotropin-releasing hormone (CRH) into the hypothalamic-hypophyseal portal vessels. The CRH then acts locally in the adjacent anterior pituitary gland to activate type 1 CRH receptors on the cell surface of pituitary corticotroph cells to induce the release of adrenocorticotropic hormone (ACTH, corticotrophin) into the systemic circulation.[7]

The ACTH binds cell surface receptors (melanocortin 2 receptor [MC2R]) on adrenocortical cells and stimulates the adrenal glands to synthesize and secrete cortisol. Five ACTH receptor types have been characterized in humans, most of which bind both the ACTH and the α-melanocyte– and γ-melanocyte–stimulating hormones (α- and γ-MSHs).[8] The MC2R is the only ACTH receptor type that is expressed in the human adrenal cortex and the only type that does not bind MSHs.[8] The MC2R is a G protein–coupled transmembrane receptor that acts via adenylate cyclase to increase cyclic AMP levels, which then activate a variety of enzymes critical for cortisol synthesis.[8] At present, melanocortin receptor subtype expression in the equine adrenal cortex has not been characterized but is presumed to be similar to that in humans.

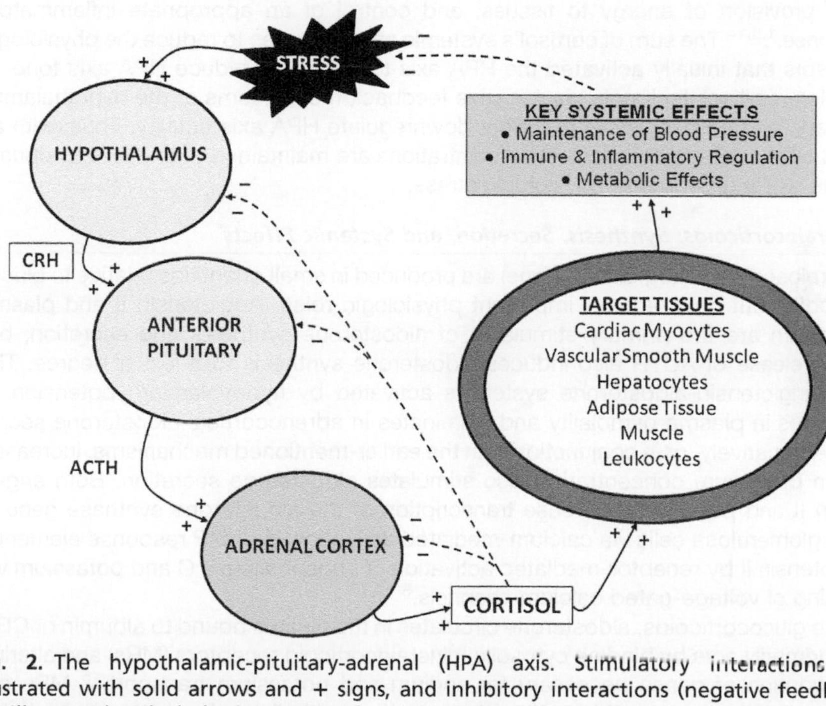

Fig. 2. The hypothalamic-pituitary-adrenal (HPA) axis. Stimulatory interactions are illustrated with solid arrows and + signs, and inhibitory interactions (negative feedback) are illustrated with dashed arrows and – signs. ACTH, adrenocorticotropic hormone; CRH, corticotropin-releasing hormone.

The critical enzymes necessary for cortisol synthesis are predominantly expressed in the zona fasciculata cells and include 3β-hydroxysteroid dehydrogenase (3β-HSD), 17α-hydroxylase, 21α-hydroxylase, and 11β-hydroxylase (see **Fig. 1**).[3] 11β-Hydroxylase catalyzes the final step in cortisol synthesis from the 11-deoxycortisol precursor molecule and is present only in glucocorticoid-producing cells.[3]

Cortisol is not stored in adrenocortical cells but rather is secreted into the systemic circulation immediately after ACTH-induced synthesis.[5] Like all steroid hormones, cortisol is lipophilic and thus is transported in the plasma predominantly bound to plasma proteins, including cortisol-binding globulin (CBG) and albumin.[9] In most adult mammals, including horses, approximately 90% of circulating cortisol is bound.[6,9–12] Because cortisol receptors are located in the cytoplasm of steroid-responsive cells, only the free unbound portion of the circulating cortisol is available to enter cells via diffusion across the plasma membrane and to bind these intracellular glucocorticoid receptors (GRs).[13]

Binding of cortisol to the cytoplasmic GR causes conformational changes in the GR that allow dissociation of regulatory heat shock proteins, permitting the cortisol-GR complex to dimerize, localize to the nucleus, bind DNA at glucocorticoid response elements (GREs), and regulate transcription of glucocorticoid-responsive genes.[1] In humans, there are 2 GR isoforms: GRα and GRβ, but GRβ seems to be transcriptionally inactive and may function as an endogenous inhibitor of GRα activity.[13] To the authors' knowledge, equine GR isoforms and their respective activities are not well characterized.

Many cell types are sensitive to glucocorticoids, permitting cortisol to exert diverse effects necessary for stress responses to both health and disease. Essential glucocorticoid-mediated physiologic responses include maintenance of blood pressure, provision of energy to tissues, and control of an appropriate inflammatory response.[1,5,14] The sum of cortisol's systemic effects serves to reduce the physiologic stressors that initially activated the HPA axis to ultimately reduce HPA axis tone. In addition, cortisol itself acts via negative feedback mechanisms at the hypothalamic, pituitary, and adrenal levels to further downregulate HPA axis activity. Thus, with an intact HPA axis, plasma cortisol concentrations are maintained at a level appropriate for the existing degree of physiologic stress.

Mineralocorticoids: Synthesis, Secretion, and Systemic Effects

Mineralocorticoids (eg, aldosterone) are produced in small quantities relative to glucocorticoids but have equally important physiologic roles. Angiotensin II and plasma potassium are the primary stimulants of aldosterone synthesis and secretion, but acute release of ACTH also induces aldosterone synthesis to a lesser degree. The renin-angiotensin-aldosterone system is activated by hypovolemia/hypotension or increases in plasma osmolality and culminates in adrenocortical aldosterone secretion. Alternatively, or in conjunction with the earlier-mentioned mechanisms, increased serum potassium concentration also stimulates aldosterone secretion. Both angiotensin II and potassium increase transcription of the aldosterone synthase gene in zona glomerulosa cells via calcium-mediated activation of cAMP response elements, angiotensin II by receptor-mediated activation of phospholipase C and potassium via opening of voltage-gated calcium channels.[5]

Like glucocorticoids, aldosterone circulates in the plasma bound to albumin or CBG and primarily acts by binding cytosolic mineralocorticoid receptors (MRs) and altering transcription of genes necessary for sodium and potassium transport.[15] MRs are predominantly expressed in sodium-transporting epithelia in the distal renal tubules and colon, with lesser expression in the rest of the intestinal tract and the heart.[5]

Aldosterone induces transcription of an aldosterone-regulated kinase that increases the activity of apical membrane sodium channels.[15] The net effect of these events is increased sodium flux across epithelial cells, resulting in increased renal and intestinal sodium and water resorption and concurrent stimulation of potassium excretion via the basolateral Na^+/K^+ ATPase.[15] Mineralocorticoids are vital for appropriate fluid and electrolyte balance, and mineralocorticoid deficiency rapidly results in hyponatremia, hyperkalemia, and hypovolemia.

Adrenal Androgens: Synthesis, Secretion, and Systemic Effects

In adult men, circulating androgens are primarily of testicular origin, but in women, more than half of plasma androgens may originate from the adrenal cortices. ACTH is necessary for the synthesis and secretion of adrenal androgens, but another factor (or factors) that is as yet unidentified is also required for adrenal androgen synthesis.[5] Like other adrenal steroids, adrenal androgens are transported in the plasma bound to albumin and CBG and act via cytosolic steroid hormone receptors to modulate gene transcription. Adrenal androgens, such as DHEA and androstenedione, can be extraglandularly metabolized to active testosterone and estrogens and play a particularly important role in early pubertal sexual development in most species. Increased adrenal androgen production is postulated to play a role in mares with estrus-related behavior problems, although this has not been definitively proven.[16]

METHODS FOR DIAGNOSIS OF ADRENOCORTICAL INSUFFICIENCY

Testing methods used to diagnose adrenocortical insufficiency in both human and veterinary medicine fall into 2 general categories: (1) assessment of endogenous basal adrenocortical activity by measurement of circulating or excreted hormone concentrations and (2) dynamic assessment of adrenocortical responsiveness by assessment of hormone production after administration of exogenous regulatory hormones.[17]

In general, measurement of basal plasma hormone concentrations offers a rapid and safe means of assessing adrenocortical function. Well-established commercial radioluminescent or chemiluminescent immunoassays are readily available for the measurement of equine cortisol and can provide results rapidly.[6,17] Commercial immunoassays are also available for most other adrenal corticosteroids, and the measurement of aldosterone and adrenal androgens has been described in horses.[18–20] However, cortisol and other adrenal steroids are typically secreted in a pulsatile fashion and plasma concentrations can vary widely during a 24-hour period in both healthy and sick individuals with time of day, season, emotional state, and moment-to-moment changes in physiologic stressors.[5,17] Thus, documentation of a single random low basal concentration of any steroid hormone should be interpreted with caution because true steroid deficiency is not always indicated.

The assessment of cortisol concentrations in conjunction with regulatory hormone (ACTH, CRH) concentrations can provide a more comprehensive picture of HPA axis function. Plasma CRH and ACTH concentrations are easily assessed in most species via commercially available immunoassays, but because CRH is predominantly secreted into the hypothalamic-hypophyseal portal vessels rather than into the systemic circulation, accurate measurement of CRH concentrations requires sophisticated sampling methodology. In addition, although in healthy individuals ACTH and cortisol concentrations are fairly closely correlated, ACTH-cortisol dissociation is not uncommon during illness.[21]

Dynamic tests are designed to circumvent some of these limitations. The most commonly used dynamic test to diagnose cortisol insufficiency is the ACTH stimulation test, during which the cortisol response to exogenous synthetic ACTH (usually cosyntropin, α1-24 corticotropin) is measured. Typically, in the classic high-dose ACTH stimulation test, serum cortisol concentration is measured just before and 30 and 90 minutes after intravenous or intramuscular administration of a supraphysiological quantity of ACTH (1.0–2.0 μg/kg, approximately 100–250 μg in people and foals). This high-dose ACTH stimulation test produces a maximal adrenal response, so an inadequate increase in cortisol concentration in this test is used to diagnose both absolute irreversible adrenal insufficiency (eg, Addison's Disease) and transient RAI/CIRCI.[5,22–24]

However, the high-dose ACTH stimulation test may be less sensitive for diagnosis of the transient reversible HPA axis suppression that occurs in RAI/CIRCI. In some patients with RAI/CIRCI, the adrenal gland fails to produce an appropriate cortisol response to physiological concentrations of ACTH but may still respond adequately to supraphysiological ACTH concentrations.[25,26] A measurable cortisol response can be produced by the administration of lower ACTH doses (0.01–0.20 μg/kg, approximately 1–10 μg in people and foals),[25,26] and such low-dose stimulation tests may more accurately diagnose RAI/CIRCI in critically ill patients.[25–27]

However, both the high-dose and low-dose ACTH stimulation tests only evaluate the adrenal component of the HPA axis. Therefore, patients with cortisol insufficiency due to impaired HPA axis function at the hypothalamic and/or pituitary levels may produce an appropriate cortisol response to exogenous ACTH and may be falsely interpreted as having intact HPA axis function. The CRH stimulation test is occasionally used to assess the function of the higher levels of the HPA axis function and is most helpful for distinguishing among adrenocortical, hypothalamic, and pituitary failure if both ACTH and cortisol concentrations are measured before and after CRH stimulation.[5] Effects of various doses of ovine CRH on cortisol concentrations in adult horses have been determined, and a CRH stimulation test protocol for use in horses has been described.[28] However, this test is expensive and, in people, is less sensitive for the diagnosis of HPA axis hypofunction than other means[29]; therefore, the CRH stimulation test is not currently recommended as a first-line means of HPA axis assessment.

The metyrapone test may be more useful for assessing the integrity of the entire HPA axis. In people, metyrapone (30 mg/kg), a specific inhibitor of the adrenocortical steroidogenic enzyme 11β-hydroxylase, is administered orally at midnight.[5,30] Because 11β-hydroxylase catalyzes the conversion of 11-deoxycortisol to cortisol in the last step of adrenocortical cortisol synthesis, metyrapone administration results in a decrease in circulating cortisol concentrations. With an intact HPA axis, this decrease in plasma cortisol stimulates increased HPA axis activity, resulting in increased CRH and ACTH secretion and attempted stimulation of adrenocortical cortisol synthesis. However, because the last step in cortisol synthesis is inhibited by metyrapone, cortisol concentrations remain low, whereas concentrations of the precursor 11-deoxycortisol increase. A decrease in cortisol concentrations to below 7.0 μg/dL 8 to 10 hours after metyrapone administration confirms that 11β-hydroxylase suppression was adequate. Increases in ACTH and 11-deoxycortisol concentrations at this time suggest an intact HPA axis, whereas low ACTH and 11-deoxycortisol concentrations suggest HPA axis dysfunction at the hypothalamic and/or pituitary levels.[5,30] However, if ACTH concentrations increase but 11-deoxycortisol remains low, primary adrenocortical dysfunction is implied. Measurement of 11-deoxycortisol is described in the horse,[31] but commercial assays are not readily available in all clinical settings, and many assays require a cumbersome extraction step. Furthermore, although intravenous infusions of metyrapone have been described in horses,[32] oral metyrapone has not been used for HPA axis function assessment in ill horses to date.

The insulin tolerance test (ITT) is currently considered the gold standard test for the diagnosis of HPA axis hypofunction[33] and has been described in both foals[34] and adult horses.[35] In the ITT, hypoglycemia is induced by the administration of exogenous insulin, and the cortisol response to the physiologic stress of this hypoglycemia is measured. A blunted or an absent increase in plasma cortisol after hypoglycemia implies HPA axis dysfunction. ACTH concentrations can also be measured in conjunction with cortisol concentrations to differentiate between adrenal and central HPA axis dysfunctions. However, given the risks associated with severe hypoglycemia as is induced in the ITT,[33] as well as the potential for preexisting glucose derangements or peripheral insulin resistance during severe illness,[36] the clinical utility of the ITT in critically ill patient is limited.

Some of the physiologic consequences of CIRCI may be associated with cortisol resistance in peripheral tissues rather than circulating cortisol insufficiency.[37–40] In such cases, the earlier-mentioned tests may suggest intact HPA axis function, with appropriate endogenous cortisol concentrations and normal responses to dynamic testing, despite clinical evidence of cortisol insufficiency, such as persistent hypotension and inflammatory dysregulation. Unfortunately, methodology for assessing cortisol activity at the tissue level is currently limited[37–40] and is not readily available for use in clinical patients with suspected RAI/CIRCI.

CURRENT UNDERSTANDING OF ADRENOCORTICAL FUNCTION IN HEALTHY FOALS AND ADULT HORSES

Horses

Basal cortisol concentrations in healthy adult horses at rest are reported in the approximate range of 1.1 to 14.3 μg/dL (30–395 nmol/L), which is consistent with resting cortisol concentrations in other domestic animal species.[19,28,41–45] In addition to the pulsatile (ultradian) rhythm to corticosteroid secretion described earlier, adult horses exhibit a circadian rhythm to cortisol secretion similar to other species, with peak secretion in the morning and the nadir in the evening.[5,32,44] However, this circadian rhythm is easily disrupted in horses by simple routine changes.[32] Cortisol responses to ACTH stimulation testing in adult horses are described and suggest that adult horses show a comparable dose-dependent effect of exogenous ACTH on cortisol concentrations as is described in other species.[5,45,46] In general, an approximate 2.5- to 5-fold increase in cortisol concentration is observed within 30 minutes after administration of a 0.1 to 1.0 μg/kg dose of exogenous ACTH (cosyntropin).[46] Administration of higher doses (2–10 μg/kg) results in a sustained and greater (5–10 fold) increase in cortisol concentration by 90 to 180 minutes after ACTH administration.[46]

Reported resting plasma concentrations of aldosterone and androstenedione in healthy adult horses have also been described. Basal aldosterone concentrations have been described within a range of approximately 14 to 50 pg/mL.[18,19,47] Androstenedione concentrations in adult horses are reported within a range of less than 0.050 to 0.986 ng/mL.[16,19] Sex and age variations in adrenal androgen concentrations may be relevant[19] but, at present, are poorly understood in horses.

Foals

HPA axis function in the fetal and neonatal foal has been investigated in several studies with a variety of methodologies and differs from both adult horses and other mammalian species in key ways that may affect the neonatal foal's ability to respond to stress. Compelling evidence shows that maturation of the HPA axis occurs in the days just before parturition and continues during the first several weeks of life in the foal, much later than is described in other species.[48–51] For example, premature foals have lower serum cortisol concentrations (<3 μg/dL) in the 2 hours after birth than full-term foals (12–14 μg/dL).[51] Concurrently, premature foals exhibit significantly higher endogenous ACTH concentrations than term foals (650 pg/mL vs 300 pg/mL at 30 minutes postpartum).[51]

These low baseline cortisol and concurrent high ACTH concentrations in premature foals imply that foals may have impaired adrenocortical sensitivity to ACTH, limited cortisol synthetic capacity, or both when compared with adult horses. ACTH stimulation testing in foals supports this theory because premature foals show a blunted cortisol response to exogenous ACTH, with only a 28% increase in plasma cortisol 30 to 60 minutes after stimulation compared with a 208% increase in normal term foals.[48] MC2R density or activity has not been described in foals or horses of any age, but there is some evidence to suggest that the fetal foal's adrenal gland may be incapable of synthesizing cortisol until very late in gestation. Immunohistochemical localization showed that key steroidogenic enzymes necessary for cortisol synthesis (p450SCC and 3β-HSD) are absent or present in very low amounts until just before parturition in the foal,[52,53] much later than is described in other species.[54]

Furthermore, adrenocortical function may not be fully mature at birth even in full-term foals. By 12 to 24 hours of age, mean basal cortisol concentrations are lower in healthy neonatal foals (approximately 2.0–3.6 μg/dL) than reported mean concentrations in healthy adult horses (approximately 3–7 μg/dL), despite comparable or higher concurrent ACTH concentrations in foals.[16,42,55–57] This apparent decreased cortisol response to endogenous ACTH in the neonatal foal is supported by further evidence of limited cortisol responses to exogenous ACTH in the same study; in neonatal foals during the first week of life, the increase in cortisol concentration after administration of both a low (10 μg) and a high (100 μg) dose of ACTH was approximately half than that seen in adult horses in response to a comparable dose of ACTH.[46,56] Insulin-induced cortisol responses in foals within 12 hours of birth are also less than half of the responses achieved in 7- to 14-day-old foals.[34] Furthermore, this decreased adrenocortical responsiveness seems to persist during the first few months of life because 12-week-old foals showed significantly greater cortisol responses to a low-dose (0.1 μg/kg) ACTH stimulation test than younger foals.[58] The specific cause of these impaired cortisol responses in neonatal foals is not known, but regardless of the causative mechanism or mechanisms, this evidence of fetal and neonatal HPA axis immaturity is certain to affect, and may possibly impair, the foal's ability to respond to physiologic stress and disease during the neonatal period.

In contrast to cortisol, newborn foals seem to be able to mount a substantial aldosterone response to hypovolemia/hyponatremia[20,59]; in fact, one study suggested that the aldosterone response in foals seems to be exaggerated when compared with that in adult horses and may reflect differences in tubular sensitivity to aldosterone between neonates and adults.[20] However, well-established reference ranges for plasma aldosterone or adrenal androgen concentrations in foals are not currently available.

ADRENOCORTICAL INSUFFICIENCY

General Mechanisms of Adrenocortical Dysfunction Resulting in Cortisol Insufficiency

Cortisol insufficiency can result from HPA axis impairment at one or several levels and may be transient or permanent.[5] Permanent HPA axis dysfunction results from the destruction of one or more glandular components of the axis and is infrequent in both human and veterinary medicine. Immune-mediated adrenocortical destruction (eg, Addison disease) is the most common manifestation of permanent HPA axis hypofunction in both human and veterinary patients[5,60] but has not been described in horses to date. Patients with Addison disease cannot mount an appropriate cortisol response to stress and thus frequently present with hemodynamic instability and collapse.[5,60] Aldosterone deficiency, in addition to cortisol deficiency, is a typical feature of Addison disease and results in fluid and electrolyte derangements that contribute to the development of hypovolemia, hypotension, and cardiovascular collapse in affected individuals.[5,60]

Irreversible adrenocortical, hypothalamic, or pituitary destruction may also result from neoplastic infiltration or from invasion of the glands by infectious organisms but are rare in all species.[60,61] Severe adrenocortical hemorrhage and necrosis resulting in adrenal insufficiency (Waterhouse-Friderichsen syndrome) is also described in both people and horses with septic and endotoxic shock and is believed to result from vascular derangements and ischemia associated with the primary disease.[62] Congenital abnormalities in CRH receptor 1, MC2R, or GR structure or function and congenital absence of synthetic enzymes necessary for pituitary or adrenocortical hormone synthesis are described in people and can also result in HPA axis hypofunction.[5]

Although irreversible HPA axis hypofunction due to destruction of HPA axis components is uncommon,[5,25,63,64] recent evidence suggests that transient HPA axis dysfunction (RAI/CIRCI) may occur in a substantial number of critically ill patients with a variety of conditions, including acute respiratory distress syndrome,[23,24] major trauma,[65] and cardiothoracic surgery.[66] However, the predominant diseases associated with the development of RAI/CIRCI in people and infants are sepsis and septic shock.[22,25,27,39,67–70] RAI/CIRCI can result from temporary suppression of HPA axis activity at one or more levels, resulting in (1) inhibition of CRH and/or ACTH secretion, (2) decreased sensitivity to CRH or ACTH at their respective target tissues, (3) exhaustion of adrenocortical cortisol synthetic capacity (loss of adrenal reserve), or (4) impaired response to cortisol in the peripheral tissue resistance.[14,23,39]

The specific mechanisms leading to the development of RAI/CIRCI are poorly understood but may involve a combination of factors, including (1) direct damage to HPA axis components from the primary disease, (2) inhibition of hormone production by medications used to treat the primary disease, and/or (3) suppression of activity of one or more components of the HPA axis by infectious organisms or the host's own immune and inflammatory responses.[23,25,26,39] Periods of hypotension associated with hypovolemic or septic shock can result in decreased adrenal perfusion and ischemic injury to the metabolically active adrenocortical cells.[62,71] If this occurs for prolonged periods or to an extreme degree the damage may be irreversible, as seen in patients with Waterhouse-Friderichsen syndrome, but milder circulatory insults may result in transient injury and dysfunction. In addition, the anesthetic agent etomidate, which is used frequently in critically ill people and animals, is known to directly inhibit adrenocortical cortisol synthesis by inhibiting 11β-hydroxylase,[72] the enzyme that catalyzes the key last step in the synthesis of active cortisol. Several antimicrobial agents, (eg, ketoconazole and rifampin), which are often used in septic people and animals, also can inhibit adrenal steroid synthesis.[23]

However, it is the patient's own immune and inflammatory responses that seem to play the most vital role in the development of RAI/CIRCI during critical illnesses such as sepsis. Bacterial components such as endotoxin (the lipopolysaccharide component of gram-negative bacterial cell walls) and host proinflammatory cytokines participate in initiating and maintaining the HPA axis response to sepsis. These factors can directly stimulate HPA axis activity at multiple levels, ultimately resulting in the stimulation of cortisol synthesis and secretion.[39,62,73–75]

However, bacterial ligands and inflammatory cytokines may also be capable of suppressing HPA axis function at one or more levels, in the face of an overwhelming bacterial infection or excessive host inflammatory response. For example, inducible nitric oxide synthase–mediated death of hypothalamic neurons in cardioregulatory centers has been described in patients who died of septic shock and may be involved in HPA axis dysfunction in such patients.[76] Bacterial endotoxin has been shown to directly decrease pituitary CRH receptor gene expression in both rats and cattle.[77,78] In addition, tumor necrosis factor α (TNF-α) can directly impair both pituitary ACTH release and adrenocortical cortisol synthesis.[23] Cholesterol availability for corticosteroid synthesis may also be limited during sepsis, as decreased levels of plasma high-density lipoproteins are reported in critically ill individuals and are correlated with blunted cortisol responses to ACTH stimulation testing.[23]

Furthermore, several studies suggest that peripheral tissue cortisol resistance may develop in some critically ill patients. Specifically, impaired GR binding affinity has been documented in an ovine model of acute lung injury[79] and in a rodent burn model.[38] This effect was partially ameliorated in the rodent model when TNF-α and interleukin 1β were reduced by neutralizing antibodies.[38] Furthermore, nuclear localization of cortisol-GR complexes was impaired in human leukocytes exposed to plasma from patients who died of acute respiratory distress syndrome.[40] Thus, the complex relationship between endocrine and immune regulation of HPA axis function determines overall cortisol production and activity during sepsis. Any imbalance in these interactions can result in absolute or functional cortisol insufficiency and may play a critical role in the pathogenesis of RAI/CIRCI.

CIRCI in Foals

Our current understanding of HPA axis function in critically ill horses and foals is limited, but several studies suggest that RAI/CIRCI may indeed occur in septic neonatal foals. One case report of transient HPA axis dysfunction, as evidenced by both a low basal cortisol concentration and an impaired cortisol response to a high-dose ACTH stimulation test, has been described in a septic neonatal foal.[80] In addition, 2 independent studies that measured basal ACTH and cortisol concentrations in healthy and septic neonatal foals found significantly increased ACTH:cortisol ratios in nonsurviving septic foals.[81,82] Such high ACTH:cortisol ratios, with high ACTH concentrations and low corresponding cortisol concentrations, suggest that HPA axis dysfunction at the level of the adrenal gland may occur in the septic full-term foal.

HPA axis function has been further characterized in hospitalized foals using ACTH stimulation tests in 2 studies.[83,84] Neither study identified a significant difference in peak or delta cortisol responses between groups of age-matched healthy and ill foals in response to a low-dose ACTH stimulation test (0.1 μg/kg)[84] or in response to a paired low-dose (10 μg)/high-dose (100 μg) ACTH stimulation test.[83] However, when human diagnostic criteria for RAI/CIRCI[24] were adapted and applied to a group of 72 hospitalized foals, approximately 50% of all hospitalized foals and approximately 40% of septic foals met these criteria.[83] Furthermore, increased disease severity and poorer prognoses were correlated with decreased cortisol responses to ACTH stimulation in foals in both studies. Specifically, nonsurviving foals had significantly lower cortisol responses to low-dose ACTH stimulation as compared with survivors,[84] and foals that met criteria for RAI/CIRCI (as characterized by an inadequate cortisol response to a high-dose ACTH stimulation test) had a significantly greater incidence of shock, multiple organ dysfunction syndrome, and nonsurvival than foals with an adequate cortisol response to ACTH.[83]

In concert, these studies provide evidence that RAI/CIRCI occurs in critically ill and septic neonatal foals with comparable frequency and effects as in septic people and suggest that the mechanisms and management of RAI/CIRCI in critically ill foals warrant further investigation. At present, cortisol replacement therapy in the form of hydrocortisone at approximately 1 to 4 mg/kg/d is recommended for the management of RAI/CIRCI in septic people and infants.[24,85] Such therapy has not been critically evaluated in neonatal foals to date, but recent evidence suggests that in healthy 2- to 6-day-old foals, a short tapering course of hydrocortisone (1.3 mg/kg/d divided every 4 hours intravenously) has potentially beneficial antiinflammatory effects without significantly impairing innate immune function (Kelsey A. Hart, DVM, PhD, Michelle H. Barton, DVM, PhD, Vandenplas M, et al, unpublished data, 2010).

Adrenocortical Insufficiency in Adult Horses

Adrenocortical insufficiency is not well described in adult horses. Transient adrenal insufficiency characterized by low basal ACTH and cortisol concentrations and impaired cortisol responses to ACTH stimulation testing has been described in one horse after abrupt cessation of long-term anabolic steroid supplementation.[86] A syndrome of adrenal exhaustion resulting in lethargy, anorexia, and poor performance is also anecdotally described in racehorses and has been attributed to adrenal insufficiency associated with long-term steroid administration or chronic stress.[64] However, measurement of basal cortisol concentrations and ACTH stimulation testing in racehorses and endurance horses has not provided convincing evidence for adrenal insufficiency in these equine athletes.[64,87] Decreased cortisol responses to ACTH are also described in mares with abnormal estrus-related behavior,[16] but the clinical significance of this behavior is not known. However, the potential for iatrogenic adrenal insufficiency associated with HPA axis suppression by exogenous steroids should be considered in horses on chronic glucocorticoid or anabolic steroid supplementation, and care should be taken to avoid abrupt cessation of such therapy.

In addition, the adrenal gland is extremely vulnerable to ischemic injury associated with endotoxic or hypovolemic shock in horses as in many other species. Adrenocortical hemorrhage, and necrosis similar to the human Waterhouse-Friderichsen syndrome, is a common finding at necropsy examination of adult horses that succumbed to acute severe gastrointestinal disease and other diseases associated with endotoxic shock.[71] In theory, such adrenal injury could contribute to long-term adrenocortical insufficiency in surviving horses, although this has not been documented to date. To the authors' knowledge, classic hypoadrenocorticism (Addison's Disease) resulting from immune-mediated adrenocortical destruction and manifesting with glucocorticoid and mineralocorticoid deficiency has not been described in horses.

Hypoaldosteronism

In people, primary hypoaldosteronism is uncommon and most frequently occurs as a result of congenital defects in some component of the aldosterone biosynthetic pathway.[5] Hypoaldosteronism is also reported in renal diseases that damage the juxtaglomerular apparatus integral to the function of the renin-angiotensin-aldosterone system, and peripheral resistance to aldosterone is also reported in people.[5] To the authors' knowledge, such syndromes have not been described in horses. However, hypoaldosteronism is a documented cause of renal tubular acidosis in people[88] and should not be overlooked as a possible cause of renal tubular acidosis in horses.[89]

Sex Steroid Insufficiency

Adrenal androgen deficiency can result in abnormal or delayed sexual development, but because of the relatively greater contribution of gonadal androgens to sexual development, clinical diseases associated with sole defects in adrenal androgen production are uncommon in all species[90] and have not been described in horses to the authors' knowledge.

REFERENCES

1. Gravanis A, Margioris A. Pharmacology of glucocorticoids: an overview. In: Margioris A, Chrousos G, editors. Contemporary endocrinology: adrenal disorders. Totowa (NJ): Humana Press; 2001. p. 59–70.
2. Alesci S, Koch C, Bornstein S, et al. Adrenal androgens regulation and adrenopause. Endocr Regul 2001;35:95–100.
3. Wiebke A, Stewart P. Adrenal corticosteroid biosynthesis, metabolism, and action. Endocrinol Metab Clin North Am 2005;34(2):293–313.
4. Kallen C, Arakane F, Sugawara T, et al. Structure, function and regulated expression of the steroidogenic acute regulatory (StAR) protein. In: Margioris A, Chrousos G, editors. Contemporary endocrinology: adrenal disorders. Totowa (NJ): Humana Press; 2001. p. 107–17.
5. Stewart P. The adrenal cortex. In: Kronenberg H, Melmed S, Polonsky K, et al, editors. Williams textbook of endocrinology. 11th edition. Philadelphia: Saunders Elsevier; 2008. p. 445–503.
6. Rijnberk A, Mol J. Adrenocortical function. In: Kaneko J, Harvey J, Bruss M, editors. Clinical biochemistry of domestic animals. 5th edition. San Diego (CA): Academic Press; 1997. p. 553–70.
7. Maier C, Kotzmann H, Luger A. CRH-receptors and their ligands. In: Gaillard R, editor. The ACTH axis: pathogenesis, diagnosis, and treatment. Boston: Kluwer Academic Publishers; 2003. p. 65–83.
8. Clark A, King P. The ACTH receptor and its mutations. In: Gaillard R, editor. The ACTH axis: pathogenesis, diagnosis, and treatment. Boston: Kluwer Academic Publishers; 2003. p. 171–90.
9. Lewis J, Bagley C, Elder P, et al. Plasma free cortisol fraction reflects levels of functioning corticosteroid-binding globulin. Clin Chim Acta 2005;359:189–94.
10. Adcock R, Kattesh H, Robert M, et al. Relationships between plasma cortisol, cortisosteroid-binding globulin (CBG) and the free cortisol index (FCI) in pigs over a 24 hours period. J Anim Vet Adv 2006;5:85–91.
11. Irvine C, Alexander S. Measurement of free cortisol and the capacity and association constant of cortisol-binding proteins in plasma of foals and adult horses. J Reprod Fertil Suppl 1987;35:19–24.
12. Meyer H, Rothuizen J. Determination of the percentage of free cortisol in plasma in the dog by ultrafiltration/dialysis. Domest Anim Endocrinol 1993;10:45–53.
13. Nicolaides N, Galata Z, Kino T, et al. The human glucocorticoid receptor: molecular basis of biologic function. Steroids 2010;75:1–12.
14. Marik P, Zaloga G. Adrenal insufficiency in the critically ill: a new look at an old problem. Chest 2002;122:1784–96.
15. Young W. Endocrine hypertension. In: Kronenberg H, Melmed S, Polonsky K, et al, editors. Williams textbook of endocrinology. 11th edition. Philadelphia: Saunders; Elsevier, Inc; 2008. p. 505–37.
16. Hedberg Y, Dalin A, Forsberg M, et al. Effect of ACTH (tetracosactide) on steroid hormone levels in the mare. Part A: effect in intact normal mares and mares with

possible estrous related behavioral abnormalities. Anim Reprod Sci 2007;100: 73–91.

17. Federman D. The endocrine patient. In: Kronenberg H, Melmed S, Polonsky K, et al, editors. Williams textbook of endocrinology. 11th edition. Philadelphia: Saunders Elsevier; 2008. p. 12–7.
18. Gehlen H, Sundermann T, Rohn K, et al. Aldosterone plasma concentration in horses with heart valve insufficiencies. Res Vet Sci 2008;85:340–4.
19. Haffner J, Fecteau K, Eiler H, et al. Blood steroid concentrations in domestic Mongolian horses. J Vet Diagn Invest 2010;22:537–43.
20. Hollis A, Boston R, Corley K. Plasma aldosterone, vasopressin, and atrial natriuretic peptide in hypovolaemia: a preliminary comparative study of neonatal and mature horses. Equine Vet J 2008;40:64–9.
21. Bornstein S, Engeland W, Erhart-Bornstein M, et al. Dissociation of ACTH and glucocorticoids. Trends Endocrinol Metab 2008;19:175–80.
22. Annane D, Maxime V, Ibrahim F, et al. Diagnosis of adrenal insufficiency in severe sepsis and septic shock. Am J Respir Crit Care Med 2006;174: 1319–26.
23. Marik P. Critical illness related corticosteroid insufficiency. Chest 2009;135(1): 181–93.
24. Marik P, Pastores S, Annane D, et al. Recommendations for the diagnosis and management of corticosteroid insufficiency in critically ill adult patients: consensus statements from an international task force by the American College of Critical Care Medicine. Crit Care Med 2008;36(6):1937–49.
25. Marik P, Zaloga G. Adrenal insufficiency during septic shock. Crit Care Med 2003;31:141–5.
26. Kozyra E, Wax R, Burry L. Can 1 ug of cosyntropin be used to evaluate adrenal insufficiency in critically ill patients? Ann Pharmacother 2005;39:691–8.
27. Siraux V, De Backer D, Yalavatti G, et al. Relative adrenal insufficiency in patients with septic shock: comparison of low-dose and conventional corticotropin tests. Crit Care Med 2005;33:2479–86.
28. Reijerkerk E, Visser E, van Reenen C, et al. Effects of various doses of ovine corticotrophin-releasing hormone on plasma and saliva cortisol concentrations in the horse. Am J Vet Res 2009;70:361–4.
29. Schmidt I, Lahner H, Mann K, et al. Diagnosis of adrenal insufficiency: evaluation of the corticotropin-releasing hormone test and basal serum cortisol in comparison to the insulin tolerance test in patients with hypothalamic-pituitary-adrenal disease. J Clin Endocrinol Metab 2003;88:4193–8.
30. Fiad T, Kirby J, Cunningham S, et al. The overnight single-dose metyrapone test is a simple and reliable index of the hypothalamic-pituitary-adrenal axis. Clin Endocrinol 1994;40:603–9.
31. Luna S, YTaylor P, Wheeler M. Cardiorespiratory, endocrine and metabolic changes in ponies undergoing intravenous or inhalation anaesthesia. J Vet Pharmacol Ther 1996;19:251–8.
32. Alexander S, Irvine C, Donald R. Dynamics of the regulation of the hypothalamic-pituitary-adrenal (HPA) axis determined using a nonsurgical method for collecting pituitary venous blood from horses. Front Neuroendocrinol 1996;17:1–50.
33. Giordano R, Picu A, Bonelli L, et al. Hypothalamus-pituitary-adrenal axis evaluation in patients with hypothalamo-pituitary disorders; comparisons of different provocative tests. Clin Endocrinol 2008;68(6):935–41.
34. Silver M, Fowden A, Know J, et al. Sympathoadrenal and other responses to hypoglycaemia in the young foal. J Reprod Fertil Suppl 1987;35:607–14.

35. Alexander S, Roud H, Irvine C. Effect of insulin-induced hypoglycemia on secretion patterns and rates of corticotropin-releasing hormone, arginine vasopressin and adrenocorticotrophin in horses. J Endocrinol 1997;153(3):401–9.
36. Langouche L, Van den Berghe G. Glucose metabolism and insulin therapy. Crit Care Clinics 2006;22(1):119–29.
37. Cohen J, Venkatesh B. Assessment of tissue cortisol activity. Crit Care Resusc 2009;11(4):287–9.
38. Liu D, Su Y, Zhang W, et al. Changes in glucocorticoid and mineralocorticoid receptors of liver and kidney cytosols after pathologic stress and its regulation in rats. Crit Care Med 2002;30(3):623–7.
39. Marik P. Mechanisms and clinical consequences of critical illness associated adrenal insufficiency. Curr Opin Crit Care 2007;13:363–9.
40. Meduri G, Muthiah M, Carratu P, et al. Nuclear factor-κb- and glucocorticoid receptor-α mediated mechanisms in the regulation of systemic and pulmonary inflammation during sepsis and acute respiratory distress syndrome. Neuroimmunomodulation 2005;12:321–38.
41. Fazio E, Medica P, Aronica V, et al. Circulating beta-endorphin, adrenocorticotrophic hormone and cortisol levels of stallions before and after short road transport: stress effect of different distances. Acta Vet Scand 2008;50:6.
42. Place N, McGowan C, Lamb S, et al. Seasonal variation in serum concentrations of selected metabolic hormones in horses. J Vet Intern Med 2010;24(3):650–4.
43. Kudielka B, Buske-Kirschbaum A, Helhammer D, et al. HPA axis responses to laboratory pyschosocial stress in healthy elderly adults, younger adults, and children: impact of age and gender. Psychoneuroendocrinology 2004;29:83–98.
44. Lefcourt A, Bitman J, Kahl S, et al. Circadian and ultradian rhythms of peripheral cortisol concentrations in lactating dairy cows. J Dairy Sci 1993;76:2607–12.
45. Martin L, Behrend E, Mealey K, et al. Effect of low doses of cosyntropin in serum cortisol concentrations in clinically normal dogs. Am J Vet Res 2007;68(5):555–60.
46. Bousquet-Melou A, Formentini E, Picard-Hagen N, et al. The adrenocorticotropin stimulation test: contribution of a physiologically based model developed in horse for its interpretation in different pathophysiologic situations encountered in man. Endocrinology 2006;147(9):4281–91.
47. McKeever K, Malinowski K. Endocrine response to exercise in young and old horses. Equine Vet J Suppl 1999;30:561–6.
48. Silver M, Ousey J, Dudan F, et al. Studies on equine prematurity 2: post natal adrenocortical activity in relation to plasma adrenocorticotrophic hormone and catecholamine levels in term and premature foals. Equine Vet J 1984;16(4):278–86.
49. Silver M, Fowden A. Prepartum adrenocortical maturation in the fetal foal: responses to ACTH. J Endocrinol 1994;142:417–25.
50. Ousey J, Rossdale P, Fowden A, et al. Effects of manipulating intrauterine growth on post natal adrenocortical development and other parameters of maturity in neonatal foals. Equine Vet J 2004;36(7):616–21.
51. Rossdale P, Ousey J. Studies on equine prematurity 6: guidelines for assessment of foal maturity. Equine Vet J 1984;16(4):300–2.
52. Han X, Fowden A, Silver M, et al. Immunohistochemical localisation of steroidogenic enzymes and phenylethanolamine-N-methyl-transferase (PNMT) in the adrenal gland of the fetal and newborn foal. Equine Vet J 1995;27(2):140–6.
53. Weng Q, Tanaka Y, Taniyama H, et al. Immunolocalization of steroidogenic enzymes in equine fetal adrenal glands during mid-late gestation. J Reprod Dev 2007;53(5):1093–8.

54. Riley S, Boshier D, Luu-The V, et al. Immunohistochemical localization of 3 beta-hydroxysteroid/delta 5-delta 4-isomerase, tyrosine hydroxylase, and phenylethanolamine N-methyl transferase in adrenal glands of sheep fetuses throughout gestation and in neonates. J Reprod Fertil 1992;96(1):127–34.
55. Donaldson M, McDonnell S, Schanbacher B, et al. Variation in plasma adrenocorticotropic hormone concentration and dexamethasone suppression test results with season, age, and sex in healthy ponies and horses. J Vet Intern Med 2005;19(2):217–22.
56. Hart K, Heusner G, Norton N, et al. Hypothalamic-pituitary-adrenal axis assessment in healthy term neonatal foals utilizing a paired low dose/high dose ACTH stimulation test. J Vet Intern Med 2009;23:344–51.
57. Irvine C, Alexander S. Factors affecting the circadian rhythm in plasma cortisol concentrations in the horse. Domest Anim Endocrinol 1994;11(2):227–38.
58. Wong D, Vo D, Alcott C, et al. Adrenocorticotropic hormone stimulation tests in healthy foals from birth to 12 weeks of age. Can J Vet Res 2009;73(1):65–72.
59. Broughton Pipkin F, Ousey J, Wallace C, et al. Studies on equine prematurity 4: effect of salt and water loss on the renin-angiotensin-aldosterone system in the newborn foal. Equine Vet J 1984;16(4):292–7.
60. Greco D. Hypoadrenocorticism in small animals. Clin Tech Small Anim Pract 2007;22(1):32–5.
61. de Herder WLS. Overview of hyper- and hypoadrencorticism. In: Margioris A, Chrousos G, editors. Contemporary endocrinology: adrenal disorders. Totowa (NJ): Humana Press; 2001. p. 143–53.
62. Levin J, Cluff L. Endotoxemia and adrenal hemorrhage. A mechanism for the Waterhouse-Friderichsen syndrome. J Exp Med 1965;1(121):247–60.
63. Loisa P, Rinne T, Kaukinen S. Adrenocortical function and multiple organ failure in severe sepsis. Acta Anaesthesiol Scand 2002;46:145–51.
64. Dybdal N, McFarlane D. Endocrine and metabolic diseases. In: Smith B, editor. Large animal internal medicine. 4th edition. Philadelphia: Mosby; 2009. p. 1345.
65. Guillamondegui O, Gunter O, Patel S, et al. Acute adrenal insufficiency may affect outcome in the trauma patient. Am Surg 2009;75(4):287–90.
66. Henzen C, Kobza R, Schwaller-Protzmann B, et al. Adrenal function during coronary artery bypass grafting. Eur J Endocrinol 2003;148(6):663–8.
67. Aneja R, Carcillo J. What is the rationale for hydrocortisone treatment in children with infection-related adrenal insufficiency and septic shock. Arch Dis Child 2007; 92:165–9.
68. Elsouri N, Bander J, Guzman J. Relative adrenal insufficiency in patients with septic shock; a close look at practice patterns. J Crit Care 2006;21:73–8.
69. Fernandez J, Escorell A, Zabalza M, et al. Adrenal insufficiency in patients with cirrhosis and septic shock: effect of treatment with hydrocortisone on survival. Hepatology 2006;44(5):1288–95.
70. Pizarro C, Troster E, Damiani D, et al. Absolute and relative adrenal insufficiency in children with septic shock. Crit Care Med 2005;33(4):855–9.
71. McGavin M, Zachary J, editors. Pathologic basis of veterinary disease. 4th edition. St Louis (MO): Mosby Elsevier; 2007. p. 370.
72. De Jong F, Mallios C, Jansen C, et al. Etomidate suppresses adrenocortical function by inhibition of 11-beta-hydroxylation. J Clin Endocrinol Metab 1984; 59(6):1143–7.
73. Beishuizen A, Thijs L. Endotoxin and the hypothalamic-pituitary-adrenal (HPA) axis. J Endotoxin Res 2003;9(1):3–24.

74. Gaillard R. Interactions between the hypothalamic-pituitary-adrenal axis and the immunological system. In: Gaillard R, editor. The ACTH axis: pathogenesis, diagnosis, and treatment. Boston: Kluwer Academic Publishers; 2003. p. 109–35.
75. Judd A, Call G, Barney M, et al. Possible function of IL-6 and TNF as intraadrenal factors in the regulation of adrenal steroid secretion. Ann N Y Acad Sci 2000;917:628–37.
76. Sharshar T, Gray F, Lorin de la Grandmaison G, et al. Apoptosis of neurons in cardiovascular autonomic centers triggered by inducible nitric oxide synthase after death from septic shock. Lancet 2003;362:1799–805.
77. Aubry J, Turnbull A, Pozzoli G, et al. Endotoxin decreases corticotropin-releasing factor receptor 1 messenger ribonucleic acid levels in the rat pituitary. Endocrinology 1997;138(4):1621–6.
78. Qahwash I, Cassar C, Radcliff R, et al. Bacterial lipopolysaccharide-induced coordinate downregulation of arginine vasopressin receptor V3 and corticotropin-releasing factor receptor 1 messenger ribonucleic acids in the anterior pituitary of endotoxemic steers. Endocrine 2002;18:13–20.
79. Liu L, Sun B, Tian Y, et al. Changes of pulmonary glucocorticoid receptor and phospholipase A2 in sheep with acute lung injury. Am Rev Respir Dis 1993;148:878–81.
80. Couetil L, Hoffman A. Adrenal insufficiency in a neonatal foal. J Am Vet Med Assoc 1998;212:1594–6.
81. Gold J, Divers T, Barton M, et al. Plasma adrenocorticotropin, cortisol, and adrenocorticotropin/cortisol ratios in septic and normal-term foals. J Vet Intern Med 2007;21:791–6.
82. Hurcombe S, Toribio R, Slovis N, et al. Blood arginine vasopressin, adrenocorticotropin hormone, and cortisol concentrations at admission in septic and critically ill foals and their association with survival. J Vet Intern Med 2008;22(3):639–47.
83. Hart K, Slovis N, Barton M. Hypothalamic-pituitary-adrenal axis dysfunction in hospitalized neonatal foals. J Vet Intern Med 2009;23:901–12.
84. Wong D, Vo D, Alcott C, et al. Baseline plasma cortisol and ACTH concentrations and response to low dose ACTH stimulation testing in ill foals. J Am Vet Med Assoc 2009;234(1):126–32.
85. Fernandez E, Watterberg K. Relative adrenal insufficiency in the preterm and term infant. J Perinatol 2009;29(Suppl 2):S44–9.
86. Dowling P, Williams M, Clark T. Adrenal insufficiency associated with long-term anabolic steroid administration in a horse. J Am Vet Med Assoc 1994;203(8):1166–9.
87. Baker H, Baker I, Epstein V, et al. Effect of stress on steroid hormone levels in racehorses. Aust Vet J 1982;58(2):70–1.
88. Unwin R, Capasso G. The renal tubular acidoses. J R Soc Med 2000;94:221–5.
89. Arroyo L, Stampfli H. Equine renal tubular disorders. Vet Clin North Am Equine Pract 2007;23(3):631–9.
90. Styne D, Grumbach M. Puberty: ontogeny, neuroendocrinology, physiology, and disorders. In: Kronenberg H, Melmed S, Polonsky K, et al, editors. Williams textbook of endocrinology. 11th edition. Philadelphia: Saunders: Elsevier, Inc; 2008. p. 969–1166.

Endocrine Dysregulation in Critically Ill Foals and Horses

Ramiro E. Toribio, DVM, MS, PhD

KEYWORDS

• Sepsis • Parathyroid • Cortisol • ACTH • Thyroid • Energy
• Somatotropic • Progesterone

THE SYMPATHETIC SYSTEM

The initial endocrine response to stress and disease is mediated by the central nervous system, secreting neurotransmitters and releasing factors into the pituitary portal and systemic circulations as well as making direct contact with endocrine organs (neurohypophysis, pancreas, adrenal gland) and effectors (liver, heart, skeletal and smooth muscles). The activation of the sympathetic system results in epinephrine secretion by the adrenal medulla, whereas most norepinephrine in circulation is released from the synaptic clefts,[1] which is likely because the main functions of epinephrine are metabolic, whereas norepinephrine is primarily a neurotransmitter. Relevant to equine disease is that the enteric nervous system is the source of up to 50% of the catecholamines in circulation,[1,2] which is becoming a major subject of research in critical care medicine. Increased epinephrine and norepinephrine concentrations have been measured in horses with colic,[3–5] and high epinephrine concentrations have been associated with nonsurvival in horses with gastrointestinal disease.[3] No association was found between norepinephrine and severity of colic.[3] Because of their negative effect on intestinal motility, it is possible that prolonged sympathetic activity in these horses could be a contributing factor to their poor outcome. Although not related to the main goal of this article, one study found that horses in line to be slaughtered had a rapid and several fold increase in catecholamine and cortisol concentrations, reflecting that horses have a rapid response to stress by the adrenal medulla and cortex.[6]

THE HYPOTHALAMUS-PITUITARY-ADRENAL AXIS

The hypothalamus-pituitary-adrenal (HPA) axis is a regulatory system that has the goal of mounting a metabolic response to stressful conditions, to guarantee survival. On

Department of Veterinary Clinical Sciences, College of Veterinary Medicine, The Ohio State University, 601 Vernon Tharp Street, Columbus, OH 43210, USA
E-mail address: toribio.1@osu.edu

Vet Clin Equine 27 (2011) 35–47
doi:10.1016/j.cveq.2010.12.011
vetequine.theclinics.com

stressful stimulation, the hypothalamus releases the corticotropin-releasing hormone into the pituitary portal system to stimulate the pituitary corticotrophs to secrete adrenocorticotropin (ACTH). In horses, arginine vasopressin (AVP) is also a secreting factor for ACTH.[7,8] The main target for ACTH is the zona fasciculata of the adrenal gland cortex to produce glucocorticoids, in particular cortisol. To a minimal extend, ACTH also induces aldosterone secretion by the zona glomerulosa of the adrenal gland.

The HPA axis activation in horses with gastrointestinal disease is anticipated because abdominal pain is the major stressful event. Horses with gastrointestinal disease are often endotoxemic,[9] and endotoxemia in mares induces AVP, oxytocin, and ACTH release.[8] Thus, endotoxins are likely to be a key stimulus for HPA activation in sick horses because they can directly and indirectly activate pituitary cells.[10]

Several studies have found increased cortisol concentrations in horses with acute abdominal pain.[3,5,11–13] Similar results have been found in pregnant mares with acute medical and surgical abdominal disease.[12] One study showed that horses with colic and high cortisol concentrations were more likely to die,[3] whereas another study found that horses with colic had elevated ACTH, β-endorphin, and cortisol concentrations, with nonsurviving animals having the highest concentrations.[13] Cortisol concentrations were elevated in horses with acute laminitis.[14]

HPA axis dysregulation seems to be a frequent problem in critically ill foals.[15–17] AVP, ACTH, and cortisol concentrations were increased in septic foals,[15–17] and foals with the highest plasma AVP and ACTH concentrations were more likely to die, indicating that excessive hypothalamic and pituitary responses are either risk factors for death or reflect the terminal stages of severe sepsis (see article by Hurcombe in this issue for more details). Many septic foals do not have an appropriate cortisol response to endogenous or exogenous ACTH (high ACTH:cortisol ratio), a concept known as relative adrenal gland insufficiency.[15–18] One study found higher ACTH:cortisol ratios in nonsurviving septic foals.[15] Hydrocortisone is being considered as a replacement therapy for foals with adrenal insufficiency.[18] For additional information on adrenal gland function in foals see the review by Hart and Barton in this issue.

THE GROWTH HORMONE AXIS

The growth hormone (GH) is released in a pulsatile pattern by the somatotrophs of the adenohypophysis in response to exercise, hunger, and stress. The effects of the GH are mediated by insulin-like growth factor 1 (IGF-1), which is secreted by the liver.[19] This is the GH/IGF-1 or somatotropic axis. Our traditional hypothalamic-pituitary understanding of GH release has been centered on GH-releasing hormone stimulating and somatostatin inhibiting GH synthesis and secretion. However, the recent discovery of ghrelin has changed our perspective on GH regulation.[20,21] Ghrelin is a GH-releasing factor secreted by the P/D1 cells of the stomach and the arcuate nucleus of the hypothalamus in response to hypoglycemia and fasting to enhance hunger (orexigenic).[20,21] Although information on the GH/IGF-1 axis in critical illness in other species has increased dramatically in recent years,[19,22–24] information in diseased horses and foals is minimal.[25] One consistent finding in critically ill humans is a loss of the GH pulsatile pattern, with high plasma GH concentrations that are not followed by increases in IGF-1, indicating GH resistance.[19,26]

Although far from elucidating the GH/IGF-1 axis response to sepsis in equine patients, Barsnick and colleagues recently documented that GH and ghrelin concentrations in septic foals are higher than in sick nonseptic foals and healthy foals.[25] It was also found that serum IGF-1 concentrations were lower in septic foals (R. Barsnick, Ramiro E. Toribio, unpublished information, 2010). The fact that IGF-1 concentrations were low despite high GH concentrations supports our theory that GH resistance is a problem that deserves further investigation in critically ill foals. IGF-1 is the main systemic negative regulator for GH release (negative feedback), and low IGF-1 levels in septic foals likely enhance GH secretion.

In addition to stress, gastric ghrelin release contributes to GH secretion in sick equine patients. It is also possible that ghrelin secretion during critical illness represents a defensive mechanism. In other species, ghrelin has protective effects against systemic inflammation and endotoxemia[27] by decreasing endothelin 1 secretion and inhibiting sympathetic activity.[28,29] Translational studies using ghrelin to reduce inflammation, increase muscle mass, and treat cachexia and anorexia are underway in other species.[30]

THE ENERGY AXIS

The energy and somatotropic axes are part of a major regulatory system, and this separation into 2 sections is purely academic. Insulin, glucagon, cortisol, and epinephrine have been considered the main components of the energy axis; however, it is clear that this is a complex functional structure with many other hormones involved. Of interest in energy regulation are also GH, ghrelin, leptin, and adiponectin. Leptin is an adipocyte-derived hormone that regulates satiety by decreasing hunger (anorexigenic) and enhances energy expenditure by increasing insulin sensitivity.[31] Ghrelin is secreted by the stomach to induce hunger.[20,21] Thus, ghrelin and leptin work in opposite ways at the hypothalamic level. Adiponectin is another adipocyte-derived hormone that participates in energy regulation by increasing insulin sensitivity and fatty acid oxidation.[32] This hormone also induces nitric oxide–mediated vasorelaxation and has antiinflammatory properties.[31–34] Leptin and adiponectin (adipokines) blood concentrations are proportional to the body condition in humans and horses.[33,34] Similar to insulin and GH during disease, resistance to leptin and adiponectin may occur in critical illness.[31]

Increased insulin, leptin, GH, and prolactin concentrations have been measured in horses with endotoxemia.[22,35,36] Endotoxemia in horses increases insulin concentrations and may induce insulin resistance.[36] Information on adiponectin and ghrelin in horses with evidence of systemic inflammation, sepsis, or endotoxemia is lacking. The association between hormones involved in energy regulation and glucose, triglycerides, severity of sepsis, and mortality was recently investigated in critically ill foals.[25,37] Blood concentrations of glucose were low, whereas triglyceride, GH, ghrelin, and glucagon concentrations were increased in septic foals.[37] Septic foals with high insulin or low leptin concentrations were more likely to die.[37]

A novel concept in endocrinology that relates to energy regulation is the gut-brain axis.[38] This axis is involved in the regulation of satiety, food intake, glucose and fat homeostasis, insulin secretion, and bone metabolism.[38] In addition, this axis has close interactions with the adipose tissue and liver, 2 central systems in energy homeostasis. Although fat has been seen as a passive player in many body functions, in reality it represents a major endocrine organ that produces endocrine, paracrine, and autocrine factors and cytokines (adipokines, inflammatory cytokines) that modulate energy metabolism and inflammation. In fact, emphasis is being placed on the importance of the cellular components of the adipose tissue in chronic and critical illness in many species, including the horse.[39]

THYROID HORMONES

As for the HPA axis, the hypothalamus-pituitary-thyroid (HPT) axis has specific functions, mostly related to metabolic activities, cell differentiation, and development. The hypothalamus releases the thyrotropin-releasing hormone (TRH) into the pituitary portal system to stimulate the pituitary thyrotrophs to release the thyroid-stimulating hormone (TSH), which in turn stimulates the thyroid gland follicular cells to synthesize and release thyroid hormones (THs; T4, T3). In general, diseases and stress have a suppressive effect on the HPT axis.

The nonthyroidal illness syndrome (NTIS; euthyroid sick syndrome) refers to the decrease in TH concentrations (T3 in particular) that occurs in people and animals with severe illness.[40] During starvation and disease, the conversion of T4 to T3 in peripheral tissues decreases. It is believed that selenium deficiency may be involved in the pathogenesis of NTIS because iodinases, responsible for T4 to T3 conversion, are selenium-dependent enzymes.[41] With more severe disease, T4 concentrations also decrease, suggesting dysfunction at the hypothalamic, pituitary, or thyroid gland level. TSH concentrations are often inappropriately low for the measured low TH values,[42] supporting hypothalamus-pituitary dysfunction (central hypothyroidism) as part of the pathogenesis of NTIS.[42] Decreased leptin and increased cytokine concentrations in severe illness participate in the development of NTIS. Leptin increases the hypothalamic release of TRH.[43] Decreased blood thyroxine-binding globulin concentrations have been proposed as a possible cause for low total T4 concentrations in disease.[42] What is important to understand with NTIS is that low concentrations of THs do not equate to hypothyroidism.

It is not unusual for horses with various chronic diseases (eg, pituitary pars intermedia dysfunction, metabolic syndrome, laminitis) to have low TH levels, indicating NTIS. Further, low TH levels have been measured in sick foals with noncritical conditions.[44–47] However, when it comes to TH levels in critically ill horses and foals, information is lacking. The author is aware of 2 studies assessing THs in septic and premature foals[48,49] but could not find information in adult sick horses. Total T4, total T3, free T4, and free T3 levels were lower in septic foals when compared with sick nonseptic foals and healthy foals, and these concentrations were even lower in nonsurviving septic foals.[49] Similar results were reported in premature foals, which had low TH levels and an exaggerated TSH response to TRH.[48] These findings confirm that NTIS is frequent in critically ill foals but also that THs are associated with severity of disease and mortality.

CALCIUM-REGULATING HORMONES

Many acute diseases are associated with calcium dysregulation. Most horses with acute intestinal disease (eg, colic, enteritis, enterocolitis) develop hypocalcemia,[50,51] which has been linked to abnormal concentrations of parathyroid hormone (PTH),[51] the main calcium-regulating hormone. The low PTH concentrations in many horses with intestinal disease, endotoxemia, and hypocalcemia suggest an impaired parathyroid gland response to low calcium. Interleukin (IL)-1β and IL-6, inflammatory mediators known to be increased in horses with enteric disease and endotoxemia,[52,53] are likely to be involved in the pathogenesis of equine hypocalcemia and impaired parathyroid gland function. It has been shown that these cytokines inhibit the messenger RNA (mRNA) expression and secretion of PTH by equine parathyroid cells.[54] The role of other endocrine factors involved in calcium regulation is less clear. No differences in calcitonin and PTH-related protein were found among septic, sick and nonseptic, and healthy foals,[55] and vitamin D has not been investigated in critically ill equine patients.

Procalcitonin (PCT), the precursor of calcitonin is being used as a marker of sepsis and a predictor of outcome in humans with sepsis.[56,57] Because calcitonin decreases blood calcium levels and is a potential candidate in the pathogenesis of equine hypocalcemia during sepsis and endotoxemia, Toribio and colleagues[58] have cloned several genes of the equine calcitonin family. In further studies, the investigators found increased PCT mRNA expression in the leukocytes of septic foals; however, using a human PCT immunoassay they could not demonstrate differences in blood PCT concentrations between healthy and endotoxemic foals and horses, likely because there are major sequence differences between human and equine PCT (Ramiro E. Toribio, unpublished data, 2007). One study found no differences in leukocyte mRNA expression for IL-1β, IL-6, and PCT between healthy and septic foals.[59] Of interest, mean PCT concentrations were several folds higher in septic foals than in controls. It is also unclear how PCT primers were designed in this study to assess PCT mRNA expression because the equine *CALC-I* gene is tricky for primer design, with common splice sites for PCT and calcitonin gene–related peptide (CGRP).[58] Thus, additional work with the calcitonin gene family may clarify its role in the pathogenesis of hypocalcemia and sepsis.

WATER, SODIUM, AND BLOOD PRESSURE

Hypotension, poor tissue perfusion, and disorders of water and sodium metabolism are common in critically ill foals and horses; however, equine-specific endocrine data in this field are limited. Hypoperfusion has been associated with foal mortality,[16] and the underlying hormonal mechanisms for vasopressor refractory hypotension in foals remain unclear.

The main function of the renin-angiotensin-aldosterone system (RAAS) is to preserve blood pressure and tissue perfusion. Renin is a renal enzyme secreted in response to hypotension, low tubular chloride concentrations (sensed by the juxtaglomerular apparatus), and sympathetic activation.[60] Renin cleaves angiotensinogen to angiotensin I, which is converted in the lungs by angiotensin-converting enzymes into angiotensin II, a potent vasoconstrictor that also induces aldosterone and AVP secretion. Aldosterone is secreted by the zona glomerulosa of the adrenal gland in response to hyperkalemia, angiotensin II, and ACTH. Aldosterone increases renal sodium retention and potassium elimination, thus affecting blood pressure and tissue perfusion. AVP is secreted by the neurohypophysis in response to hypotension, hyperosmolality, and angiotensin II to induce vasoconstriction and increase renal water retention.

Most equine information on the RAAS has been generated from adult horses under different exercise conditions.[61–63] Abnormally high plasma AVP concentrations have been measured in septic foals with evidence of hypotension.[16] AVP and atrial natriuretic peptide concentrations were elevated in horses with acute abdominal disease and evidence of hypotension[64]; however, no differences before and after fluid resuscitation were found in sick foals, indicating differences between neonates and adult horses.[64] The role or association of brain natriuretic peptide with equine disease remains to be determined. Aldosterone concentrations were elevated in foals and horses admitted to a veterinary hospital with evidence of hypovolemia.[64] Renin activity and aldosterone concentrations were increased in horses with experimental laminitis.[14] Because many of these horses with laminitis developed hyponatremia, it was speculated that the increases in renin and aldosterone represented a homeostatic response. There is evidence that newborn septic foals have a high aldosterone response to systemic inflammation that parallels AVP, ACTH, and cortisol secretion, which is inverse to potassium concentrations (K. Dembek, K. Onasch, Ramiro E. Toribio, unpublished data, 2010).

As previously mentioned, refractory hypotension and poor tissue perfusion are serious complications in septic foals.[65] There is no question that inflammatory mediators, receptor downregulation, and the interplay between vasoconstrictors and vasodilators are involved in the pathogenesis of these processes. See "Other Endocrine Factors" later.

Nitric oxide mediates the action of most vasodilators, and excessive nitric oxide production during sepsis has been proposed as the main cause of hypotension refractory to vasopressors.[66] This phenomenon remains to be proven in foals but should be considered. The fact that most septic foals have increased AVP concentrations[16] backs the receptor downregulation theory. However, several hypotensive foals respond to AVP therapy (vasopressin, desmopressin), indicating that this phenomenon is quite complex. There are also those foals with a poor response to norepinephrine, which only improves after AVP treatment, supporting synergistic actions between these hormones. Although there is no specific data for foals, treatment with glucocorticoids enhances the response to vasopressors in hypotensive human neonates.[67,68] This treatment could be relevant in hypotensive foals with relative adrenal insufficiency that do not respond to vasopressors and in which hydrocortisone (or dexamethasone) should be considered. Data on blood catecholamine concentrations in septic foals are absent, and valuable information on the clinical benefits of AVP and AVP-catecholamine infusions in equine patients is not readily available.

REPRODUCTIVE HORMONES

It is valid to assume that severe disease results in reproductive hormone dysregulation. Because reproductive success is primarily measured as the ability of a mare to get pregnant or carry a pregnancy to term, it should not be surprising that most information available is from mares.[69–72] Endotoxemia is frequent in horses with gastrointestinal disease,[9] often associated with mortality. One retrospective study of 115 pregnant mares found an abortion rate of 20.5% for surgical colics, 40% for uterine torsions, and 10.8% for medical colics, with an average abortion rate of 16.4%.[73]

Several studies have shown that endotoxemia leads to prostaglandin (PG) release, luteolysis, early embryonic death, and abortion in mares.[69–72] Endotoxin infusion to healthy mares during the estrus cycle causes PG F2α release, luteolysis, lowering of progesterone concentrations, and shortening of the cycle.[72] *Salmonella* endotoxin administration to pregnant mares in early gestation resulted in a rapid increase of PG F2α concentrations that was associated with a decrease in progesterone concentrations and fetal death (days 23–55 of gestation).[71] Abortion due to endotoxemia was less likely in mares after day 60. However, gastrointestinal disease and endotoxin remain a major risk for equine fetal loss and should be taken seriously. These studies support the administration of progestogens (eg, altrenogest) to critically ill mares in early gestation.[69] As important is the prompt treatment with flunixin meglumine to prevent PG F2α release, luteolysis, and fetal loss.[70]

Because it is claimed that progestogens maintain myometrial quiescence, one study assessed their concentrations in late gestating mares with normal and compromised pregnancies, including placentitis, uterine torsion, colic, and laminitis.[74] Mares with placentitis had higher progesterone and pregnenolone concentrations, indicating increased fetal/placental metabolic activity in response to stress. In mares with non-placental pathologies, progestogens were lower than in controls. No association was found between progestogens concentrations and maintenance of pregnancy.[74]

Prolactin concentrations increased in mares and geldings after endotoxin administration[22]; however, the clinical implications of this finding are unclear. Endotoxemia induces AVP, oxytocin, and ACTH release in mares[8] and could be another process leading to embryonic death or abortion because ACTH induces cortisol secretion, a key event to end gestation.[75]

OTHER ENDOCRINE FACTORS

It is of interest that when it comes to endocrine factors that are involved in inflammation and regulation of blood pressure and that have been associated with sepsis and mortality in other species, data to better understand these processes in severely ill equine patients are lacking.

Endothelin 1

Endothelin (ET-1) is a strong vasoconstrictor released by the endothelium under physiologic and pathologic conditions. ET-1 is involved in the pathogenesis of microcirculatory dysfunction during sepsis and endotoxemia.[76,77] ET-1 is also central to the development of pulmonary hypertension in critical disease.[76] Increased ET-1 concentrations have been measured in septic neonates from other species,[78] and it is reasonable to assume a similar response in septic foals. High ET-1 concentrations were measured in horses with endotoxemia,[79] and ET-1 has been implicated in the pathogenesis of equine laminitis.[79–81] Being relevant to many pathologic processes, it is not surprising that ET-1 receptor antagonists (bosentan, sitaxsentan, tezosentan) have been developed to treat myocardial ischemia, pulmonary hypertension, and systemic inflammation in humans.[77,82] Although it may sound impractical or expensive, antagonism to ET-1 has promising clinical applications to equine patients with endotoxemia, laminitis, and pulmonary hypertension. For example, tezosentan improved splanchnic and intestinal circulation and the acid base status in endotoxemic pigs.[77] Endotoxemia and laminitis are frequent complications in horses with gastrointestinal disease and foals with sepsis.

CGRP

CGRP is a product of the calcitonin gene family synthesized by the central and peripheral nervous systems.[58] Considered one of the most potent endogenous vasodilators, CGRP is also a neurotransmitter involved in pain and nociception.[58] Increased CGRP concentrations have been measured in different diseases, including sepsis and endotoxemia.[83,84] CGRP also seems to have antiinflammatory actions during endotoxemia by inhibiting cytokine production by macrophages.[85] Although information on CGRP and acute equine disease is minimal,[86] it can be assumed that CGRP participates in the development of pain and hypotension in foals and horses with sepsis and gastrointestinal disease. After all, the equine respiratory, gastrointestinal, and urinary tracts are rich in CGRP innervation.[58,87,88]

Adrenomedullin

Adrenomedullin (ADM), another vasodilator of the calcitonin gene family, is produced by the adrenal medulla and many cell types. Increased ADM concentrations have been found during sepsis and endotoxemia.[89] ADM has antiapoptotic properties, attenuates ischemia and reperfusion injury, enhances microcirculatory function, reduces gut mucosa permeability, and has been proposed as a molecule to improve cardiovascular function during sepsis.[89–91] The ratio between ET-1 and ADM, 2 counteracting peptides, was associated with mortality in human septic patients.[92] The author could not find any information in ADM in equids.

Erythropoietin

Although problems associated with erythropoietin (EPO) production has not been reported in critically ill equine patients, it is important for the reader to know that the administration of human recombinant EPO (rhEPO) to performance horses to enhance erythropoiesis has led to catastrophic results.[93] An elevation in the hematocrit is the initial response to rhEPO in horses; however, a number of these animals develop anti-rhEPO antibodies that can neutralize equine EPO, leading to aplastic anemia and often death. This problem was reported several years ago,[93] and the author has seen many of these cases, in some instances with more than one horse affected from the same trainer.

SUMMARY

In severe illness, various endocrine homeostatic systems react to overcome adverse conditions. An appropriate response requires coordination among different systems and their effectors. In many instances, abnormal levels of endocrine factors and refractoriness of the effectors to hormonal stimulation complicates outcome. Understanding the endocrinology of acute disease has benefits from a therapeutic and prognostic perspective. Many drugs that improve survival have been developed from this kind of information and have the potential to be used in equine practice. This article provides an overview on the equine endocrine response to critical illness and sepsis from the available data.

REFERENCES

1. Asfar P, Hauser B, Radermacher P, et al. Catecholamines and vasopressin during critical illness. Crit Care Clin 2006;22:131–49.
2. Aneman A, Eisenhofer G, Olbe L, et al. Sympathetic discharge to mesenteric organs and the liver. Evidence for substantial mesenteric organ norepinephrine spillover. J Clin Invest 1996;97:1640–6.
3. Hinchcliff KW, Rush BR, Farris JW. Evaluation of plasma catecholamine and serum cortisol concentrations in horses with colic. J Am Vet Med Assoc 2005; 227:276–80.
4. Zierz J, Wintzer HJ. Acute pain in the horse and one possibility for its objective evaluation. Tierarztl Prax 1996;24:108–12.
5. Hodson NP, Wright JA, Hunt J. The sympatho-adrenal system and plasma levels of adrenocorticotropic hormone, cortisol and catecholamines in equine grass sickness. Vet Rec 1986;118:148–50.
6. Micera E, Albrizio M, Surdo NC, et al. Stress-related hormones in horses before and after stunning by captive bolt gun. Meat Sci 2010;84:634–7.
7. Alexander SL, Irvine CH, Donald RA. Dynamics of the regulation of the hypothalamo-pituitary-adrenal (HPA) axis determined using a nonsurgical method for collecting pituitary venous blood from horses. Front Neuroendocrinol 1996;17:1–50.
8. Alexander SL, Irvine CH. The effect of endotoxin administration on the secretory dynamics of oxytocin in follicular phase mares: relationship to stress axis hormones. J Neuroendocrinol 2002;14:540–8.
9. King JN, Gerring EL. Detection of endotoxin in cases of equine colic. Vet Rec 1988;123:269–71.
10. Whitlock BK, Daniel JA, Wilborn RR, et al. Comparative aspects of the endotoxin- and cytokine-induced endocrine cascade influencing neuroendocrine

control of growth and reproduction in farm animals. Reprod Domest Anim 2008;43(Suppl 2):317–23.
11. Edner AH, Nyman GC, Essen-Gustavsson B. Metabolism before, during and after anaesthesia in colic and healthy horses. Acta Vet Scand 2007;49:34–49.
12. Santschi EM, LeBlanc MM, Weston PG. Progestagen, oestrone sulphate and cortisol concentrations in pregnant mares during medical and surgical disease. J Reprod Fertil Suppl 1991;44:627–34.
13. Niinisto KE, Korolainen RV, Raekallio MR, et al. Plasma levels of heat shock protein 72 (HSP72) and beta-endorphin as indicators of stress, pain and prognosis in horses with colic. Vet J 2010;184:100–4.
14. Clarke LL, Garner HE, Hatfield D. Plasma volume, electrolyte, and endocrine changes during onset of laminitis hypertension in horses. Am J Vet Res 1982; 43:1551–5.
15. Gold JR, Divers TJ, Barton MH, et al. Plasma adrenocorticotropin, cortisol, and adrenocorticotropin/cortisol ratios in septic and normal-term foals. J Vet Intern Med 2007;21:791–6.
16. Hurcombe SD, Toribio RE, Slovis N, et al. Blood arginine vasopressin, adrenocorticotropin hormone, and cortisol concentrations at admission in septic and critically ill foals and their association with survival. J Vet Intern Med 2008;22: 639–47.
17. Hart KA, Slovis NM, Barton MH. Hypothalamic-pituitary-adrenal axis dysfunction in hospitalized neonatal foals. J Vet Intern Med 2009;23:901–12.
18. Hart KA, Ferguson DC, Heusner GL, et al. Synthetic adrenocorticotropic hormone stimulation tests in healthy neonatal foals. J Vet Intern Med 2007;21:314–21.
19. Mesotten D, Van den BG. Changes within the GH/IGF-I/IGFBP axis in critical illness. Crit Care Clin 2006;22:17–28.
20. Kojima M, Hosoda H, Date Y, et al. Ghrelin is a growth-hormone-releasing acylated peptide from stomach. Nature 1999;402:656–60.
21. Nakazato M, Murakami N, Date Y, et al. A role for ghrelin in the central regulation of feeding. Nature 2001;409:194–8.
22. Huff NK, Thompson DL Jr, Mitcham PB, et al. Hyperleptinemia in horses: responses to administration of a small dose of lipopolysaccharide endotoxin in mares and geldings. J Anim Sci 2010;88:926–36.
23. Marquardt DJ, Knatz NL, Wetterau LA, et al. Failure to recover somatotropic axis function is associated with mortality from pediatric sepsis-induced multiple organ dysfunction syndrome. Pediatr Crit Care Med 2010;11:18–25.
24. Onenli-Mungan N, Yildizdas D, Yapicioglu H, et al. Growth hormone and insulin-like growth factor 1 levels and their relation to survival in children with bacterial sepsis and septic shock. J Paediatr Child Health 2004;40:221–6.
25. Barsnick RJ, Hurcombe SD, Slovis NM, et al. Hormones of the energy metabolism in septic foals: insulin, glucagon, leptin, adiponectin, ghrelin, and growth hormone [Research Abstract Program of the 2010 ACVIM Forum]. J Vet Intern Med 2010;24:708–9.
26. Balcells J, Moreno A, Audi L, et al. Growth hormone/insulin-like growth factors axis in children undergoing cardiac surgery. Crit Care Med 2001;29:1234–8.
27. Wang W, Bansal S, Falk S, et al. Ghrelin protects mice against endotoxemia-induced acute kidney injury. Am J Physiol Renal Physiol 2009;297:F1032–7.
28. Wu R, Dong W, Zhou M, et al. Ghrelin improves tissue perfusion in severe sepsis via downregulation of endothelin-1. Cardiovasc Res 2005;68:318–26.
29. Wu R, Zhou M, Das P, et al. Ghrelin inhibits sympathetic nervous activity in sepsis. Am J Physiol Endocrinol Metab 2007;293:E1697–702.

30. Ueno H, Shiiya T, Nakazato M. Translational research of ghrelin. Ann N Y Acad Sci 2010;1200:120–7.
31. Dyck DJ. Adipokines as regulators of muscle metabolism and insulin sensitivity. Appl Physiol Nutr Metab 2009;34:396–402.
32. Beltowski J, Jamroz-Wisniewska A, Widomska S. Adiponectin and its role in cardiovascular diseases. Cardiovasc Hematol Disord Drug Targets 2008;8: 7–46.
33. Galic S, Oakhill JS, Steinberg GR. Adipose tissue as an endocrine organ. Mol Cell Endocrinol 2010;316:129–39.
34. Kearns CF, McKeever KH, Roegner V, et al. Adiponectin and leptin are related to fat mass in horses. Vet J 2006;172:460–5.
35. Toribio RE, Kohn CW, Hardy J, et al. Alterations in serum parathyroid hormone and electrolyte concentrations and urinary excretion of electrolytes in horses with induced endotoxemia. J Vet Intern Med 2005;19:223–31.
36. Toth F, Frank N, Elliott SB, et al. Effects of an intravenous endotoxin challenge on glucose and insulin dynamics in horses. Am J Vet Res 2008;69:82–8.
37. Barsnick RJ, Hurcombe SD, Smith PA, et al. Insulin, glucagon and leptin in critically ill foals. J Vet Intern Med. DOI:10.1111/j.1939-1676.2010.0636.x. [Epub ahead of print].
38. Romijn JA, Corssmit EP, Havekes LM, et al. Gut-brain axis. Curr Opin Clin Nutr Metab Care 2008;11:518–21.
39. Burns TA, Geor RJ, Mudge MC, et al. Proinflammatory cytokine and chemokine gene expression profiles in subcutaneous and visceral adipose tissue depots of insulin-resistant and insulin-sensitive light breed horses. J Vet Intern Med 2010;24:932–9.
40. De Groot LJ. Dangerous dogmas in medicine: the nonthyroidal illness syndrome. J Clin Endocrinol Metab 1999;84:151–64.
41. Berger MM, Reymond MJ, Shenkin A, et al. Influence of selenium supplements on the post-traumatic alterations of the thyroid axis: a placebo-controlled trial. Intensive Care Med 2001;27:91–100.
42. De Groot LJ. Non-thyroidal illness syndrome is a manifestation of hypothalamic-pituitary dysfunction, and in view of current evidence, should be treated with appropriate replacement therapies. Crit Care Clin 2006;22:57–86.
43. Warner MH, Beckett GJ. Mechanisms behind the non-thyroidal illness syndrome: an update. J Endocrinol 2010;205:1–13.
44. Boosinger TR, Brendemuehl JP, Bransby DL, et al. Prolonged gestation, decreased triiodothyronine concentration, and thyroid gland histomorphologic features in newborn foals of mares grazing Acremonion coenophialum-infected fescue. Am J Vet Res 1995;56:66–9.
45. Furr MO, Murray MJ, Ferguson DC. The effects of stress on gastric ulceration, T3, T4, reverse T3 and cortisol in neonatal foals. Equine Vet J 1992;24:37–40.
46. McLaughlin BG, Doige CE. A study of ossification of carpal and tarsal bones in normal and hypothyroid foals. Can Vet J 1982;23:164–8.
47. McLaughlin BG, Doige CE, McLaughlin PS. Thyroid-hormone levels in foals with congenital musculoskeletal lesions. Can Vet J 1986;27:264–7.
48. Breuhaus BA, LaFevers DH. Thyroid function in normal, sick and premature Foals [abstract]. J Vet Intern Med 2005;19:445.
49. Himler M, Cattaneo A, Barsnick RJ, et al. Thyroid hormones in healthy, sick non-septic and septic foals [Research Abstract Program of the 2010 ACVIM Forum]. J Vet Intern Med 2010;24:784.

50. Garcia-Lopez JM, Provost PJ, Rush JE, et al. Prevalence and prognostic importance of hypomagnesemia and hypocalcemia in horses that have colic surgery. Am J Vet Res 2001;62:7–12.
51. Toribio RE, Kohn CW, Chew DJ, et al. Comparison of serum parathyroid hormone and ionized calcium and magnesium concentrations and fractional urinary clearance of calcium and phosphorus in healthy horses and horses with enterocolitis. Am J Vet Res 2001;62:938–47.
52. Bueno AC, Seahorn TL, Cornick-Seahorn J, et al. Plasma and urine nitric oxide concentrations in horses given below a low dose of endotoxin. Am J Vet Res 1999;60:969–76.
53. Seethanathan P, Bottoms GD, Schafer K. Characterization of release of tumor necrosis factor, interleukin-1, and superoxide anion from equine white blood cells in response to endotoxin. Am J Vet Res 1990;51:1221–5.
54. Toribio RE, Kohn CW, Capen CC, et al. Parathyroid hormone (PTH) secretion, PTH mRNA and calcium-sensing receptor mRNA expression in equine parathyroid cells, and effects of interleukin (IL)-1, IL-6, and tumor necrosis factor-alpha on equine parathyroid cell function. J Mol Endocrinol 2003;31:609–20.
55. Hurcombe SD, Toribio RE, Slovis NM, et al. Calcium regulating hormones and serum calcium and magnesium concentrations in septic and critically ill foals and their association with survival. J Vet Intern Med 2009;23:335–43.
56. Oberhoffer M, Karzai W, Meier-Hellmann A, et al. Sensitivity and specificity of various markers of inflammation for the prediction of tumor necrosis factor-alpha and interleukin-6 in patients with sepsis. Crit Care Med 1999;27:1814–8.
57. Whicher J, Bienvenu J, Monneret G. Procalcitonin as an acute phase marker. Ann Clin Biochem 2001;38:483–93.
58. Toribio RE, Kohn CW, Leone GW, et al. Molecular cloning and expression of equine calcitonin, calcitonin gene-related peptide-I, and calcitonin gene-related peptide-II. Mol Cell Endocrinol 2003;199:119–28.
59. Pusterla N, Magdesian KG, Mapes S, et al. Expression of molecular markers in blood of neonatal foals with sepsis. Am J Vet Res 2006;67:1045–9.
60. Bie P, Damkjaer M. Renin secretion and total body sodium: pathways of integrative control. Clin Exp Pharmacol Physiol 2010;37:34–42.
61. Masri M, Freestone JF, Wolfsheimer KJ, et al. Alterations in plasma volume, plasma constituents, renin activity and aldosterone induced by maximal exercise in the horse. Equine Vet J Suppl 1990;9:72–7.
62. McKeever KH, Hinchcliff KW, Schmall LM, et al. Renal tubular function in horses during submaximal exercise. Am J Physiol 1991;261:R553–60.
63. Cooley JL, Hinchcliff KW, McKeever KH, et al. Effect of furosemide on plasma atrial natriuretic peptide and aldosterone concentrations and renin activity in running horses. Am J Vet Res 1994;55:273–7.
64. Hollis AR, Boston RC, Corley KT. Plasma aldosterone, vasopressin and atrial natriuretic peptide in hypovolaemia: a preliminary comparative study of neonatal and mature horses. Equine Vet J 2008;40:64–9.
65. Corley KT. Inotropes and vasopressors in adults and foals. Vet Clin North Am Equine Pract 2004;20:77–106.
66. Kotsovolis G, Kallaras K. The role of endothelium and endogenous vasoactive substances in sepsis. Hippokratia 2010;14:88–93.
67. Noori S, Siassi B, Durand M, et al. Cardiovascular effects of low-dose dexamethasone in very low birth weight neonates with refractory hypotension. Biol Neonate 2006;89:82–7.

68. Russell JA, Walley KR, Gordon AC, et al. Interaction of vasopressin infusion, corticosteroid treatment, and mortality of septic shock. Crit Care Med 2009; 37:811–8.
69. Daels PF, Stabenfeldt GH, Hughes JP, et al. Evaluation of progesterone deficiency as a cause of fetal death in mares with experimentally induced endotoxemia. Am J Vet Res 1991;52:282–8.
70. Kindahl H, Daels P, Odensvik K, et al. Experimental models of endotoxaemia related to abortion in the mare. J Reprod Fertil Suppl 1991;44:509–16.
71. Daels PF, Starr M, Kindahl H, et al. Effect of salmonella typhimurium endotoxin on PGF-2 alpha release and fetal death in the mare. J Reprod Fertil Suppl 1987;35: 485–92.
72. Fredriksson G, Kindahl H, Stabenfeldt G. Endotoxin-induced and prostaglandin-mediated effects on corpus luteum function in the mare. Theriogenology 1986;25: 309–16.
73. Boening KJ, Leendertse IP. Review of 115 cases of colic in the pregnant mare. Equine Vet J 1993;25:518–21.
74. Ousey JC, Houghton E, Grainger L, et al. Progestagen profiles during the last trimester of gestation in thoroughbred mares with normal or compromised pregnancies. Theriogenology 2005;63:1844–56.
75. Fowden AL, Forhead AJ, Ousey JC. The endocrinology of equine parturition. Exp Clin Endocrinol Diabetes 2008;116:393–403.
76. Rossi P, Persson B, Boels PJ, et al. Endotoxemic pulmonary hypertension is largely mediated by endothelin-induced venous constriction. Intensive Care Med 2008;34:873–80.
77. Andersson A, Fenhammar J, Frithiof R, et al. Mixed endothelin receptor antagonism with tezosentan improves intestinal microcirculation in endotoxemic shock. J Surg Res 2008;149:138–47.
78. Figueras-Aloy J, Gomez-Lopez L, Rodriguez-Miguelez JM, et al. Plasma endothelin-1 and clinical manifestations of neonatal sepsis. J Perinat Med 2004;32: 522–6.
79. Menzies-Gow NJ, Bailey SR, Stevens K, et al. Digital blood flow and plasma endothelin concentration in clinically endotoxemic horses. Am J Vet Res 2005;66: 630–6.
80. Stokes AM, Venugopal CS, Hosgood G, et al. Comparison of 2 endothelin-receptor antagonists on in vitro responses of equine palmar digital arterial and venous rings to endothelin-1. Can J Vet Res 2006;70:197–205.
81. Keen JA, Hillier C, McGorum BC, et al. Endothelin mediated contraction of equine laminar veins. Equine Vet J 2008;40:488–92.
82. Plusczyk T, Witzel B, Menger MD, et al. ETA and ETB receptor function in pancreatitis-associated microcirculatory failure, inflammation, and parenchymal injury. Am J Physiol Gastrointest Liver Physiol 2003;285:G145–53.
83. Joyce CD, Fiscus RR, Wang X, et al. Calcitonin gene-related peptide levels are elevated in patients with sepsis. Surgery 1990;108:1097–101.
84. Berg RM, Strauss GI, Tofteng F, et al. Circulating levels of vasoactive peptides in patients with acute bacterial meningitis. Intensive Care Med 2009;35:1604–8.
85. Gomes RN, Castro-Faria-Neto HC, Bozza PT, et al. Calcitonin gene-related peptide inhibits local acute inflammation and protects mice against lethal endotoxemia. Shock 2005;24:590–4.
86. Moore RM, Charalambous AC, Masty J. Alterations in colonic arterial and venous plasma neuropeptide concentrations in horses during low-flow ischemia and reperfusion of the large colon. Am J Vet Res 1996;57:1200–5.

87. Sonea IM, Bowker RM, Robinson NE, et al. Distribution of SP- and CGRP-like immunoreactive nerve fibers in the lower respiratory tract of neonatal foals: evidence for loss during development. Anat Embryol (Berl) 1994;190:469–77.
88. Russo D, Bombardi C, Grandis A, et al. Sympathetic innervation of the ileocecal junction in horses. J Comp Neurol 2010;518:4046–66.
89. Temmesfeld-Wollbruck B, Hocke AC, Suttorp N, et al. Adrenomedullin and endothelial barrier function. Thromb Haemost 2007;98:944–51.
90. Temmesfeld-Wollbruck B, Brell B, zu Dohna C, et al. Adrenomedullin reduces intestinal epithelial permeability in vivo and in vitro. Am J Physiol Gastrointest Liver Physiol 2009;297:G43–51.
91. Shah KG, Rajan D, Jacob A, et al. Attenuation of renal ischemia and reperfusion injury by human adrenomedullin and its binding protein. J Surg Res 2010;163:110–7.
92. Schuetz P, Christ-Crain M, Morgenthaler NG, et al. Circulating precursor levels of endothelin-1 and adrenomedullin, two endothelium-derived, counteracting substances, in sepsis. Endothelium 2007;14:345–51.
93. Piercy RJ, Swardson CJ, Hinchcliff KW. Erythroid hypoplasia and anemia following administration of recombinant human erythropoietin to two horses. J Am Vet Med Assoc 1998;212:244–7.

Endocrinology of the Equine Neonate Energy Metabolism in Health and Critical Illness

Rosa J. Barsnick, Dr. med. vet., MS[a], Ramiro E. Toribio, DVM, MS, PhD[b,*]

KEYWORDS

• Foal • Insulin • Glucagon • Leptin • Adiponectin
• Ghrelin • Growth hormone

Hormonal control of energy metabolism plays an important role in the peripartum development and health of the equine neonate. The endocrine system is generally functional at the time of birth, but the maturation of the endocrine system and the associated energy metabolism is delayed and continues during the postnatal period. During this time, the energy metabolism is highly susceptible to disturbances, especially when illness occurs. Hormones involved in energy metabolism, including insulin, glucagon, leptin, adiponectin, ghrelin, growth hormone (GH), and insulin-like growth factor-1 (IGF-1), have recently been studied in healthy and critically ill neonatal foals. Understanding these hormones in the equine neonate will support appropriate therapeutic interventions as well as prognostic assessment of the sick foal.

ENERGY METABOLISM IN THE FETAL AND NEWBORN FOAL

During fetal development, nutrients are exchanged across the placenta. Glucose and lactate are the main energy substrates for the mammalian fetus.[1] Little is known about equine fetal energy metabolism, but it has been shown that placental transfer of fatty acids and oxidation of amino acids are lower in equine fetuses compared with other species.[2] The epitheliochorial placenta is permeable to amino and fatty acids.[3] Sufficient gluconeogenesis occurs only in late gestation in equine fetuses, and is likely dependent on the prepartum increase of cortisol;[4] therefore, transplacental glucose

No disclosures.
[a] Pferdeklinik in Kirchheim (Kirchheim Equine Hospital), Nürtinger Street 200, 73230 Kirchheim/Teck, Germany
[b] Department of Veterinary Clinical Sciences, College of Veterinary Medicine, The Ohio State University, 601 Vernon L. Tharp Street, Columbus, OH 43210, USA
* Corresponding author.
E-mail address: toribio.1@osu.edu

Vet Clin Equine 27 (2011) 49–58
doi:10.1016/j.cveq.2010.12.001 vetequine.theclinics.com
0749-0739/11/$ – see front matter

supply is the main energy source for the fetus. Compared with fetal lambs and piglets, equine fetuses use a greater proportion of umbilical oxygen uptake for glucose oxidation, and overall dependence on glucose as a metabolic substrate is higher in fetal foals than in other species.[2,5] In addition, the newborn foal has almost no hepatic fat stores,[3] and little adipose tissue. Consequently, foals are highly dependent on glucose intake and could rapidly develop hypoglycemia when caloric intake decreases.

Maturation of the endocrine system and the associated energy metabolism in the equine neonate is delayed and continues in the postnatal period.[2,6–8] In particular, endocrine glucoregulatory mechanisms are not fully competent at birth; thus, hypoglycemia is common in critically ill foals, because of anorexia or inability to nurse.[8–11] In these cases, energy has to be delivered by enteral or parenteral routes. A major complication of parenteral nutrition in foals is the development of hyperglycemia (glucose intolerance).[12] Hyperglycemia causes oxidative stress, glucotoxicity and β-cell dysfunction,[13] and has been associated with increased mortality in critically ill humans and foals.[11,14] However, more commonly, changes in energy metabolism in critically ill foals are characterized by hypoglycemia and hypertriglyceridemia.[11,15–18] Septic foals have significantly lower blood glucose concentrations than sick nonseptic or healthy foals, and nonsurvivors have lower glucose concentrations than survivors.[11,15,16]

Serum triglyceride concentrations are often increased in hospitalized foals.[16] Because carbohydrate stores in foals are limited, these are quickly depleted, leading to mobilization of fat depots. Ultimately, when the liver cannot maintain glucose production from fatty acids, blood triglyceride concentrations increase. In calves, glucose concentrations decrease and triglyceride concentrations increase in response to administration of endotoxin or tumor necrosis factor α (TNF-α).[19] A similar mechanism may contribute to hypoglycemia and hypertriglyceridemia in septic foals.[20]

INSULIN

Insulin is a peptide hormone produced by the β-cells of the pancreas. Insulin secretion increases in response to increased blood glucose concentrations to maintain normoglycemia by stimulating cellular glucose uptake, glycogenesis, and fatty acid synthesis, as well as reducing glucose production by decreasing gluconeogenesis, lipolysis, and proteinolysis.[21]

The insulin receptor belongs to the tyrosine kinase family of transmembrane receptors, which exert their function by phosphorylating various target proteins. Glucose transporter (GLUT) proteins permit the concentration-dependent movement of glucose from the extracellular to the intracellular compartment. Of the GLUTs (GLUT1, GLUT2, GLUT3, and GLUT4), GLUT4 is the only one regulated by insulin. In skeletal muscle and adipose tissue, insulin binding to its receptor leads to the translocation of GLUT4 from intracellular vesicles to the cell membrane. Physical activity also promotes GLUT4 translocation, in various species, including horses.[22] Further, GLUT4 activity is central to the pathogenesis of insulin resistance in humans and horses.

The endocrine pancreas is functional before birth; however, newborn and premature foals have a lower insulin response to increased blood glucose concentrations than older foals and foals born at term,[6,23] suggesting that β-cell responsiveness adapts to enteral feeding during the first week of life. Based on the slower glucose clearance in newborn foals, transient insulin resistance has been proposed to occur in the first day after birth.[10]

Insulin resistance has been assessed only in healthy neonatal foals, and seems to be associated with maternal diet during late gestation.[24] Insulin resistance as a response to systemic inflammation has not been evaluated in critically ill foals by means of dynamic studies (glucose clamp or frequently sampled intravenous glucose tolerance test), and many assumptions are made by extrapolation from other species. Insulin resistance and hyperglycemia are common manifestations of endocrine dysregulation in people with sepsis or endotoxemia,[25–28] and tight glycemic control using insulin therapy has been shown to increase survival in these patients.[29] Insulin also has antiinflammatory properties by decreasing inflammatory cytokines and enhancing antiinflammatory mediators,[26] which may confer some therapeutic benefit in patients in a proinflammatory state (eg, septicemia/endotoxemia). As in humans, insulin is frequently used in equine neonates when hyperglycemia occurs,[30] although controlled studies for this type of intervention are lacking.

The investigators measured insulin and glucose concentrations of septic and sick nonseptic newborn foals on admission, and found that insulin was significantly lower in these foals compared with healthy foals. Further, insulin and glucose concentrations were positively correlated in all groups of the study population.[31] This finding was interpreted as an appropriate physiologic response of insulin to glycemia. These findings contrasted with other studies, in which insulin concentrations were increased during sepsis or endotoxemia in adult horses and calves.[19,32] Sepsis and endotoxemia induce insulin resistance in humans,[25] adult horses,[32,33] and mice,[34] but insulin resistance remains to be documented in critically ill foals. Although we do not have an explanation for these species and age differences, it is possible that insulin signaling and GLUT4 activity may be less sensitive to inflammatory mediators in newborn foals.

GLUCAGON

Glucagon is a peptide hormone secreted by the α cells of the pancreas and has opposing physiologic roles to insulin because it stimulates gluconeogenesis, glycogenolysis, and lipolysis.

The pancreatic α cells of the equine fetus are responsive to stimuli associated with stress like anesthesia or parturition and arginine administration, but glucagon concentrations are not affected by variations in glycemia until after birth.[35] Compared with other mammalian species, equine fetuses have higher plasma glucagon concentrations, resulting in an insulin/glucagon ratio that favors gluconeogenesis in utero. However, hepatic glycogen and gluconeogenic enzyme levels are comparably low, likely limiting gluconeogenesis. Possibly, high glucagon concentrations help maintain the glucose supply when placental glucose delivery is compromised.[35] Similarly, glucagon is believed to be important for maintaining or enhancing gluconeogenesis in the catabolic state of critical illness in humans.[36]

Hyperglucagonemia has been reported in septic and endotoxemic humans, dogs, rats, and recently in septic foals.[31,36–38] High glucagon concentrations in septic foals are likely a physiologic response to decreased energy uptake and hypoglycemia. They could also represent a response to systemic inflammation. This finding, as well as the earlier described relationship between glucose and insulin, supports the supposition that healthy and most critically ill neonatal foals have an appropriate endocrine response to glycemia. That is, pancreatic α and β-cells are responsive to blood glucose in newborn foals.

LEPTIN

Leptin, an adipocyte-derived hormone (adipokine), is considered the main regulator of satiety (anorexigenic), and its blood concentrations are correlated with total body fat in horses, humans, dogs, and other species.[39–42] Leptin concentrations decrease in feed-restricted mares[43] and increase after a high-carbohydrate meal.[44] Leptin increases insulin sensitivity in humans.[42] Leptin is present in mare's milk, with high concentrations in the colostrum.[45,46] In the newborn foal, blood leptin concentrations increase after birth and decline to concentrations similar to mare's milk within a few days.[47] In is unclear whether this increase in foal leptin concentrations is from endogenous sources or leptin absorbed from the colostrum.

Blood leptin concentrations were not different between healthy foals and sick or septic foals.[15] However, septic foals that died had lower leptin concentrations than septic foals that survived.[15] Leptin decreases during anorexia, just as in healthy feed-restricted adult horses,[43,44] but low leptin concentrations do not seem to allow sufficient stimulation of hunger in septic foals. The difference in leptin concentrations between septic survivor and nonsurvivor foals is in agreement with a study in which high leptin concentrations in adult septic humans were associated with survival.[48] Other studies in septic or endotoxemic children,[49] rodents,[50] and dogs[51,52] have found the opposite, with increased leptin concentrations being associated with severity of disease and mortality. No association between leptin concentrations and systemic inflammation was found in other studies.[48,49,51,53–57]

A proportional relationship between leptin and glucose has been reported in horses that had an increase in insulin first, followed by an increase in leptin after feeding, indicating that insulin may be driving this increase in leptin.[58] However, the investigators did not find a correlation between insulin and leptin concentrations in healthy or sick neonatal foals.[31]

The role of leptin in neonatal energy metabolism varies among species, including their response to systemic inflammation. Age and sex also influence regulation and function of leptin.[59] Not enough information on leptin in the equine neonate is available to determine its role in energy metabolism during health and disease.

ADIPONECTIN

Adiponectin is another adipocyte-derived peptide hormone, which is negatively correlated with body fat mass in horses and other species,[39,42] yet also increases insulin sensitivity.[60] Adiponectin promotes the cell membrane translocation GLUT4 and increases glycolysis and fatty acid oxidation.[45] Adiponectin has been studied in healthy horses, but an immediate adiponectin response to feeding or fasting has not been documented.[39,61,62] No information on adiponectin is available in horses with pathologic conditions. Adiponectin increases in human endotoxemia,[53,60] but decreases in rats with sepsis.[63] In neonatal foals, blood adiponectin concentrations were not different between healthy, sick nonseptic, and septic foals.[15] Studies in mice and humans indicate that adiponectin may have antiinflammatory and lipopolysaccharide-neutralizing properties.[60,63,64]

GHRELIN

Ghrelin is produced in the gastric mucosa by oxyntic cells that are characterized by round, compact, electron-dense secretory granules (P/D_1 cells in humans, A-like cells in rats, and X/A-like cells in dogs).[65,66] Ghrelin promotes food intake (orexigenic), and exerts several metabolic, neuroendocrine, and also nonendocrine actions.[67] Ghrelin is also synthesized by the hypothalamic arcuate nucleus to stimulate the secretion of GH from the pituitary gland.

Ghrelin secretion increases with anorexia. Serum ghrelin concentrations decrease after carbohydrate challenge and hyperglycemia (eg, grain, intravenous dextrose).[68]

It is unclear whether glucose or insulin mediates the inhibition of ghrelin secretion.[67] A possibility may be indirect inhibition via somatostatin. Somatostatin is produced in the hypothalamus, stomach, intestine, and pancreatic δ cells and its main function is to inhibit GH release. However, it also inhibits ghrelin secretion and can be released in response to hyperglycemia and endotoxemia.[69] Ghrelin concentrations are increased in septic foals.[31] Reduced ghrelin clearance caused by hepatorenal injury in sepsis and endotoxemia[52,70] could contribute to the ghrelin increase in critically ill foals.

The association between glucose and ghrelin concentrations in newborn foals is inverse,[31] which seems appropriate because ghrelin is released in response to hypoglycemia. Ghrelin concentrations were increased in septic foals and associated with severity of sepsis.[31,71] Likewise, ghrelin concentrations were higher in human and dogs with sepsis and endotoxemia.[52,72,73]

Ghrelin has recently been called "a signal of insufficient energy intake,"[74] and negative energy balance and anorexia provide an explanation for increased ghrelin concentrations in diseased foals.

In humans, ghrelin induces lipolysis.[75] Assuming that ghrelin increase from hypoglycemia promotes lipolysis, it is likely that ghrelin is involved in the development of hypertriglyceridemia in septic foals. In mice, triglycerides and fasting promote the transport of ghrelin across the blood-brain barrier.[76] Thus, it is possible that hypertriglyceridemia contributes to ghrelin transport to induce hunger and GH release in sick foals. Nevertheless, in most critically ill foals, these mechanisms do not seem to overcome anorexia.

GH

GH (somatotropin) is predominantly an anabolic peptide hormone that stimulates cell proliferation, amino acid uptake, protein synthesis, and growth. GH also has catabolic effects by enhancing lipolysis and inhibiting insulin signaling and cellular glucose transport.[77]

Hypothalamic GH-releasing hormone stimulates pituitary somatotrophs to secrete GH, whereas somatostatin from the hypothalamus and gastrointestinal tract inhibits GH release. Most effects of GH on musculoskeletal growth are mediated through IGF-1, whereas its effects in adipose tissue are direct. IGF-1 inhibits GH secretion in a negative feedback mechanism. GH and IGF-1 are the main components of the somatotropic axis.

GH increases in horses during exercise, feed deprivation, and stress.[78–80] The association between GH secretion and sepsis or endotoxemia has been studied in several species,[81–83] and recently in foals.[31,71] GH concentrations were higher in septic foals and associated with low serum glucose and high serum triglyceride concentrations.[31,71] Similarly, increased GH secretion occurs during sepsis and endotoxemia in humans and rodents.[81–83] GH hypersecretion in septic foals could be explained in part by hypoglycemia and high ghrelin concentrations, although in the cited study the investigators found no association between ghrelin and GH. This finding suggests that other factors are involved in GH secretion in critically ill foals. We recently found that IGF-1 concentrations were lower in septic foals and negatively correlated with GH concentrations (Barsnick RJ, Toribio RE, unpublished information, 2010). We consider this an inappropriate IGF-1 response to GH stimulation (GH resistance), which likely contributes to additional GH synthesis and secretion.

Recombinant bovine TNF-α has been shown to increase GH secretion in dairy heifers.[84] Interleukin 1 (IL-1) and endotoxin directly stimulate the pituitary to release

GH in pigs, sheep, and humans.[85] Septic foals and horses with gastrointestinal disease often have detectable concentrations of endotoxin in blood,[20] and IL-1 and TNF-α concentrations are often increased in these animals.[86–88]

High GH concentration is a good predictor of mortality in septic children[82] and adult critically ill patients.[83] However, the usefulness of GH as a prognostic indicator in septic foals has yet to be determined.

SUMMARY

Many aspects of the hormonal control of the energy metabolism in neonatal foals still need to be elucidated. The endocrine pancreas is functional before birth, but glucoregulatory mechanisms are not fully matured at the time of birth. Insulin, glucagon, leptin, and adiponectin as well as ghrelin and GH seem to respond in a physiologically expected fashion to changes in the energy state (eg, hypoglycemia caused by anorexia). However, neonatal sepsis leads to endocrine dysregulation in certain individuals. Leptin responses in particular vary substantially between species; thus, one has to be careful when extrapolating from other species. Future work on hormones of the energy metabolism may have clinical implications (eg, the prognostic value of insulin and leptin in septic foals, or the value of therapeutic intervention with insulin).

REFERENCES

1. Pere MC. Materno-foetal exchanges and utilisation of nutrients by the foetus: comparison between species. Reprod Nutr Dev 2003;43(1):1–15.
2. Fowden AL, Silver M. Glucose and oxygen metabolism in the fetal foal during late gestation. Am J Physiol 1995;269(6 Pt 2):R1455–61.
3. Stammers JP, Hull D, Leadon DP, et al. Maternal and umbilical venous plasma lipid concentrations at delivery in the mare. Equine Vet J 1991;23(2):119–22.
4. Fowden AL, Mijovic J, Ousey JC, et al. The development of gluconeogenic enzymes in the liver and kidney of fetal and newborn foals. J Dev Physiol 1992;18(3):137–42.
5. Fowden AL. Comparative aspects of fetal carbohydrate metabolism. Equine Vet J Suppl 1997;24:19–25.
6. Fowden AL, Ellis L, Rossdale PD. Pancreatic beta cell function in the neonatal foal. J Reprod Fertil Suppl 1982;32:529–35.
7. Gold JR, Divers TJ, Barton MH, et al. Plasma adrenocorticotropin, cortisol, and adrenocorticotropin/cortisol ratios in septic and normal-term foals. J Vet Intern Med 2007;21(4):791–6.
8. Silver M, Fowden AL. Prepartum adrenocortical maturation in the fetal foal: responses to ACTH1-24. J Endocrinol 1994;142(3):417–25.
9. Fowden AL, Silver M. Comparative development of the pituitary-adrenal axis in the fetal foal and lamb. Reprod Domest Anim 1995;30(4):170–7.
10. Holdstock NB, Allen VL, Bloomfield MR, et al. Development of insulin and proinsulin secretion in newborn pony foals. J Endocrinol 2004;181(3):469–76.
11. Hollis AR, Furr MO, Magdesian KG, et al. Blood glucose concentrations in critically ill neonatal foals. J Vet Intern Med 2008;22(5):1223–7.
12. Krause JB, McKenzie HC III. Parenteral nutrition in foals: a retrospective study of 45 cases (2000–2004). Equine Vet J 2007;39(1):74–8.
13. Poitout V. Glucolipotoxicity of the pancreatic beta-cell: myth or reality? Biochem Soc Trans 2008;36(Pt 5):901–4.
14. Finfer S, Chittock DR, Su SY, et al. Intensive versus conventional glucose control in critically ill patients. N Engl J Med 2009;360(13):1283–97.

15. Barsnick RJ, Hurcombe SD, Saville WJ, et al. Endocrine energy response in septic foals: insulin, leptin and adiponectin [abstract]. Proceedings of the 27th Annual ACVIM Forum [abstract #117]. Montreal (Canada), June 2009.
16. Barsnick RJ, Hurcombe SD, Smith PA, et al. Insulin, glucagon and leptin in critically ill foals. J Vet Intern Med 2010. [Epub ahead of print]. Available at: http://www.ncbi.nlm.nih.gov/pubmed/21092004. Accessed December 11, 2010.
17. Brewer BD, Koterba AM. Development of a scoring system for the early diagnosis of equine neonatal sepsis. Equine Vet J 1988;20(1):18–22.
18. Paradis MR. Update on neonatal septicemia. Vet Clin North Am Equine Pract 1994;10(1):109–35.
19. Kenison DC, Elsasser TH, Fayer R. Tumor necrosis factor as a potential mediator of acute metabolic and hormonal responses to endotoxemia in calves. Am J Vet Res 1991;52(8):1320–6.
20. Barton MH, Morris DD, Norton N, et al. Hemostatic and fibrinolytic indices in neonatal foals with presumed septicemia. J Vet Intern Med 1998;12(1):26–35.
21. Bansal P, Wang Q. Insulin as a physiological modulator of glucagon secretion. Am J Physiol Endocrinol Metab 2008;295(4):E751–61.
22. McCutcheon LJ, Geor RJ, Hinchcliff KW. Changes in skeletal muscle GLUT4 content and muscle membrane glucose transport following 6 weeks of exercise training. Equine Vet J Suppl 2002;34:199–204.
23. Fowden AL, Silver M, Ellis L, et al. Studies on equine prematurity 3: insulin secretion in the foal during the perinatal period. Equine Vet J 1984;16(4):286–91.
24. George LA, Staniar WB, Treiber KH, et al. Insulin sensitivity and glucose dynamics during pre-weaning foal development and in response to maternal diet composition. Domest Anim Endocrinol 2009;37(1):23–9.
25. Agwunobi AO, Reid C, Maycock P, et al. Insulin resistance and substrate utilization in human endotoxemia. J Clin Endocrinol Metab 2000;85(10):3770–8.
26. Das UN. Insulin in the critically ill with focus on cytokines, reactive oxygen species, HLA-DR expression. J Assoc Physicians India 2007;55(Suppl):56–65.
27. Langouche L, Vanhorebeek I, Van den Berghe G. The role of insulin therapy in critically ill patients. Treat Endocrinol 2005;4(6):353–60.
28. Van Cromphaut SJ, Vanhorebeek I, Van den Berghe G. Glucose metabolism and insulin resistance in sepsis. Curr Pharm Des 2008;14(19):1887–99.
29. Brierre S, Kumari R, Deboisblanc BP. The endocrine system during sepsis. Am J Med Sci 2004;328(4):238–47.
30. Beuchner-Maxwell VA. Hyperglycemia in the neonatal foal: management with continuous insulin infusion. Equine Pract 1994;16(8):13–6.
31. Barsnick RJ, Hurcombe SD, Saville WJ, et al. Hormones of energy metabolism in septic foals: associations between insulin, glucagon, leptin, adiponectin, ghrelin and growth hormone [abstract]. Proceedings of the 28th Annual ACVIM Forum [abstract #124]. Anaheim (CA), June 2010.
32. Toribio RE, Kohn CW, Hardy J, et al. Alterations in serum parathyroid hormone and electrolyte concentrations and urinary excretion of electrolytes in horses with induced endotoxemia. J Vet Intern Med 2005;19(2):223–31.
33. Toth F, Frank N, Elliott SB, et al. Effects of an intravenous endotoxin challenge on glucose and insulin dynamics in horses. Am J Vet Res 2008;69(1):82–8.
34. Matsuda N, Yamamoto S, Yokoo H, et al. Nuclear factor-kappaB decoy oligodeoxynucleotides ameliorate impaired glucose tolerance and insulin resistance in mice with cecal ligation and puncture-induced sepsis. Crit Care Med 2009;37(10):2791–9.

35. Fowden AL, Forhead AJ, Bloomfield M, et al. Pancreatic alpha cell function in the fetal foal during late gestation. Exp Physiol 1999;84(4):697–705.
36. Lang CH, Bagby GJ, Blakesley HL, et al. Importance of hyperglucagonemia in eliciting the sepsis-induced increase in glucose production. Circ Shock 1989; 29(3):181–91.
37. Ishida K. The significance of plasma gastrointestinal glucagon in endotoxemia. Circ Shock 1985;16(4):317–23.
38. Meinz H, Lacy DB, Ejiofor J, et al. Alterations in hepatic gluconeogenic amino acid uptake and gluconeogenesis in the endotoxin treated conscious dog. Shock 1998;9(4):296–303.
39. Kearns CF, McKeever KH, Roegner V, et al. Adiponectin and leptin are related to fat mass in horses. Vet J 2006;172(3):460–5.
40. Maffei M, Halaas J, Ravussin E, et al. Leptin levels in human and rodent: measurement of plasma leptin and ob RNA in obese and weight-reduced subjects. Nat Med 1995;1(11):1155–61.
41. Sagawa MM, Nakadomo F, Honjoh T, et al. Correlation between plasma leptin concentration and body fat content in dogs. Am J Vet Res 2002;63(1):7–10.
42. Staiger H, Tschritter O, Machann J, et al. Relationship of serum adiponectin and leptin concentrations with body fat distribution in humans. Obes Res 2003;11(3): 368–72.
43. McManus CJ, Fitzgerald BP. Effects of a single day of feed restriction on changes in serum leptin, gonadotropins, prolactin, and metabolites in aged and young mares. Domest Anim Endocrinol 2000;19(1):1–13.
44. Steelman SM, Michael-Eller EM, Gibbs PG, et al. Meal size and feeding frequency influence serum leptin concentration in yearling horses. J Anim Sci 2006;84(9):2391–8.
45. Radin MJ, Sharkey LC, Holycross BJ. Adipokines: a review of biological and analytical principles and an update in dogs, cats, and horses. Vet Clin Pathol 2009;38(2):136–56.
46. Salimei E, Varisco G, Rosi F. Major constituents, leptin, and non-protein nitrogen compounds in mares' colostrum and milk. Reprod Nutr Dev 2002;42(1):65–72.
47. Berg EL, McNamara DL, Keisler DH. Endocrine profiles of periparturient mares and their foals. J Anim Sci 2007;85(7):1660–8.
48. Arnalich F, Lopez J, Codoceo R, et al. Relationship of plasma leptin to plasma cytokines and human survival in sepsis and septic shock. J Infect Dis 1999; 180(3):908–11.
49. Blanco-Quiros A, Casado-Flores J, Arranz E, et al. Influence of leptin levels and body weight in survival of children with sepsis. Acta Paediatr 2002;91(6):626–31.
50. Finck BN, Kelley KW, Dantzer R, et al. In vivo and in vitro evidence for the involvement of tumor necrosis factor-alpha in the induction of leptin by lipopolysaccharide. Endocrinology 1998;139(5):2278–83.
51. Waelput W, Brouckaert P, Broekaert D, et al. A role for leptin in the systemic inflammatory response syndrome (SIRS) and in immune response, an update. Curr Med Chem 2006;13(4):465–75.
52. Yilmaz Z, Ilcol YO, Ulus IH. Endotoxin increases plasma leptin and ghrelin levels in dogs. Crit Care Med 2008;36(3):828–33.
53. Anderson PD, Mehta NN, Wolfe ML, et al. Innate immunity modulates adipokines in humans. J Clin Endocrinol Metab 2007;92(6):2272–9.
54. Koc E, Ustundag G, Aliefendioglu D, et al. Serum leptin levels and their relationship to tumor necrosis factor-alpha and interleukin-6 in neonatal sepsis. J Pediatr Endocrinol Metab 2003;16(9):1283–7.

55. Soliman M, Abdelhady S, Fattouh I, et al. No alteration in serum leptin levels during acute endotoxemia in sheep. J Vet Med Sci 2001;63(10):1143–5.
56. Soliman M, Ishioka K, Kimura K, et al. Plasma leptin responses to lipopolysaccharide and tumor necrosis factor alpha in cows. Jpn J Vet Res 2002;50(2–3): 107–14.
57. Tzanela M, Orfanos SE, Tsirantonaki M, et al. Leptin alterations in the course of sepsis in humans. In Vivo 2006;20(4):565–70.
58. Cartmill JA, Thompson DL Jr, Storer WA, et al. Effect of dexamethasone, feeding time, and insulin infusion on leptin concentrations in stallions. J Anim Sci 2005; 83(8):1875–81.
59. Cebulj-Kadunc N, Kosec M, Cestnik V. Serum leptin concentrations in Lipizzan fillies. Reprod Domest Anim 2009;44(1):1–5.
60. Keller P, Moller K, Krabbe KS, et al. Circulating adiponectin levels during human endotoxaemia. Clin Exp Immunol 2003;134(1):107–10.
61. Gordon ME, McKeever KH. Diurnal variation of ghrelin, leptin, and adiponectin in Standardbred mares. J Anim Sci 2005;83(10):2365–71.
62. Pratt SE, Geor RJ, McCutcheon LJ. Effects of dietary energy source and physical conditioning on insulin sensitivity and glucose tolerance in standardbred horses. Equine Vet J Suppl 2006;36:579–84.
63. Tsuchihashi H, Yamamoto H, Maeda K, et al. Circulating concentrations of adiponectin, an endogenous lipopolysaccharide neutralizing protein, decrease in rats with polymicrobial sepsis. J Surg Res 2006;134(2):348–53.
64. Uji Y, Yamamoto H, Tsuchihashi H, et al. Adiponectin deficiency is associated with severe polymicrobial sepsis, high inflammatory cytokine levels, and high mortality. Surgery 2009;145(5):550–7.
65. Hayashida T, Murakami K, Mogi K, et al. Ghrelin in domestic animals: distribution in stomach and its possible role. Domest Anim Endocrinol 2001;21(1):17–24.
66. Rindi G, Necchi V, Savio A, et al. Characterisation of gastric ghrelin cells in man and other mammals: studies in adult and fetal tissues. Histochem Cell Biol 2002; 117(6):511–9.
67. Ghigo E, Broglio F, Arvat E, et al. Ghrelin: more than a natural GH secretagogue and/or an orexigenic factor. Clin Endocrinol (Oxf) 2005;62(1):1–17.
68. Gordon ME, McKeever KH. Oral and intravenous carbohydrate challenges decrease active ghrelin concentrations and alter hormones related to control of energy metabolism in horses. J Anim Sci 2006;84(7):1682–90.
69. Yelich MR, Umporowicz DM, Drolet BA. Role of somatostatin in glucose regulation during endotoxicosis in the rat. Am J Physiol 1993;264(2 Pt 2):R254–61.
70. Wu R, Zhou M, Cui X, et al. Ghrelin clearance is reduced at the late stage of polymicrobial sepsis. Int J Mol Med 2003;12(5):777–81.
71. Barsnick RJ, Hurcombe SD, Saville WJ, et al. Association of growth hormone and ghrelin with the energy metabolism and mortality in septic foals [abstract]. Proceedings of the 27th Annual ACVIM Forum [abstract #323]. Montreal (Canada), June 2009.
72. Maruna P, Gurlich R, Frasko R, et al. Ghrelin and leptin elevation in postoperative intra-abdominal sepsis. Eur Surg Res 2005;37(6):354–9.
73. Vila G, Maier C, Riedl M, et al. Bacterial endotoxin induces biphasic changes in plasma ghrelin in healthy humans. J Clin Endocrinol Metab 2007;92(10):3930–4.
74. Wolls T. Ghrelin–defender of fat. Prog Lipid Res 2009;48(5):257–74.
75. Vestergaard ET, Gormsen LC, Jessen N, et al. Ghrelin infusion in humans induces acute insulin resistance and lipolysis independent of growth hormone signaling. Diabetes 2008;57(12):3205–10.

76. Banks WA, Burney BO, Robinson SM. Effects of triglycerides, obesity, and starvation on ghrelin transport across the blood-brain barrier. Peptides 2008; 29(11):2061–5.
77. Bhatti SF, Van Ham LM, Mol JA, et al. Ghrelin, an endogenous growth hormone secretagogue with diverse endocrine and nonendocrine effects. Am J Vet Res 2006;67(1):180–8.
78. Christensen RA, Malinowski K, Massenzio AM, et al. Acute effects of short-term feed deprivation and refeeding on circulating concentrations of metabolites, insulin-like growth factor I, insulin-like growth factor binding proteins, somatotropin, and thyroid hormones in adult geldings. J Anim Sci 1997;75(5):1351–8.
79. Huff NK, Thompson DL Jr, Mitcham PB, et al. Hyperleptinemia in horses: responses to administration of a small dose of lipopolysaccharide endotoxin in mares and geldings. J Anim Sci 2010;88(3):926–36.
80. Thompson DL Jr, DePew CL, Ortiz A, et al. Growth hormone and prolactin concentrations in plasma of horses: sex differences and the effects of acute exercise and administration of growth hormone-releasing hormone. J Anim Sci 1994; 72(11):2911–8.
81. Maxime V, Siami S, Annane D. Metabolism modulators in sepsis: the abnormal pituitary response. Crit Care Med 2007;35(Suppl 9):S596–601.
82. Onenli-Mungan N, Yildizdas D, Yapicioglu H, et al. Growth hormone and insulin-like growth factor 1 levels and their relation to survival in children with bacterial sepsis and septic shock. J Paediatr Child Health 2004;40(4):221–6.
83. Schuetz P, Muller B, Nusbaumer C, et al. Circulating levels of GH predict mortality and complement prognostic scores in critically ill medical patients. Eur J Endocrinol 2009;160(2):157–63.
84. Kushibiki S, Hodate K, Ueda Y, et al. Administration of recombinant bovine tumor necrosis factor-alpha affects intermediary metabolism and insulin and growth hormone secretion in dairy heifers. J Anim Sci 2000;78(8):2164–71.
85. Whitlock BK, Daniel JA, Wilborn RR, et al. Comparative aspects of the endotoxin- and cytokine-induced endocrine cascade influencing neuroendocrine control of growth and reproduction in farm animals. Reprod Domest Anim 2008;43(Suppl 2): 317–23.
86. Morris DD, Crowe N, Moore JN. Correlation of clinical and laboratory data with serum tumor necrosis factor activity in horses with experimentally induced endotoxemia. Am J Vet Res 1990;51(12):1935–40.
87. Seethanathan P, Bottoms GD, Schafer K. Characterization of release of tumor necrosis factor, interleukin-1, and superoxide anion from equine white blood cells in response to endotoxin. Am J Vet Res 1990;51(8):1221–5.
88. Winchell WW, Hardy J, Levine DM, et al. Effect of administration of a phospholipid emulsion on the initial response of horses administered endotoxin. Am J Vet Res 2002;63(10):1370–8.

Equine Hyperlipidemias

Harold C. McKenzie III, DVM, MS

KEYWORDS

• Triglyceride • Energy • Metabolism • Nutrition • Hyperlipemia
• Azotemia

Hyperlipidemias are defined by the presence of elevated lipid concentrations in the blood and are typically associated with periods of negative energy balance and physiologic stress. This increase in circulating lipids represents a normal physiologic response that serves to mobilize the energy reserves present in the fat depots of the body, but under certain circumstances, this response can become exaggerated and inappropriate. In increased concentrations, circulating lipids typically occur in the triglyceride form, and moderate increases in serum triglyceride concentration can lead to minor complications, with the most common being anorexia and depression. Increasing triglyceride concentrations can interfere with numerous normal physiologic functions, particularly in regard to reducing insulin sensitivity. This interference can result in the exacerbation of hyperlipidemia by impairing the ability of the body to limit fat mobilization, leading to worsening of lipid accumulation and severe complications, including renal and hepatic lipidosis and even death. Insulin-resistant individuals are at risk for hyperlipidemia, with the most commonly affected animals being ponies, miniature horses, and donkeys. The true incidence of hyperlipidemias in large-breed horses is not known, but these conditions seem to be increasingly encountered in the clinical setting, perhaps in relation to the increasing degree of obesity in the equine population.

DISORDERS OF EQUINE FAT METABOLISM

Dyslipidemias are disorders of lipid metabolism associated with abnormal amounts of circulating lipids. In horses, dyslipidemias present as hyperlipidemias, characterized by accumulation of circulating lipids in the form of triglycerides. Hyperlipidemias are most common in miniature horses, ponies, and donkeys but are uncommon in horses.[1] Several terms are used to describe equine dyslipidemias, including hyperlipemia, hyperlipidemia, hypertriglyceridemia, and severe hypertriglyceridemia

---

The author has nothing to disclose.
Marion duPont Scott Equine Medical Center, Virginia/Maryland Regional College of Veterinary Medicine, Virginia Polytechnic and State University, 17690 Old Waterford Road, Leesburg, VA 20176, USA
E-mail address: hmckenzi@vt.edu

Vet Clin Equine 27 (2011) 59–72
doi:10.1016/j.cveq.2010.12.008 vetequine.theclinics.com

(**Table 1**). Hypertriglyceridemia is present when serum triglyceride concentrations exceed the normal range (100 mg/dL) but is not associated with the evidence of clinical disease.[2] Hyperlipidemia is characterized by serum triglyceride concentrations from 100 to 500 mg/dL without gross lipemia.[3] Lipemia describes the presence of gross turbidity in a blood sample because of the presence of high concentrations of triglycerides but does not refer to a clinical syndrome (**Fig. 1**). Severe hypertriglyceridemia is defined as serum triglyceride concentrations exceeding 500 mg/dL, but in the absence of gross lipemia, which differentiates this condition from hyperlipemia.[3] Hyperlipemia is defined as a serum triglyceride concentration more than 500 mg/dL with visible lipemia and fatty infiltration of the liver or multiple organ systems.[2]

NORMAL ENERGY METABOLISM IN HORSES

Having evolved in sparse grassland environments, equine energy metabolism is based on the continuous intake of energy-poor diets, with roughage representing the primary feed source. Roughages contain variable amounts of nonstructural carbohydrates (sugars, starches), large quantities of structural carbohydrates (cellulose, lignin), and small amounts of protein and fat. Following ingestion, most of the nonstructural carbohydrates, proteins, and fats are absorbed in the small intestine. After absorption into the circulation, glucose can be used by tissues as an energy source or can be converted to either glycogen, for energy storage in the liver, or triglycerides, for energy storage in body fat. Insoluble carbohydrates, however, must undergo bacterial digestion in the hindgut to be absorbed in the form of volatile fatty acids (VFAs), and this process is shared by any soluble carbohydrates or proteins that reach the large intestine.[4] The primary VFAs are acetate, propionate, and butyrate. After absorption, these VFAs have different metabolic fates. Propionate is taken up by the liver and can be used for gluconeogenesis. Acetate and butyrate cannot be used for gluconeogenesis but can be used directly by some tissues as an energy source or are directed toward the synthesis of fatty acids, which occurs primarily in adipose tissue depots rather than in the liver.[5] Interestingly, because of their organization as hindgut

Table 1
Distinguishing characteristics of the various types of hyperlipidemias that have been described in horses

Equine Hyperlipidemias	Serum Triglyceride Concentration (mg/dL)	Gross Lipemia	Fatty Infiltration of Organs	Clinical Disease	Breeds Affected
Hypertriglyceridemia	>100	No	No	No	All
Hyperlipidemia	<500	No	No	No	All
Severe Hypertriglyceridemia	>500	No	Rare	Rare	Large-breed horses
Hyperlipemia	>500	Yes	Yes	Yes	Predisposed: ponies, miniature horses, donkeys Rare: large-breed horses

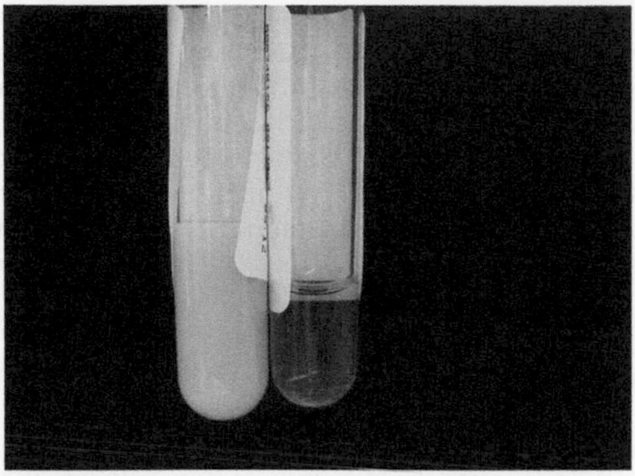

Fig. 1. Gross lipemia in a serum sample (*left*) as compared with a normal sample (*right*). (*Courtesy of* Dr Ramiro E. Toribio, College of Veterinary Medicine, The Ohio State University, Columbus, OH.)

fermenters, equids readily shift between the glucose-oriented metabolic pattern of the nonruminants when fed with diets high in soluble carbohydrates and a VFA-oriented metabolism similar to the ruminants when fed with a roughage-based diet.[6]

The normal metabolic response to intestinal glucose absorption is the release of insulin from the pancreas. Insulin clears glucose from the bloodstream and maintains serum blood glucose concentrations in a tight range (60–90 mg/dL). This function is achieved by increasing the tissue uptake of glucose, but if additional glucose is not currently needed as an energy source, it is converted into hepatic or muscle glycogen or depot fat. Insulin also suppresses the activity of hormone-sensitive lipase (HSL). HSL initiates the breakdown of triglycerides in adipose tissues, resulting in the release of glycerol, which is readily metabolized or converted to glucose, and free fatty acids (FFAs), which are metabolized via beta oxidation. HSL represents the rate-limiting step in the breakdown of fat, and if not regulated effectively, then excessive amounts of FFAs are released. FFAs not taken up by the peripheral tissues are normally removed from circulation by the liver and metabolized for energy, converted into ketone bodies, or esterified to form triglycerides. The liver processes the triglycerides into very-low-density lipoproteins (VLDLs) for export into the circulation. VLDLs are then transported to the peripheral tissues, where lipoprotein lipase (LPL) hydrolyzes the triglycerides from the VLDL, and the triglycerides are taken up by the cells of the peripheral tissues. LPL activity is stimulated by insulin and glucose-dependent insulinotropic polypeptide (GIP), which is a gastrointestinal hormone secreted in response to the ingestion of carbohydrates and fats.[7]

If a negative energy balance develops, several signals interact to maintain normoglycemia. First, the metabolic rate slows to decrease the consumption of glucose. Second, glucagon secretion increases and insulin secretion decreases, with the net effect being catabolic. Gluconeogenesis, glycogenolysis, and peripheral lipolysis ensue. In order to preserve the limited supply of glucose, there is a shift toward the use of fatty acids as a primary energy source. The release of leptin, a hormone expressed in adipose tissue, may increase as well, resulting in further energy release from fat stores. Because equids have limited stores of glycogen, maintenance of blood glucose concentrations is heavily dependent on gluconeogenesis, and protein catabolism increases to provide amino acids as precursors for glucose synthesis.

The response to a negative energy balance is increased in the presence of physiologic stress, such as that associated with illness or recovery from surgery. Increased endogenous glucocorticoid production is a normal response to physiologic stress, which leads to increased plasma cortisol concentrations and a loss of the normal circadian rhythm of cortisol production.[8] Cortisol inhibits insulin secretion and insulin actions but promotes catabolism and energy substrate mobilization. Increased catecholamine production in stress and illness upregulates the activity of HSL via stimulation of β-adrenoreceptors.[9]

DISTURBANCES OF ENERGY METABOLISM

Several factors can contribute to abnormalities of energy metabolism in equids, with the most common apparent cause being insulin resistance. Fasting has been shown to induce a state of insulin resistance in normal ponies,[10] whereas diets high in sugars and starches decrease insulin sensitivity in Thoroughbred weanlings and geldings.[11,12] Physical inactivity and increasing age also contribute to the development of insulin resistance.[13–15] Moreover, obese ponies and horses as well as ponies that have had laminitis are insulin resistant as compared with normal ponies or horses.[12,16,17] The association of obesity, insulin resistance, hyperinsulinemia, and hypertriglyceridemia with laminitis, particularly in ponies, has led to the characterization of the equine metabolic syndrome.[18,19] Pituitary pars intermedia dysfunction (PPID) has also been associated with hyperinsulinemia[13] and increased lipolysis in horses.[20] Complicating the management of clinically ill equine patients is the fact that systemic inflammation is associated with the development of insulin resistance, because several studies have shown that endotoxin administration induces an insulin-resistant state in horses.[21,22]

In animals with any or all of the aforementioned risk factors, the development of a negative energy balance can induce an inappropriate and excessive mobilization of peripheral fat stores. The liberated FFAs are converted into triglycerides within the liver, and the exported VLDLs accumulate within the circulation to excessive levels.[23] The increased circulating concentrations of FFAs and triglycerides can further complicate the normal homeostatic mechanisms that regulate energy metabolism, primarily by interfering with the actions of insulin. By preventing insulin from suppressing the activity of HSL, the rate of tissue lipolysis increases, worsening the hypertriglyceridemia. It has been shown that increased circulating FFA concentrations lead to the accumulation of lipid metabolites in muscle and hepatic tissue.[24] This accumulation disrupts the normal pathways that are responsible for insulin-induced glucose uptake in skeletal muscles and interferes with gluconeogenesis in the liver.[25] The result of all these interactions can be a fulminant self-perpetuating hyperlipidemia.

The accumulation of circulating lipids poses substantial risks to the patient, with the most severe being the possibility of tissue fat accumulation. The liver uses little FFAs for energy, and the pathway for ketone body formation is not well developed in horses, with the result that large amounts of triglycerides are produced. Excessive fat mobilization may overwhelm the capacity of the liver to process triglycerides into VLDL, leading to triglyceride accumulation and hepatic lipidosis. The kidneys are at risk of lipidosis as well, with renal lipidosis and/or azotemia reported in ponies and horses in association with hypertriglyceridemia.[3,26,27] The presence of azotemia may worsen hyperlipidemias by downregulating LPL activity.[28,29] Although the liver and kidneys seem to be at the greatest risk, there is evidence in other species that the pancreas may be damaged by fat accumulation as well, potentially contributing to the development of diabetes mellitus.[30]

DIAGNOSIS OF HYPERLIPIDEMIAS

The clinical signs of hyperlipidemias are nonspecific but most commonly include depression, anorexia, and decreased water intake.[3,31] More severe signs may include colic, fever, diarrhea, cachexia, and ventral edema.[2,26,31–34] Definitive diagnosis of hyperlipidemia requires documentation of increased levels of circulating lipids. Gross observation of a blood sample represents a simple means of ascertaining if lipemia is present (see **Fig. 1**), but lipemia is not present in all types of hyperlipidemias and is actually uncommon in large-breed horses affected with severe hypertriglyceridemia.[3] Serum triglyceride concentration should be measured as part of a routine serum biochemical evaluation in ponies, miniature horses, or donkeys because of their predisposition to hyperlipidemias and in hospitalized horses of all breeds because stress, illness, and hypophagia are common in the hospitalized population.

Hematologic changes are nonspecific and typically related to underlying disease processes but may include hemoconcentration, neutrophilia, neutropenia, left shift, and hyperfibrinogenemia.[3,35–37] Hyperlipemic ponies and donkeys are often hypoglycemic, although they are typically insulin resistant.[1] Metabolic acidosis is common in affected animals.[26,38] Azotemia is also frequent and may reflect either prerenal azotemia and/or renal dysfunction secondary to renal lipidosis.[3,26,34,39] Hepatic involvement may be demonstrated by increases in the serum bilirubin concentration as well as the hepatocellular and biliary enzyme levels.[3,26,31,34,35] Measurement of serum bile acid levels can be used to confirm the presence of hepatic dysfunction.

INCIDENCE OF HYPERLIPIDEMIAS

Hypertriglyceridemia, hyperlipemia, and hyperlipidemia are much more common in pony breeds, miniature horses, and donkeys, with Shetland ponies and donkeys being especially predisposed.[26,28,32] In one report, the incidence of hyperlipemia in ponies was 5.1 affected animals per 100 ponies per year.[33] Historically, the prognosis for affected ponies and donkeys has been reported to be grave, with mortality rates of 43% to 80%,[26,33,39,40] although recent reports showed mortality rates as low as 0% to 33% with aggressive treatment.[27,31,34,41]

Less is known regarding the frequency of hyperlipidemias in large-breed horses. Hypertriglyceridemia seems to occur more frequently in lactating or pregnant mares, and insulin resistance is reported to be more common in obese animals or in those with equine Cushing syndrome (ie, PPID) or the equine metabolic syndrome, but the actual rates of occurrence of hyperlipidemias in these groups are unknown. One retrospective study reported severe hypertriglyceridemia in 13 hospitalized horses in a 2-year period, which represented 0.57% of the hospitalized patient population.[3] The prevalence of obesity in large-breed horses seems to be increasing, particularly in pleasure riding horses that are fed high-grain diets but do not receive frequent high-intensity exercise.[42] This observation is supported by a recent publication from the United Kingdom, in which 45% of 319 pleasure riding horses were fat or very fat.[43] This trend toward increasing obesity is likely to contribute to insulin resistance and may result in an increased incidence of hyperlipidemias in large-breed horses, which argues for an increase in surveillance for hypertriglyceridemia in hospitalized horses.

PREVENTION OF HYPERLIPIDEMIAS

The most effective preventive approach is to avoid situations of stress and negative energy balance in animals likely to be susceptible to hyperlipidemias. Stressors can include transport, changes in management, and endoparasitism, all of which can be avoided or controlled by appropriate management.[32,44] The avoidance of negative energy balance can be more difficult to achieve, especially in mares, because pregnancy and lactation represent unavoidable periods of negative energy balance. Similar challenges arise in attempting to prevent negative energy balance in hospitalized animals, particularly in those with gastrointestinal diseases that require enteral rest. In the clinical setting, early enteral feeding has been shown to be beneficial in humans and horses following intestinal surgery, and this approach is increasingly used in equine patients.[45] Since the first encounter of severe hypertriglyceridemia in the author's clinic, there has been an increased appreciation of the need for early nutritional support and the incidence of severe hypertriglyceridemia in hospitalized patients has decreased to near zero.

It may be possible to decrease the risk of hyperlipidemias in susceptible animals by taking measures to improve their insulin sensitivity. Because obesity is clearly linked with insulin resistance, there should be a benefit to normalizing the body weight of susceptible animals. Great care should be taken with this approach because dietary restriction is often the first step in reducing body weight. By definition, reductions of caloric intake induce a state of negative energy balance, however, and could induce the onset of the very hyperlipidemic conditions one is trying to avoid.[46] Careful application of dietary restriction can be effective in resolving obesity and restoring insulin sensitivity, as demonstrated by the study of Van Weyenberg and colleagues[47] in Shetland ponies. Although caloric restriction was effective, there was an increase in serum triglyceride concentrations throughout the study period, from a mean of 30 mg/dL to a mean of approximately 120 mg/dL.

Exercise may represent a more effective means of reducing body weight and adiposity. Even moderate increases in activity result in an increased metabolic rate and decreased adiposity, but short-term exercise is unlikely to improve insulin sensitivity for more than a few days.[14,48] One recent study concluded that exercise of higher intensity or longer duration induces greater decreases in body weight and adiposity and is likely necessary for improvement in insulin sensitivity in overweight or obese, insulin-resistant horses.[48] The optimal approach is likely to combine careful dietary restriction with an appropriate increase in physical activity, similar to what is prescribed in humans.

Feeding fat-enriched diets to both ponies and horses has been shown to increase the activity of LPL and improve tissue clearance of plasma triglycerides, likely by increasing the activity of GIP.[7,49] It has been suggested that feeding fat-enriched diets might be beneficial in animals susceptible to hyperlipidemias because of improvement in triglyceride clearance, but this approach should be considered with caution because of concurrent decreases in glucose tolerance and insulin sensitivity.[1,7]

The pharmacologic approach may improve insulin sensitivity in at-risk animals. Agents that have been reported to improve insulin sensitivity in horses include metformin and a synthetic thyroid hormone (levothyroxine). Metformin is an oral biguanide that is widely used in human medicine as an insulin-sensitizing agent, and it has been used in the management of insulin-resistant horses.[50] Metformin primarily controls blood glucose concentrations by inhibiting hepatic gluconeogenesis and glycogenolysis, but it also enhances peripheral tissue insulin sensitivity.[51] Although there is some evidence of efficacy in the literature, the drug is not well absorbed following oral administration in horses and is not recommended for use pending further information regarding pharmacodynamics in horses.[51]

The administration of levothyroxine sodium has been shown to induce weight loss and improve insulin sensitivity in horses.[19] This supplementation increases circulating thyroxine concentrations above the normal range, but signs of clinical hyperthyroidism are not reported.[52] The current recommendation is that levothyroxine sodium should be administered to horses and large ponies at a dosage of 48 mg/d in the feed for 3 to 6 months along with modifications of diet and exercise, whereas smaller ponies and miniature horses should be given 24 mg of levothyroxine sodium daily.[19] Treated horses should be weaned from levothyroxine sodium therapy after the desired body weight is achieved, first by reducing the dosage to 24 mg/d for 2 weeks and then 12 mg/d for 2 weeks.[19]

MANAGEMENT OF HYPERLIPIDEMIAS

Effective management requires that clinicians identify the affected animals as early as possible to institute therapy before the hypertriglyceridemia becomes severe. The first line of surveillance is recognition of animals at risk by identifying the predisposing factors for hyperlipidemias. Gross observation of the blood for lipemia is not sensitive and should not be relied on in the clinical setting, and it is recommended that serum triglycerides be measured as part of the routine serum biochemical evaluation in clinically ill horses, and this evaluation is mandatory when evaluating any pony, miniature horse, or donkey.

Once hyperlipidemia is identified, the most important component of management is correction of the underlying condition that has resulted in a negative energy balance. Some conditions, such as pregnancy or lactation, are not easily addressed, but any primary disease process should be addressed as rapidly as possible. The second component of management is the correction of the patient's negative energy balance. If there is a lack of voluntary intake in a patient capable of tolerating enteral nutrition, then enteral supplementation is indicated. If the enteral route is unavailable, parenteral nutritional (PN) support is required.

Correction of Negative Energy Balance

The ultimate goal of dietary supplementation is the correction of the negative energy balance by meeting the patient's resting energy requirement (RER); however, there is some debate regarding the actual RER of the hospitalized equine patient. Hospitalized horses are stall-confined and inactive, thus consuming less energy than a horse at pasture or in routine work. In one study, the RER of stall-confined horses was 30% lower than that of horses at pasture.[53] More strikingly, the energy requirements of hospitalized premature foals or foals with hypoxic-ischemic encephalopathy were one-third of the energy requirement of healthy age-matched foals.[54] The determination of the RER is further complicated by the potential influence of physiologic stress or illness, which is demonstrated by the fact that anesthesia and experimental exploratory laparotomy in normal horses were associated with a 10% increase in resting caloric demand.[55] Given all these potential influences, a definitive RER value cannot be provided for all patients, but a reasonable RER value for most hospitalized mature equids is 22 to 23 kcal/kg/d.[56,57]

In reality, it can be challenging, particularly in the critically ill patient, to deliver the amount of energy required to meet the patient's estimated RER. Provision of excessive enteral nutrition may result in the development of diarrhea, which can be severe and even life threatening.[58] Provision of excessive PN can contribute to hyperglycemia, hypertriglyceridemia, or hyperlipemia, as well as electrolyte derangements.[57] For all these reasons, one should be conservative when initiating nutritional support, and a maximal target of 60% of RER is recommended.[41]

Indeed, in most cases it is not necessary to entirely correct the negative energy balance by meeting the patient's RER because the excessive lipid liberation is related to the decrease in insulin secretion that accompanies decreased feed intake. This reduction in insulin secretion, particularly in horses conditioned to diets high in soluble carbohydrates, removes the normal suppressive effect of insulin on HSL. The increase in HSL activity leads to rapid liberation of large amounts of FFAs, and this response is exaggerated in the obese patient. To address this situation in the clinical setting, the solution may be as simple as providing small amounts of carbohydrates (5–10 kcal/kg/d) to stimulate endogenous insulin production. Despite providing less than one-fourth of the daily RER, this solution was effective in correcting hypertriglyceridemia in some large-breed horses.[3] Insulin resistance is likely to be present in any equid with hyperlipidemia, and in these patients, the administration of carbohydrates alone is likely to result in hyperglycemia. Insulin therapy is often required to overcome peripheral insulin resistance, allow for appropriate tissue uptake of glucose from the circulation, and restore normal HSL activity.

Enteral Nutritional Support

Provision of nutritional support by the enteral route is generally preferred because it is the most natural and physiologic means of nutrient delivery and the intestinal mucosa is partially dependent on the products of digestion for energy and nutrients. In addition, enteral nutrition is less expensive. If there is any question about the ability of the animal to tolerate feeding, then a thorough evaluation of the gastrointestinal function is needed before institution of enteral nutritional support. This evaluation should include abdominal auscultation, nasogastric intubation to evaluate for gastric reflux, and abdominal ultrasonographic examination. Horses with evidence of gastrointestinal dysfunction, such as gastric reflux, bowel distension, increased bowel wall thickness, or ileus, are unlikely to tolerate enteral feeding and should receive intravenous nutritional support. All efforts to encourage the voluntary intake of feed should be exhausted before instituting forced feeding.

A positive response may be observed with the oral administration of even small amounts (5 kcal/kg/d) of simple sugars. High-fructose corn syrup can be used as an oral carbohydrate source, but care must be taken not to feed excessive amounts to avoid carbohydrate overload. This product provides energy of approximately 4 kcal/mL, and horses typically accept it readily when administered orally using a dosage syringe. A 60-mL dose of corn syrup given orally every 2 hours delivers approximately 5 kcal/kg/d to a 500-kg horse and is well tolerated clinically. If more complete nutritional supplementation is required in the inappetant animal, the only alternative for the administration of enteral feedstuffs is the use of nasogastric intubation. Intermittent nasogastric intubation is often used for this purpose and can be effective. However, large-bolus feedings may overwhelm digestive capacity, and repeated intubation can be a stress for some patients. The primary advantage of intermittent intubation is that the large bore of the tube permits feeding slurry feeds, which more closely mimic the horse's normal diet. Use of small-bore indwelling nasogastric feeding tubes and feeding small volumes of liquid feedstuffs at frequent intervals (eg, every 1–2 hours) may be preferred over repeated passage of a nasogastric tube because the former decreases the risk of pharyngeal trauma and improves patient comfort. Another advantage of small-bore indwelling tubes is that they do not interfere with voluntary water or feed intake. Correct placement of small-bore feeding tubes should be confirmed by endoscopy because the flexible nature of these tubes makes it difficult to be certain of placement based on feel alone.

PN Support

Although the enteral route is generally preferred to provide nutritional support, there are a variety of situations in which a horse may be unable to receive enteral nutrition or is unable to tolerate the required volume of enteral nutrition. In these circumstances, PN aids in delivering the appropriate caloric and nutritional support in a controlled manner and eliminates concerns regarding intestinal absorption and intestinal volume overload. The limitations of PN support primarily include the expense of this therapy and the risk of secondary complications. These complications may include hyperglycemia, hypertriglyceridemia, thrombophlebitis, and an increased risk of bloodstream infections.[59] Electrolyte abnormalities, such as hypokalemia, may develop with PN.

Short-term caloric supplementation

Carbohydrate solutions represent the simplest means of providing intravenous caloric support. After initial fluid resuscitation, electrolyte solutions containing added dextrose may be used as the primary fluids for maintenance therapy in horses with minimal ongoing fluid losses. The caloric content of a 5% dextrose solution is 0.17 kcal/mL, so an infusion rate of 5 mL/kg/h would be required to deliver approximately 20 kcal/kg/d. Unfortunately, this rate of infusion is up to 5 times that which is considered to be a maintenance rate for an adult horse (1–2 mL/kg/h), so a 5% dextrose solution cannot be depended on as a primary form of PN. However, electrolyte solutions containing 5% dextrose can be used to provide moderate amounts of carbohydrates to stimulate endogenous insulin production because an infusion rate of 1 mL/kg/h delivers 4 kcal/kg/d. Alternatively, a 50% dextrose solution can be delivered using an infusion pump, as long as additional isotonic fluids are being administered concurrently to avoid endothelial injury caused by the hypertonic nature of this solution. However, the use of a 50% dextrose solution should be avoided if an infusion pump is not available. The caloric content of a 50% dextrose solution is 1.7 kcal/mL, so an infusion rate of 0.5 mL/kg/h of this solution delivers approximately 20 kcal/kg/d. In patients that are likely to be incapable of enteral feeding for more than 24 hours, PN solutions containing carbohydrates and amino acids should be used rather than simple carbohydrate solutions. The provision of amino acids provides amino acid precursors for gluconeogenesis and limits endogenous protein catabolism. Lipid-containing PN solutions are typically only needed in patients likely to require prolonged parenteral support or those that are unable to tolerate carbohydrates. There is some concern that lipid-containing solutions could exacerbate preexisting hypertriglyceridemia, and for this reason, these solutions should be avoided in patients with very high serum triglyceride levels (>1000 mg/dL or gross lipemia).[57]

Insulin Therapy

The frequent presence of insulin resistance makes it difficult to achieve even a conservative rate of administration of intravenous nutrition in hyperlipidemic patients, and this difficulty can be addressed only by the administration of exogenous insulin. However, the administration of insulin to any patient requires diligent management to prevent profound hypoglycemia. Intermittent depot administration of subcutaneous insulin may offer some advantages in terms of simplicity of administration and moderation of effects, but this route of administration does not allow for changes in dosage over the short term. Subcutaneous administration may result in periods of hypoglycemia several hours after administration, but the simultaneous administration of oral carbohydrates can help ameliorate this effect. Close monitoring of blood glucose levels is required while determining the most appropriate doses of insulin and oral carbohydrates in each patient. In one report, 0.15 IU/kg of insulin zinc suspension was administered subcutaneously twice daily to ponies and donkeys, in conjunction with enteral or PN support, and the dosage of insulin was increased in increments of 0.05 IU/kg if hyperglycemia occurred.[41]

Insulin can also be administered as a continuous rate infusion (CRI), but patients receiving insulin should receive intravenous dextrose concomitantly to avoid hypoglycemia. The use of CRI insulin allows for a rapid onset of action while providing a timely means of adjustment of the dose. Because of the apparent gradual saturation of insulin receptors, the maximal effect of CRI insulin is not typically seen until approximately 90 minutes after initiation of therapy. The response to changing rates of infusion occurs over a similar time frame, so it is recommended to avoid altering the rate of infusion of PN solutions too rapidly after changing the rate of insulin infusion.

An initial insulin infusion rate of 0.07 IU/kg/h is generally well tolerated and represents a reasonable starting point for most patients. Simultaneous alterations should be avoided in both the insulin and the PN infusion rates because this can lead to a "roller-coaster ride," wherein the blood glucose concentration increases and decreases because of the delay in the body's response to these changes. Using a protocol in which changes in blood glucose concentration are primarily addressed by altering the insulin infusion rate can minimize dramatic alterations in blood glucose concentration.[60] Blood glucose monitoring should be performed at least hourly for the first 2 to 3 hours after initiation of the insulin CRI, and if hyperglycemia (blood glucose level >180 mg/dL) persists after the first 2 hours, the insulin infusion rate may be increased by 50%, followed by hourly blood glucose monitoring for a further 2 to 3 hours. This procedure may be repeated if hyperglycemia persists. Conversely, if hypoglycemia (blood glucose level <60 mg/dL) is noted, then a bolus of 0.25 mL/kg of 50% dextrose solution should be administered intravenously over 3 to 5 minutes. The blood glucose level should then be reassessed every 30 minutes for at least 90 minutes to ensure that hypoglycemia does not recur. If hypoglycemia does recur, then a second bolus of dextrose is administered, and the insulin infusion rate is decreased by 50%. Close monitoring is required for a further 60 to 90 minutes to ensure that hypoglycemia does not recur and hyperglycemia does not develop. Further changes to the insulin infusion rate are not usually necessary once a steady state has been achieved. Blood glucose monitoring should be done every 3 to 6 hours for the first day of therapy. The ongoing frequency of blood glucose monitoring depends on patient stability; blood glucose may not need to be monitored more frequently than every 12 hours in the stable patient. Patient reassessment is indicated if the patient has become even more insulin resistant (requiring additional insulin administration to avoid hyperglycemia), because this may be an early indicator of an overall deterioration in the patient's condition accompanied by increasing systemic inflammation. When PN is to be discontinued, it is recommended that the PN and insulin infusion rates be gradually reduced by 25% to 50% increments every 4 to 6 hours while gradually increasing enteral feeding. It is important that blood glucose monitoring is continued during this weaning process to prevent the development of severe hypoglycemia.

OTHER TREATMENTS FOR HYPERLIPIDEMIAS

Apart from correction of the primary disease and the provision of appropriate nutritional support, there does not seem to be any single specific therapy that is effective in resolving equine hyperlipidemias. The most widely discussed therapies include insulin and heparin administration. Inherently, insulin administration seems to be a logical therapy even in insulin-resistant individuals because it both suppresses HSL and activates LPL. The literature is conflicted, however, regarding insulin therapy as a primary treatment of hyperlipidemias in ponies, horses, and donkeys. Historically, the use of insulin was not associated with any apparent improvement in outcomes, and it was considered that insulin therapy might be ineffective because excessive fat mobilization was secondary to insulin resistance.[31] Alternatively, it seems possible that there was an inherent selection bias, wherein the animals most likely to receive insulin therapy were those with profound insulin resistance and refractory hyperglycemia, and these individuals seemed to have more severe hyperlipidemia and were less likely to survive. Recent studies have reported that insulin, when administered concurrently with appropriate nutritional support, seems to aid in the resolution of hypertriglyceridemia.[27,41]

Heparin has been used in the treatment of hyperlipidemias because it promotes peripheral triglyceride use and stimulates LPL activity.[31,32,39,61] The efficacy of this treatment has been questioned because the activity of LPL was not deficient in hyperlipemic ponies but was, in fact, increased 2-fold.[23] Heparin therapy has also been questioned because of the risk of heparin-induced thrombocytopenia and bleeding disorders.[31,62] On the other hand, heparin has been shown to be effective in both equine and human patients in rapidly reducing plasma triglyceride concentrations and may be useful in managing the severely hypertriglyceridemic (>1000 mg/dL) or lipemic patient.[41,62] If used, treatment with heparin should be for a very short term to minimize the risk of side effects.

SUMMARY

Although the risk of hyperlipidemias is greatest in ponies, miniature horses, and donkeys, all equids are potentially at risk if they are in a situation involving a negative energy balance. The sedentary lifestyle of many modern horses and the frequent feeding of high-carbohydrate diets mean that increasing numbers of animals are at risk of obesity and insulin resistance. Both these factors contribute substantially to the risk of excessive fat mobilization and the development of hyperlipidemias. Veterinarians can decrease the risk to their patients by being vigilant for those individuals most likely to be insulin resistant and instituting appropriate monitoring, prevention, and management strategies.

REFERENCES

1. Hughes KJ, Hodgson DR, Dart AJ. Equine hyperlipaemia: a review. Aust Vet J 2004;82(3):136–42.
2. Naylor JM. Hyperlipemia and hyperlipidemia in horses, ponies and donkeys. Comp Cont Educ Pract Vet 1982;4:321–6.
3. Dunkel B, McKenzie HC 3rd. Severe hypertriglyceridaemia in clinically ill horses: diagnosis, treatment and outcome. Equine Vet J 2003;35(6):590–5.
4. Bergman EN. Energy contributions of volatile fatty acids from the gastrointestinal tract in various species. Physiol Rev 1990;70(2):567–90.
5. Suagee JK, Corl BA, Crisman MV, et al. De novo fatty acid synthesis and NADPH generation in equine adipose and liver tissue. Comp Biochem Physiol B Biochem Mol Biol 2010;155(3):322–6.
6. Argenzio RA, Hintz HF. Effect of diet on glucose entry and oxidation rates in ponies. J Nutr 1972;102(7):879–92.
7. Schmidt O, Deegen E, Fuhrmann H, et al. Effects of fat feeding and energy level on plasma metabolites and hormones in Shetland ponies. J Vet Med A Physiol Pathol Clin Med 2001;48(1):39–49.
8. Lavery GG, Glover P. The metabolic and nutritional response to critical illness. Curr Opin Crit Care 2000;6(4):233–8.

9. Langin D. Adipose tissue lipolysis as a metabolic pathway to define pharmacological strategies against obesity and the metabolic syndrome. Pharmacol Res 2006;53(6):482–91.
10. Argenzio RA, Hintz HF. Volatile fatty acid tolerance and effect of glucose and VFA on plasma insulin levels in ponies. J Nutr 1971;101(6):723–9.
11. Treiber KH, Boston RC, Kronfeld DS, et al. Insulin resistance and compensation in Thoroughbred weanlings adapted to high-glycemic meals. J Anim Sci 2005; 83(10):2357–64.
12. Hoffman RM, Boston RC, Stefanovski D, et al. Obesity and diet affect glucose dynamics and insulin sensitivity in Thoroughbred geldings. J Anim Sci 2003; 81(9):2333–42.
13. McGowan CM, Frost R, Pfeiffer DU, et al. Serum insulin concentrations in horses with equine Cushing's syndrome: response to a cortisol inhibitor and prognostic value. Equine Vet J 2004;36(3):295–8.
14. Powell DM, Reedy SE, Sessions DR, et al. Effect of short-term exercise training on insulin sensitivity in obese and lean mares. Equine Vet J Suppl 2002;34:81–4.
15. Pratt SE, Geor RJ, McCutcheon LJ. Effects of dietary energy source and physical conditioning on insulin sensitivity and glucose tolerance in standardbred horses. Equine Vet J Suppl 2006;36:579–84.
16. Jeffcott LB, Field JR, McLean JG, et al. Glucose tolerance and insulin sensitivity in ponies and Standardbred horses. Equine Vet J 1986;18(2):97–101.
17. Frank N, Elliott SB, Brandt LE, et al. Physical characteristics, blood hormone concentrations, and plasma lipid concentrations in obese horses with insulin resistance. J Am Vet Med Assoc 2006;228(9):1383–90.
18. Geor R, Frank N. Metabolic syndrome—from human organ disease to laminar failure in equids. Vet Immunol Immunopathol 2009;129(3–4):151–4.
19. Frank N, Geor RJ, Bailey SR, et al. Equine metabolic syndrome. J Vet Intern Med 2010;24(3):467–75.
20. van der Kolk JH, Wensing T, Kalsbeek HC, et al. Lipid metabolism in horses with hyperadrenocorticism. J Am Vet Med Assoc 1995;206(7):1010–2.
21. Vick MM, Murphy BA, Sessions DR, et al. Effects of systemic inflammation on insulin sensitivity in horses and inflammatory cytokine expression in adipose tissue. Am J Vet Res 2008;69(1):130–9.
22. Toth F, Frank N, Chameroy KA, et al. Effects of endotoxaemia and carbohydrate overload on glucose and insulin dynamics and the development of laminitis in horses. Equine Vet J 2009;41(9):852–8.
23. Watson TD, Burns L, Love S, et al. Plasma lipids, lipoproteins and post-heparin lipases in ponies with hyperlipaemia. Equine Vet J 1992;24(5):341–6.
24. Shulman GI. Cellular mechanisms of insulin resistance. J Clin Invest 2000;106(2): 171–6.
25. Morino K, Petersen KF, Shulman GI. Molecular mechanisms of insulin resistance in humans and their potential links with mitochondrial dysfunction. Diabetes 2006; 55(Suppl 2):S9–15.
26. Watson TD, Murphy D, Love S. Equine hyperlipaemia in the United Kingdom: clinical features and blood biochemistry of 18 cases. Vet Rec 1992;131(3): 48–51.
27. Waitt LH, Cebra CK. Characterization of hypertriglyceridemia and response to treatment with insulin in horses, ponies, and donkeys: 44 cases (1995–2005). J Am Vet Med Assoc 2009;234(7):915–9.
28. Naylor JM, Kronfeld DS, Acland H. Hyperlipemia in horses: effects of undernutrition and disease. Am J Vet Res 1980;41(6):899–905.

29. Sato T, Liang K, Vaziri ND. Down-regulation of lipoprotein lipase and VLDL receptor in rats with focal glomerulosclerosis. Kidney Int 2002;61(1):157–62.
30. Gan SI, Edwards AL, Symonds CJ, et al. Hypertriglyceridemia-induced pancreatitis: a case-based review. World J Gastroenterol 2006;12(44):7197–202.
31. Moore BR, Abood SK, Hinchcliff KW. Hyperlipemia in 9 miniature horses and miniature donkeys. J Vet Intern Med 1994;8(5):376–81.
32. Jeffcott LB, Field JR. Current concepts of hyperlipaemia in horses and ponies. Vet Rec 1985;116(17):461–6.
33. Jeffcott LB, Field JR. Epidemiological aspects of hyperlipaemia in ponies in south eastern Australia. Aust Vet J 1985;62(4):140–1.
34. Oikawa S, McGuirk S, Nishibe K, et al. Changes of blood biochemical values in ponies recovering from hyperlipemia in Japan. J Vet Med Sci 2006;68(4):353–9.
35. Field JR. Hyperlipemia in a quarter horse. Comp Cont Educ Pract Vet 1988;10:218–21.
36. Gilbert RO. Congenital hyperlipaemia in a Shetland pony foal. Equine Vet J 1986;18(6):498–500.
37. Mair TS. Hyperlipaemia and laminitis secondary to an injection abscess in a donkey. Equine Vet Educ 1995;7:8–11.
38. Hughes KJ, Hodgson DR, Dart AJ. Hyperlipaemia in a 7-week-old miniature pony foal. Aust Vet J 2002;80(6):350–1.
39. Gay CC, Sullivan ND, Wilkinson JS, et al. Hyperlipaemia in ponies. Aust Vet J 1978;54(10):459–62.
40. Love S. Hyperlipaemia comes of age. Equine Vet Educ 1990;2:171–2.
41. Durham AE. Clinical application of parenteral nutrition in the treatment of five ponies and one donkey with hyperlipaemia. Vet Rec 2006;158(5):159–64.
42. Johnson PJ, Wiedmeyer CE, Messer NT, et al. Medical implications of obesity in horses—lessons for human obesity. J Diabetes Sci Technol 2009;3(1):163–74.
43. Wyse CA, McNie KA, Tannahill VJ, et al. Prevalence of obesity in riding horses in Scotland. Vet Rec 2008;162(18):590–1.
44. Watson TD, Love S. Equine hyperlipidemia. Comp Cont Educ Pract Vet 1994;16:89–97.
45. Lewis SJ, Andersen HK, Thomas S. Early enteral nutrition within 24 h of intestinal surgery versus later commencement of feeding: a systematic review and meta-analysis. J Gastrointest Surg 2009;13(3):569–75.
46. Geor RJ, Harris P. Dietary management of obesity and insulin resistance: countering risk for laminitis. Vet Clin North Am Equine Pract 2009;25(1):51–65, vi.
47. Van Weyenberg S, Hesta M, Buyse J, et al. The effect of weight loss by energy restriction on metabolic profile and glucose tolerance in ponies. J Anim Physiol Anim Nutr (Berl) 2008;92(5):538–45.
48. Carter RA, McCutcheon LJ, Valle E, et al. Effects of exercise training on adiposity, insulin sensitivity, and plasma hormone and lipid concentrations in overweight or obese, insulin-resistant horses. Am J Vet Res 2010;71(3):314–21.
49. Geelen SN, Sloet van Oldruitenborgh-Oosterbaan MM, Beynen AC. Dietary fat supplementation and equine plasma lipid metabolism. Equine Vet J Suppl 1999;30:475–8.
50. Durham AE, Rendle DI, Newton JE. The effect of metformin on measurements of insulin sensitivity and beta cell response in 18 horses and ponies with insulin resistance. Equine Vet J 2008;40(5):493–500.
51. Hustace JL, Firshman AM, Mata JE. Pharmacokinetics and bioavailability of metformin in horses. Am J Vet Res 2009;70(5):665–8.

52. Frank N, Sommardahl CS, Eiler H, et al. Effects of oral administration of levothyroxine sodium on concentrations of plasma lipids, concentration and composition of very-low-density lipoproteins, and glucose dynamics in healthy adult mares. Am J Vet Res 2005;66(6):1032–8.
53. Pagan JD, Hintz HF. Equine energetics. I. Relationship between body weight and energy requirements in horses. J Anim Sci 1986;63:815–21.
54. Ousey JC, Holdstock NB, Rossdale PD, et al. How much energy do sick neonatal foals require compared with healthy foals? Pferdeheilkunde 1996;12:231–7.
55. Cruz AM, Cote N, McDonell WN, et al. Postoperative effects of anesthesia and surgery on resting energy expenditure in horses as measured by indirect calorimetry. Can J Vet Res 2006;70(4):257–62.
56. Magdesian KG. Nutrition for critical gastrointestinal illness: feeding horses with diarrhea or colic. Vet Clin North Am Equine Pract 2003;19(3):617–44.
57. Magdesian KG. Parenteral nutrition in the mature horse. Equine Vet Educ 2010; 22(7):364–71.
58. Dunkel BM, Wilkins PA. Nutrition and the critically ill horse. Vet Clin North Am Equine Pract 2004;20(1):107–26.
59. Krause JB, McKenzie HC 3rd. Parenteral nutrition in foals: a retrospective study of 45 cases (2000–2004). Equine Vet J 2007;39(1):74–8.
60. McKenzie HC 3rd, Geor RJ. Feeding management of sick neonatal foals. Vet Clin North Am Equine Pract 2009;25(1):109–19, vii.
61. Mogg TD, Palmer JE. Hyperlipidemia, hyperlipemia, and hepatic lipidosis in American miniature horses: 23 cases (1990–1994). J Am Vet Med Assoc 1995; 207(5):604–7.
62. Cole RP. Heparin treatment for severe hypertriglyceridemia in diabetic ketoacidosis. Arch Intern Med 2009;169(15):1439–41.

Equine Metabolic Syndrome

Nicholas Frank, DVM, PhD[a,b,*]

KEYWORDS

- Obesity • Regional adiposity • Hyperinsulinemia
- Insulin resistance • Laminitis

Veterinarians have long recognized that obese horses and ponies are prone to laminitis, but the concept of an equine metabolic syndrome (EMS) was first proposed by Johnson[1] in 2002. This concept has developed over time, and EMS was recently described in a consensus statement released by the American College of Veterinary Internal Medicine.[2] In human medicine, metabolic syndrome (MetS) refers to a set of risk factors that predict the risk of cardiovascular disease,[3] including obesity, glucose intolerance and insulin resistance (IR), dyslipidemia, microalbuminuria, and hypertension. Associated conditions in humans include nonalcoholic fatty liver disease and polycystic ovary syndrome. EMS shares some of the features of MetS, including obesity, IR, and dyslipidemia, but differs in that laminitis is the primary disease of interest.

COMPONENTS OF THE SYNDROME

EMS is not a specific disease entity, but rather a clinical syndrome associated with laminitis.[4,5] Increased adiposity, hyperinsulinemia, and IR are the 3 principal components of this syndrome, and it is difficult to separate these factors from one another. Hyperinsulinemia is detected in most insulin resistant horses and affected animals are usually obese or exhibit regional adiposity (**Fig. 1**). One or all of these factors may determine laminitis susceptibility, but it is also conceivable that another, as yet unidentified, factor predisposes horses with EMS to laminitis. Other components of EMS include dyslipidemia,[4–6] altered blood adipokine concentrations,[5,7,8] systemic inflammation,[9] and seasonal arterial hypertension.[10] In contrast to MetS in humans, atherosclerosis and coronary heart disease are not detected in horses with EMS, and this may be explained by the herbivorous diet of horses or lipoprotein composition

[a] Department of Large Animal Clinical Sciences, University of Tennessee College of Veterinary Medicine, 2407 River Drive, Knoxville, TN 37996, USA
[b] Division of Medicine, School of Veterinary Medicine and Science, University of Nottingham, Sutton Bonington Campus, Leicestershire LE12 5RD, UK
* Department of Large Animal Clinical Sciences, University of Tennessee College of Veterinary Medicine, 2407 River Drive, Knoxville, TN 37996.
E-mail address: nfrank@utk.edu

Vet Clin Equine 27 (2011) 73–92
doi:10.1016/j.cveq.2010.12.004 vetequine.theclinics.com
0749-0739/11/$ – see front matter

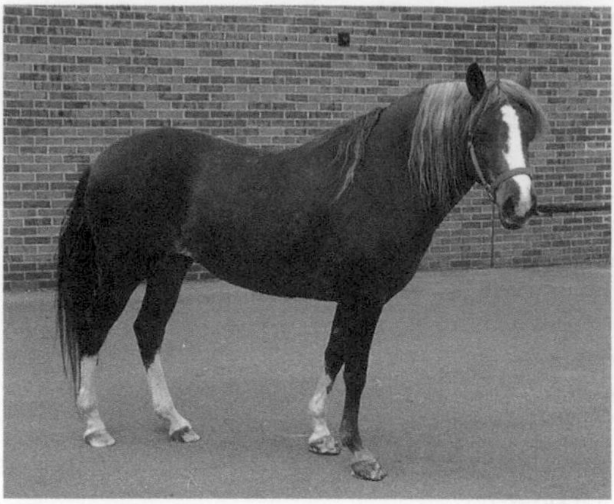

Fig. 1. A 7-year-old Morgan horse mixed breed mare with physical characteristics of equine metabolic syndrome.

of equine blood. Most circulating cholesterol is carried within high-density lipoproteins in horses, rather than low-density lipoproteins, which are atherogenic.[11]

BREED PREDISPOSITION

EMS occurs most commonly in pony breeds, Morgan horses, Paso Finos, Arabians, Saddlebreds, Quarter horses, and Tennessee Walking horses. Most horses and ponies with EMS are obese, and owners often describe them as "easy keepers." Environmental issues such as overfeeding and lack of exercise contribute to obesity, and these problems are increasing with modern management practices.

CLINICAL PRESENTATION

Laminitis

Horses and ponies with EMS are predisposed to laminitis, so this is the most common presenting complaint. Laminitis typically develops after animals have been grazing on pasture, which is referred to as pasture-associated laminitis.[12] Episodes of laminitis often occur after heavy rains and abundant sunlight, when grasses have been growing rapidly and accumulating water-soluble carbohydrates (WSC) through increased photosynthesis.[13] Grazing on rapidly growing pastures increases total energy intake and promotes obesity, while also increasing WSC consumption. Resting insulin concentrations increase as a result, and this alters proxy measures of insulin sensitivity and pancreatic output.[4,5] However, proxy measures used for blood samples have been collected under fed conditions in previous studies, so it is difficult to determine whether insulin sensitivity per se progressively decreases in response to pasture grazing. This distinction is an important one because laminitis has been experimentally induced in ponies and horses by infusing insulin intravenously, suggesting that hyperinsulinemia is the trigger for disease.[14,15] One challenge for researchers in the future is to conduct studies in which the effects of obesity, IR, and hyperinsulinemia on laminitis development are evaluated independently.

Pasture grazing also raises the risk of intestinal carbohydrate overload, particularly when animals are moved onto new pastures without gradual transition.[12] In these situations, the amount of WSC entering the intestinal tract exceeds the digestive and absorptive capacities of the small intestine and increases the amount of substrate available for fermentation within the large intestine. Increased fermentation raises lactic acid concentrations, lowers pH, and increases mucosal permeability.[16] Movement of gut-derived factors including exotoxins, endotoxins, and vasoactive amines into the circulation induces a systemic inflammatory response and activates platelets.[17] Evidence for an intestinal trigger for pasture-associated laminitis comes from studies in which oligofructose has been administered to horses as a model for carbohydrate overload on pasture. Treated horses exhibit clinical signs consistent with a systemic inflammatory response, followed by laminitis.[18–20]

Laminitis is typically thought of as a catastrophic event causing severe lameness, but a milder form of laminitis is often detected in horses and ponies with EMS. Divergent growth rings (founder lines) are sometimes recognized in horses that are walking soundly, indicating that hoof growth has been disrupted by a previous laminitis episode (**Fig. 2**). A growth ring is considered divergent when the distance to the coronary band is shorter at the dorsum than the heel. These findings suggest that horses develop laminitis that goes unnoticed by the owner, particularly when animals are kept on pasture. A full diagnostic evaluation should therefore include lateral radiographs of the feet and placement of hoof testers. Mild lameness associated with laminitis can sometimes be detected by tightly circling the horse on a hard surface.

Complications of Hospitalization

There are anecdotal reports of horses and ponies with EMS showing greater susceptibility to laminitis triggered by grain overload, retained fetal membranes, and colitis. It is therefore important to recognize the EMS phenotype and alert owners to the potential risk of laminitis. Obese horses are also susceptible to colic caused by lipomas. A pedunculated lipoma can lead to strangulation of the small intestine and moderate to severe colic, accompanied by intestinal distension and reflux.

Problems with IR are sometimes recognized for the first time when hypertriglyceridemia develops in hospitalized patients that enter negative energy balance. Insulin-resistant horses mobilize lipids more readily and are more susceptible to equine hyperlipemia.[11] Hyperglycemia and glucosuria may also be detected in affected horses when dextrose is administered intravenously to provide partial parenteral nutrition. Exogenous insulin is often required in these cases to maintain plasma glucose concentrations below renal threshold while dextrose is administered. Of interest, there

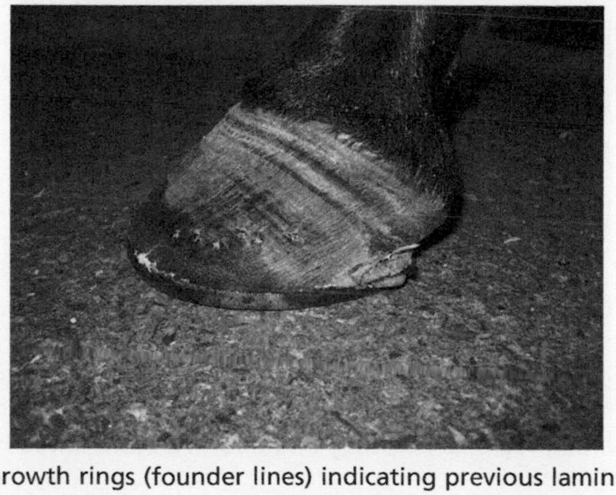

Fig. 2. Divergent growth rings (founder lines) indicating previous laminitis.

have been no reports of laminitis developing as a result of intravenous insulin infusion to manage hyperglycemia.

Obesity and Regional Adiposity

As more owners and veterinarians have become aware of EMS, obesity and regional adiposity are increasingly identified as abnormal states during routine health examinations. Severely affected horses have a body condition score (BCS) of 8 or 9 on the 1 (poor) to 9 (extremely fat) scale developed by Henneke and colleagues[21] and marked expansion of the neck crest, which may fall to one side. Enlargement of adipose tissues within the neck region is a common manifestation of regional adiposity and is commonly referred to as a cresty neck (**Fig. 3**) Carter and colleagues[22] created a scoring system to assess horses with this form of regional adiposity using a 0 to 5 range, and scores of 3 or more are often detected in horses or ponies with EMS (**Fig. 4**). The description provided for a score of 3 is "Crest enlarged and thickened, so fat is deposited more heavily in middle of the neck than toward poll and withers, giving a mounded appearance. Crest fills cupped hand and begins losing side-to-side flexibility." Neck circumference can also be measured by dividing the distance along a line from the poll to the cranial aspect of the withers (x) by 4 and measuring the circumference of the neck at 3 equidistant points (0.25x, 0.50x, and 0.75x). These measurements can be used to assess progress after management plans are implemented.

Preputial or Mammary Gland Swelling

Obese geldings affected by EMS sometimes present with the complaint of preputial swelling (**Fig. 5**), with insect bites or trauma suspected. However, further examination reveals adipose tissue expansion and edema secondary to reduced lymphatic return. Owners should be questioned about the body condition of their horse and whether obesity has developed in the past few months. Because edema can be a component of this preputial swelling, it is exacerbated by stall confinement and addressed by increasing exercise. Horses with this problem respond well to weight loss, indicating that expanded adipose tissue is the primary problem. Mares with EMS sometimes present with adipose tissue expansion in the mammary gland region.

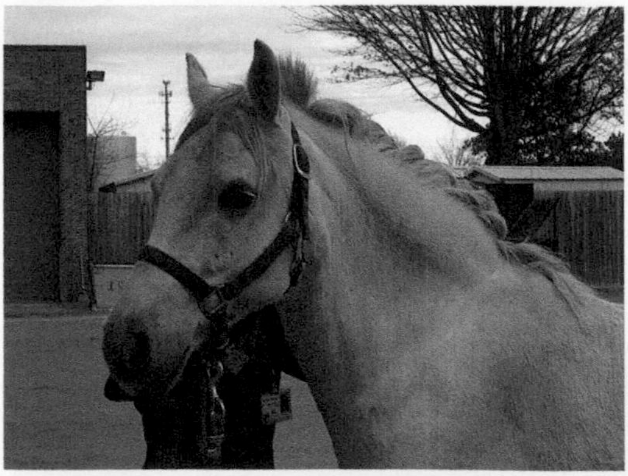

Fig. 3. A horse exhibiting regional adiposity in the form a pronounced neck crest, which is referred to as a cresty neck.

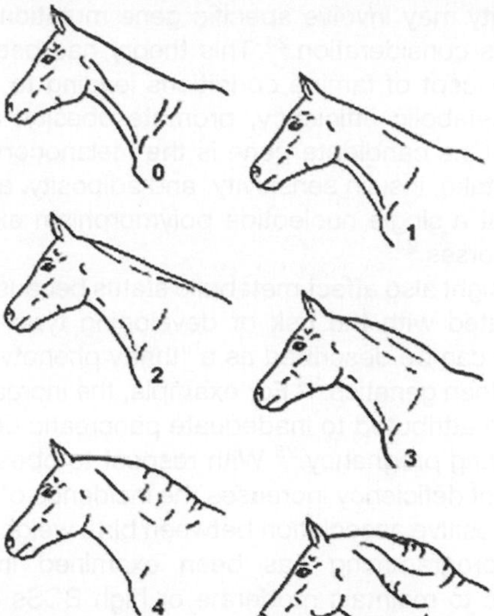

Fig. 4. Crest neck scoring system. (*Reprinted from* Carter RA, Geor RJ, Burton SW, et al. Apparent adiposity assessed by standardised scoring systems and morphometric measurements in horses and ponies. Vet J 2009;179:204; with permission.)

PATHOPHYSIOLOGY

Predisposition

Some horses and ponies appear to be genetically predisposed to EMS, and this is the focus of ongoing study at the University of Minnesota (www.cvm.umn.edu/equinegenetics/ems). There are numerous anecdotal reports of EMS in related horses and ponies, and Treiber and colleagues[4] detected a dominant inheritance pattern for laminitis in ponies with EMS. Many animals with EMS appear to require fewer calories to maintain body weight, indicating enhanced metabolic efficiency. Genetic

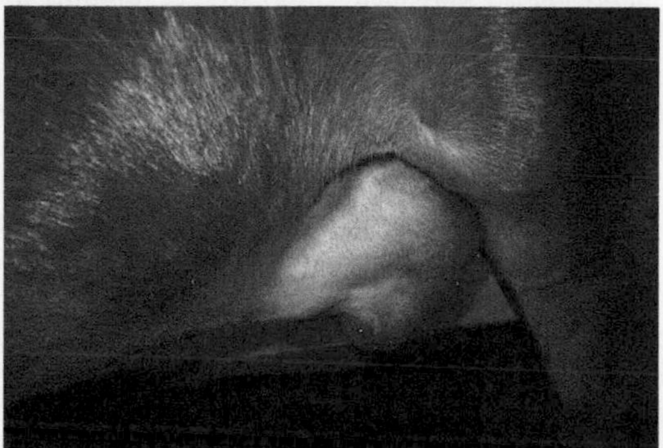

Fig. 5. Adipose tissue expansion around the prepuce of a 16-year-old Tennessee Walking horse gelding.

predisposition to obesity may involve specific gene mutations, and the concept of "thrifty genes" warrants consideration.[23] This theory has been applied to humans, and focuses on the concept of famine conditions leading to selection of metabolic genes that improve metabolic efficiency, promote obesity, and increase appetite when food is plentiful. One candidate gene is the melanocortin-4 receptor (MC4R), which regulates feed intake, insulin sensitivity, and adiposity, and results of a preliminary study indicate that a single nucleotide polymorphism exists within the coding region of this gene in horses.[24]

Fetal programming might also affect metabolic status because fetal birth weight has been inversely associated with the risk of developing type 2 diabetes mellitus in humans.[25] This feature can be described as a "thrifty phenotype" that is determined by environment rather than genetics.[23] For example, the increased risk of type 2 diabetes mellitus has been attributed to inadequate pancreatic development caused by nutrient deprivation during pregnancy.[25] With respect to obesity, some reports indicate that in utero nutrient deficiency increases the incidence of this problem, whereas others demonstrate a positive association between birth weight and body mass index later in life.[24] Fetal programming has been examined in horses. Ousey and colleagues[26] fed mares to maintain moderate or high BCSs during pregnancy, but all horses inadvertently lost approximately 10% of body mass at mid-gestation as a result of *Streptococcus equi* infection. When intravenous glucose tests were performed in foals at 2 to 4 days of age, insulin concentrations were higher in foals from moderate BCS mares. These results suggest that acute nutrient restriction at mid-gestation affected foals in utero and altered β-cell responsiveness or insulin sensitivity. Feeding mares a high starch diet during pregnancy has also been shown to affect glucose concentrations and insulin sensitivity in preweaned foals.[27] A trend toward lower insulin sensitivity was detected in foals at 160 days of age. Further studies are therefore required to determine whether nutrient deficiency or excess during gestation contribute to the development of EMS. It is possible that epigenetics plays a role in EMS if environmental conditions induce heritable changes in gene expression without altering the DNA sequence.[3] Epigenetic effects are mediated by alterations in DNA methylation or histone configuration, and might explain why in utero conditions during one pregnancy affect subsequent generations.

Hyperinsulinemia

It is assumed that hyperinsulinemia results from increased pancreatic insulin secretion in response to reduced insulin sensitivity, and this is referred to as compensated insulin resistance.[28] Values for insulin sensitivity and the acute insulin response to glucose (AIRg) provide evidence of compensated IR in insulin-resistant horses and ponies. These values are estimated from minimal model analysis of frequently-sampled intravenous glucose tolerance test (FSIGTT) data, with AIRg representing pancreatic insulin secretion. Treiber and colleagues[29] reported higher AIRg values in horses and ponies with lower insulin sensitivity, and Carter and colleagues[30] demonstrated that mean AIRg increased by 408% as insulin sensitivity decreased by 71% when obesity was induced in Arabian geldings. In contrast, uncompensated insulin resistance refers to inadequate insulin secretion in response to IR, with higher glucose concentrations detected. This situation has been described in clinically laminitic ponies, and should be suspected whenever hyperglycemia is detected in an animal with the physical characteristics of EMS.[4] A dynamic test is recommended in these cases because hyperinsulinemia may be absent. Diabetes mellitus also occurs in horses and is characterized by persistent hyperglycemia, with glucosuria detected in some cases. This condition may be more common than previously thought, and has been detected in horses with pituitary pars intermedia dysfunction.[31] Inadequate pancreatic insulin secretion results in hyperglycemia with concurrent IR in some, but not all, cases.

Recent evidence suggests that higher blood insulin concentrations also result from reduced hepatic insulin clearance.[32] Pancreatic insulin secretion can be assessed by measuring serum connecting peptide (C-peptide) concentrations because this molecule is released with insulin as the hormone is secreted. Approximately 70% of insulin secreted by the pancreas is cleared by the liver, whereas C-peptide remains in circulation.[32] The C-peptide to insulin ratio therefore reflects hepatic insulin clearance. Obese horses have high insulin and C-peptide concentrations, yet lower C-peptide to insulin ratios, indicating both increased insulin secretion and reduced hepatic clearance.[32]

Hepatic Insulin Resistance

Higher plasma γ-glutamyl transferase (GGT) and aspartate aminotransferase (AST) activities are detected in some horses with EMS, and lipid accumulation within hepatocytes is a common postmortem finding. This feature suggests that hepatic lipidosis develops in some horses with EMS in the same way that nonalcoholic fatty liver syndrome has been associated with MetS in humans.[3] Reduced insulin clearance by the liver in horses with EMS is a manifestation of hepatic IR. This problem reflects the impact of obesity on liver function and includes upregulation of inflammatory pathways.[33] Results of a preliminary study indicate that Toll-like receptor pathways are upregulated in the liver of obese insulin-resistant horses.[34] Impaired hepatic function might also increase the risk of laminitis by reducing the clearance of gut-derived triggers for laminitis or altering the metabolism of dietary carbohydrates.

Peripheral Insulin Resistance

Insulin resistance is defined as a reduction in the action of insulin on target tissues.[35] Normal actions of insulin include inhibition of gluconeogenesis and lipolysis and stimulation of glycogen synthesis.[33] Mechanisms of IR include defects in the insulin receptor, insulin signaling pathways, or glucose transporter 4 (GLUT4) synthesis, translocation, or function. One important action of insulin is to stimulate glucose transport into cells, and this occurs rapidly as GLUT4 proteins translocate to cell membranes. Vesicles containing preformed GLUT4 are present within the cytoplasm, and transporters move to the plasma membrane after activation by the insulin signaling cascade. Results of a recent study indicate that GLUT4 translocation is impaired in insulin-resistant horses. Waller and colleagues[36] demonstrated that GLUT4 translocation to the cell surface is significantly reduced in skeletal muscle from insulin-resistant horses, despite normal protein abundance. Results of this preliminary study provide the first information regarding mechanisms of IR in horses.

Obesity

Obesity develops as animals consume more energy than they expend. Studies have not been performed to measure metabolic efficiency or compare rates of weight gain among different breeds of horse, but increased awareness of EMS has led clinicians to recognize that some horses and ponies develop obesity more readily, and this problem is difficult to reverse in the same animals. When obesity has been induced in horses, the breed of horse has affected outcomes. Quinn and colleagues[37] failed to detect a decrease in insulin sensitivity associated with weight gain in Thoroughbred geldings whereas Carter and colleagues[30] induced IR in Arabian geldings by providing 200% of daily digestible energy requirement for 16 weeks. Body weight increased by

20% and insulin sensitivity decreased by 71% in the latter study as obesity was induced. These findings suggest that obesity has a greater impact on insulin sensitivity in certain animals, which corresponds with clinical observations that some obese horses are insulin resistant whereas others have normal insulin sensitivity. There is also evidence that obesity is more difficult to reverse in individual animals. In a study of obese Shetland ponies, it was necessary to lower feed amounts to 35% of maintenance energy requirement to maintain weight loss equivalent to 1% of ideal body weight per week across a 16-week study period.[38]

Lipotoxicity

Increased adiposity and IR are associated in animals and humans, and several mechanisms have been proposed to explain this finding, including (1) intracellular lipid accumulation, (2) inflammatory mediator production by adipose tissues, and (3) altered adipokine secretion by adipose tissues. The first mechanism is referred to as lipotoxicity and involves repartitioning of fatty acids to skeletal muscle and other tissues, including the liver and pancreas. As adipose tissues reach their capacity for lipid storage, fatty acid uptake by other tissues increases. Randle and colleagues[39] demonstrated in a series of classic studies that a glucose fatty acid cycle exists in which fatty acids compete with glucose for oxidation within muscle. As fatty acid influx increases, intracellular lipid metabolites such as diacylglycerol, fatty acid coenzyme A, and ceramide accumulate, and this increases phosphorylation of serine/threonine sites on insulin receptor substrates 1 and 2, which reduces phosphatidylinositol 3-kinase activity.[40] This disruption in the insulin signaling pathway results in IR.

Inflammation

Adipokines are released from adipocytes and include leptin, resistin, adiponectin, visfatin, apelin, and macrophage chemoattractant proteins.[41] Proinflammatory cytokines such as tumor necrosis factor α (TNFα) and interleukins 1 (IL-1β) and 6 (IL-6) are also released from macrophages residing within adipose tissues. Vick and colleagues[9] provided evidence of systemic inflammation in obese horses by detecting increased expression of TNFα and IL-1β within the blood. However, no differences in proinflammatory cytokine expression were detected in adipose tissues when Burns and colleagues[42] compared insulin-resistant horses with control animals. It is interesting that the same study revealed higher mRNA expression of IL-1β and IL-6 mRNA in nuchal ligament adipose tissue when compared with omental, retroperitoneal, mesocolic, and tail head depots, which supports assertions that the cresty neck is an important phenotypic marker for IR.[6,22] More recently, the same research group reported increased macrophage chemoattractant protein-2 (MCP-2) mRNA expression within omental adipose tissue samples.[43] Omental adipose tissues had greater MCP-2 expression than other adipose tissue depots, and mRNA abundance was significantly higher in insulin-resistant horses.

Omental adipose tissue depots warrant close examination because visceral adiposity is an important component of MetS in humans.[44] Waist circumference is often measured to assess adiposity and abdominal obesity is predictive for IR in humans.[45] Potential explanations for this association include (1) increased release of fatty acids into the portal circulation leading to hepatic IR, (2) higher adipokine and inflammatory cytokine secretion by visceral adipose tissues, and (3) greater expansion of omental adipose tissues compared with subcutaneous tissues in response to overall adipose tissue dysfunction.[44] The first explanation centers on the findings that omental tissues have higher rates of lipolysis and that fatty acids are carried to the liver by the portal circulation. As explained earlier, hepatic IR results in decreased insulin clearance and therefore hyperinsulinemia, increased glucose production, and very low-density lipoprotein (VLDL) secretion. Higher VLDL-triglyceride concentrations have been detected in obese insulin-resistant horses.[6]

Abdominal obesity might also be connected with IR through altered cortisol production within visceral adipose tissues; specifically, increased 11-β hydroxysteroid dehydrogenase 1 (11βHSD1) activity.[1] Preadipocytes within adipose tissue are converted to adipocytes under the influence of corticosteroids, and these cells produce 11βHSD1, which locally amplifies glucocorticoid action. Diet-induced obesity leads to increased visceral fat preadipocyte differentiation in wild-type but not 11βHSD1 (−/−) mice, and this suggests that 11βHSD1 (ketoreductase) activity is augmented in mouse mesenteric preadipocytes, where it contributes to visceral fat accumulation.[46] In humans, mesenteric and omental adipose tissues are thought to play a more important role in the development of type 2 diabetes mellitus.[47] Only one published study[48] describes the measurement of 11βHSD1 activity in adipose tissues collected from horses, and omental fat was not examined. The results suggested that some horses with EMS had higher 11βHSD1 activity within subcutaneous adipose tissues, but groups did not differ significantly. Further studies are therefore required to examine 11βHSD1 activity within omental adipose tissues collected from insulin-resistant horses.

Adipokines

Two adipokines have been examined to date in horses: leptin and adiponectin. Leptin is sometimes referred to as the satiety factor because this adipokine is released by adipose tissues when energy supplies are plentiful.[49] Receptors on neurons found within the arcuate nucleus of the hypothalamus respond to circulating leptin concentrations, with both appetite-stimulating (orexigenic) and satiety (anorexigenic) neurons expressing leptin receptors. Activation of leptin receptors on orexigenic neurons causes downregulation and suppressed appetite. Leptin signaling also increases pro-opiomelanocortin synthesis and therefore the production of α melanocyte-stimulating hormone, which is an agonist for MC4R. As explained earlier, MC4R is involved in appetite and body weight regulation, and defects in the gene for this receptor are monogenic causes of obesity and body fat distribution in humans.[50]

Higher leptin concentrations are detected in insulin-resistant horses and ponies,[5,6,8,51] and this might represent a state of leptin resistance. Hyperleptinemia has been associated with obesity,[6,8] but horses with leaner BCSs are also affected.[51] Cut-off values for defining hyperleptinemia have differed among studies, depending on whether concentrations are measured as a diagnostic test or are used to define study groups. Carter and colleagues[5] determined a cut-off value of 7.3 ng/mL to predict the occurrence of laminitis in ponies using receiver operating characteristic plots, whereas horses were allocated to normoleptinemic (<5 ng/mL) or hyperleptinemic (>12 ng/mL) groups in another report.[52] In the latter study, hyperleptinemic horses were insulin resistant when compared with horses of the same body condition that had low leptin concentrations. These findings suggest that leptin concentrations can be measured to detect IR in horses and that hyperleptinemia is a component of EMS. Leptin resistance is a concept that warrants consideration, because owners have subjectively observed that horses and ponies with EMS show greater appetite and consume more grass when allowed to graze freely. Leptin resistance might also affect metabolic efficiency, because concentrations of this hormone increase in the late summer as horses accumulate body fat mass and then decline again in the winter.[51] It is therefore conceivable that horses with EMS maintain a state of leptin resistance throughout the year and gain weight as a result.

Adiponectin is considered an insulin-sensitizing adipokine, and blood concentrations are positively correlated with insulin sensitivity in humans and animals.[41,53] This protein is secreted as a homotrimer and circulates as trimers, hexamers, and high molecular weight (HMW) multimers composed of 4 to 6 noncovalently bonded trimers. Kearns and colleagues[8] used a murine/rat enzyme-linked immunosorbent assay (ELISA) to measure total adiponectin, and found that blood concentrations were inversely proportional to body fat mass in horses. A validated assay for total adiponectin is no longer available for horses, but results of a preliminary study using a commercially available ELISA for human HMW adiponectin have recently been reported.[54] Lower concentrations were detected in obese horses and those with evidence of systemic inflammation.

HMW adiponectin is the metabolically active form of adiponectin, but results of studies performed in humans have been mixed with respect to the importance of measuring this isoform. One group reported that HMW adiponectin concentrations are an independent predictor of insulin sensitivity, whereas another concluded that HMW and total adiponectin were equally useful for diagnosing IR.[55,56] Additional studies are required to determine whether HMW concentrations can be used to diagnose IR in horses.

DIAGNOSIS

Screening Tests

Screening testing for EMS is outlined in **Box 1**. EMS should be suspected when an obese horse with regional adiposity presents for examination, particularly if laminitis is also detected. Most owners describe their horses as easy keepers when providing a history, and sometimes report that related horses have suffered from obesity and

Box 1
Screening diagnostic testing for EMS

Screening tests

Historical information

- Owner reports that the horse is an easy keeper (high metabolic efficiency)

Physical examination findings

- Obese (BCS $\geq$7/9)
- Pronounced neck crest (score $\geq$3/5)
- Other evidence of regional adiposity (tail head, prepuce, mammary gland region)
- Divergent growth rings (founder lines) or lameness associated with laminitis

Blood testing (leave only one flake of hay after 10:00 PM; collect blood in the morning)

- Fasting glucose concentration above reference range (>110 mg/dL)
- Fasting insulin concentration >20 μU/mL
- Fasting leptin concentration >7 ng/mL

Data from Henneke DR, Potter GD, Kreider JL, et al. Relationship between condition score, physical measurements and body fat percentage in mares. Equine Vet J 1983;15:371–2; Carter RA, Geor RJ, Burton SW, et al. Apparent adiposity assessed by standardised scoring systems and morphometric measurements in horses and ponies. Vet J 2009;179:204–10; Coat-A-Count insulin radioimmunoassay, Siemens Medical Solutions Diagnostics, Los Angeles, CA; Multi-species leptin radioimmunoassay, Millipore Inc, St Charles, MO.

laminitis. Fasting blood glucose and insulin concentrations should be measured to screen for hyperglycemia and hyperinsulinemia, which serve as indicators of IR. It is also advisable to measure plasma adrenocorticotropin hormone in horses older than 10 years because pituitary pars intermedia dysfunction (PPID) can develop in EMS horses as they age. Leptin measurements are not currently offered by commercial laboratories, but it is expected that testing will be introduced soon. Plasma triglyceride concentrations are currently available and can be requested as part of a plasma biochemistry analysis. Hypertriglyceridemia is more commonly detected in ponies with EMS[4,5] than in horses.[6]

Resting glucose and insulin concentrations are usually measured in a single blood sample to screen for hyperglycemia and hyperinsulinemia, but analysis of multiple samples increases the accuracy of testing. A standardized approach is recommended, which consists of leaving only one flake of hay with the horse after 10:00 PM the night before and then collecting blood the next morning. Blood samples should be kept cool using ice packs or a refrigerator and then sent to an established laboratory.

Blood glucose concentrations are within reference range in most insulin-resistant horses because euglycemia is maintained through increased pancreatic insulin secretion. However, glucose concentrations should always be measured to detect uncompensated IR or diabetes mellitus. Some of these patients can only be identified by detecting hyperglycemia because insulin concentrations have returned to reference range as a result of pancreatic insufficiency.

At present, the most useful screening test for IR is the resting insulin concentration, which must be performed after a short fast to minimize the impact of feeding. As with many tests, the result is more likely to be a true positive the further it falls outside of reference range. A markedly elevated (>100 μU/mL) fasting insulin concentration therefore serves as a good indication of IR. However, it is more difficult to interpret results that are closer to reference range, and breed-specific ranges are needed to improve accuracy. At present, a cut-off value of 20 μU/mL is recommended for the radioimmunoassay (Coat-A-Count insulin radioimmunoassay, Siemens Medical Solutions Diagnostics, Los Angeles, CA, USA) commonly used by commercial laboratories, with blood collected under fasting conditions. However, reference ranges for other types of insulin assay should be used where appropriate.

The glucose-to-insulin ratio can also be calculated by dividing the glucose concentration in mg/dL by the insulin concentration in μU/mL (or mU/L). Proponents of this test consider a ratio below 10 to indicate IR and refer to horses with ratios less than 4.5 as severely insulin-resistant or decompensated. This test is not recommended because results are confounded by stress-induced hyperglycemia and glucose consumption by erythrocytes when samples are collected improperly. Furthermore, the ratio does not take into account differences in insulin assays, whereas hyperinsulinemia can be defined by the individual laboratory.

Proxy measurements have also been used to assess insulin sensitivity and pancreatic insulin secretion in horses.[29] The 2 proxies used are the reciprocal of the square root of insulin (RISQI) and the modified insulin to glucose ratio (MIRG). The RISQI represents the degree of insulin sensitivity (a low number indicates IR) and the MIRG represents the ability of the pancreas to secrete insulin. Horses with compensated IR have higher MIRG values. The RISQI value is more important, and can be easily calculated by dividing 1 by the square root of the insulin concentration. A RISQI less than 0.29 indicates IR, which is equivalent to a serum insulin concentration of 12 μU/mL. This method is not recommended, because values were established for a specific group of animals and 20 μU/mL is a more appropriate cut-off value for hyperinsulinemia.

Dynamic Tests

Dynamic tests for EMS are listed in **Box 2**. It is necessary to perform a dynamic test (see **Box 2**) when the animal exhibits physical characteristics of EMS, but screening test results are equivocal. Testing is also recommended to assess the degree of IR and monitor progress. The combined glucose-insulin test (CGIT) was established by Eiler and colleagues[57] and can be performed under field conditions. Euglycemic-hyperinsulinemic clamp and FSIGTT procedures are used in research studies, but the CGIT is a more practical test that requires fewer samples.[58]

When the CGIT is performed, insulin sensitivity is assessed by measuring the time for blood glucose concentrations to return to baseline and the insulin concentration at 45 minutes. Blood glucose concentrations are measured at each time point with a hand-held glucometer until a concentration below baseline is detected, and then this time is recorded for future reference. A blood sample is also collected at 45 minutes and is submitted for the measurement of insulin. An alternative approach is to collect 2 blood samples (0 and 45 minutes) and submit them to a commercial laboratory for glucose and insulin measurements. When this test is used, IR is diagnosed by detecting a blood glucose concentration higher than baseline at 45 minutes[6] or an insulin concentration greater than 100 μU/mL at the same time point. Hypoglycemia is a rare complication of testing, and can be addressed by injecting 50% dextrose (120 mL) intravenously and feeding the horse.

An oral sugar test has recently been developed to assess horses in the field.[59] This oral glucose tolerance test is performed using corn syrup (Karo Light Syrup, Ach Food

Box 2
Dynamic diagnostic testing for EMS

Combined glucose-insulin test

Method

- Perform under fasting conditions (leave one flake of hay after 10:00 PM)
- Obtain a preinfusion blood sample to measure the baseline glucose concentration
- Inject 150 mg/kg body weight 50% dextrose solution intravenously, immediately followed by 0.10 U/kg body weight regular insulin. For a horse weighing 500 kg, inject 150 mL 50% dextrose and 0.50 mL of 100 U/mL insulin
- Collect blood at 1, 5, 15, 25, 35, 45, 60, 75, 90, 105, 120, 135, and 150 minutes
- Measure insulin concentration at 45 minutes

Interpretation

- Insulin resistant if the blood glucose concentration is above baseline or insulin concentration is greater than100 μU/mL at 45 minutes

Oral sugar test

Method

- Fast horse before testing (leave one flake of hay after 10:00 PM)
- Owner administers Karo Light Corn Syrup orally using two 60-mL catheter-tip syringes at a dosage of 15 mL per 100 kg (75 mL for a 500-kg horse)
- Collect one blood sample 60–90 minutes later

Interpretation

- Insulin concentration greater than 60 μU/mL at either time point indicates insulin resistance

Companies Inc, Cordova, TN, USA), which can be purchased and administered by the owner. Corn syrup contains glucose, maltose, maltotriose, and other sugars, and 1 mL syrup provides 1 g total glucose-based digestible carbohydrates. A dose of 150 mg/kg is used, which is equivalent to 0.15 mL/kg or 15 mL per 100 kg body weight (75 mL for a 500-kg horse). Results of a preliminary study indicate that blood insulin concentrations exceed 60 μU/mL at 60, 75, and 90 minutes in insulin-resistant horses. It is therefore recommended that the veterinarian arrive at the farm in time to collect a blood sample 60 to 90 minutes after the test dose has been administered by the owner. Corn syrup can be administered with a dose syringe and is very palatable to horses. This test was developed to address concerns that current screening tests fail to detect horses with more pronounced glucose and insulin responses to feeding.

MANAGEMENT

EMS is a disorder that should be managed with diet, housing, and exercise interventions. The 2 principal strategies for addressing IR in horses are to induce weight loss in obese horses and improve insulin sensitivity through dietary management and exercise.

Weight Reduction

Obese horses should be placed on a weight reduction diet consisting of hay plus protein/vitamin/mineral supplement. Horses should initially receive hay in amounts equivalent to 1.5% of ideal body weight per day (ie, 7.5 kg for a 500-kg horse), and this amount should be lowered to 1% of initial body weight after 1 month if the horse or pony fails to lose weight. Sweet feed should be eliminated from the diet, and horses cannot be allowed to graze on pasture during the weight loss period. In a recent study, restriction of dry matter intake to 1% of initial body mass for 16 weeks was shown to be an effective strategy for inducing weight loss in overweight and obese ponies.[60] The minimum amount of hay recommended for horses is 1% of body weight per day.[61] Increased physical activity promotes weight loss by increasing energy expenditure, so obese horses that are free of laminitis should be exercised as frequently as possible. It is recommended that obese horses be exercised under saddle (or on a lounge line) 4 to 7 days a week for a minimum of 30 minutes at a trot or canter, excluding the time required for warm up and cool down.

Analysis of hay is recommended to ensure that the nonstructural carbohydrate (NSC) content of the forage is low. Equi-analytical Laboratories (Ithaca, NY; www.equi-analytical.com) analyzes hay and provides starch, ethanol-soluble carbohydrate (ESC), and WSC content as percentages of dry matter. ESCs include simple sugars such as monosaccharides and disaccharides, whereas the WSC measurement includes the same sugars plus long-chain fructans. The NSC content of the hay is calculated by taking the sum of WSC and starch values. Some nutritionists consider it more appropriate to exclude long-chain fructans and take the sum of ESC and starch values to calculate NSC, because long-chain fructans are primarily digested in the large intestine and are not expected to elicit postprandial glucose and insulin responses.

A general recommendation is to select hay with NSC content of less than 10% (dry matter basis) for insulin-resistant horses and ponies. However, the importance of NSC content depends on the severity of IR and hyperinsulinemia in the individual animal. Acquiring hay with less than 10% NSC content is very important for horses and ponies with marked fasting hyperinsulinemia (>100 μU/mL), but greater flexibility can be shown when managing mildly affected animals. Most horses with EMS suffer from obesity, and the reversal of this condition has the greatest influence on insulin sensitivity. Because low-NSC hay usually contains less digestible energy, it can also be selected to promote weight loss.

This review has primarily focused on the obese phenotype because this is the most common manifestation of EMS. However, some affected animals exhibit a leaner body condition, with expanded adipose tissue deposits in specific regions of the body. Examples include (1) previously obese horses that have lost weight after effective management and (2) older animals that have developed PPID, yet remain affected by EMS. In the first situation, IR remains present or will develop again if the patient is allowed to gain weight again. In the case of PPID, anecdotal reports suggest that the layering of this endocrinopathy on top of preexisting EMS exacerbates IR and increases the risk of laminitis. Pergolide treatment is warranted in these cases. Leaner horses that are insulin resistant or have a history of this problem must receive sufficient energy for maintenance without inducing obesity or exacerbating IR; this can be achieved by increasing the amount of hay fed or providing a low-NSC pelleted feed designed for insulin-resistant horses. Each individual horse must be fed according to its body condition and rate of weight gain. Most low-NSC feeds are palatable, but it may take several weeks for the horse to accept a new feed.

Pasture Access

Obesity often develops in horses that are predisposed to EMS when they are given free access to pasture and rarely exercised. Feed intake can be very high when horses are permitted to graze on large pastures or after grass quality increases as a result of reseeding and fertilization. This form of overfeeding is difficult to explain to owners, and represents an important interaction between the metabolism of the individual horse and its diet. Because energy intake cannot be controlled when horses are grazing freely, access to pasture must be limited while inducing weight loss. Strategies for limiting grass consumption on pasture include short (<1 hour) turnout periods twice daily, confinement in a small paddock, round pen, or area enclosed with electric fence, or use of a grazing muzzle. Horses should be housed in dirt paddocks or small grass lots the rest of the time, and addition of a companion to the enclosure increases exercise. Pasture access should also be restricted because affected animals are predisposed to laminitis.[12]

Pasture access should be incrementally increased by 1 hour per turnout per week once obesity and IR have resolved, but body condition should be monitored closely because genetically predisposed animals will return to an obese insulin-resistant state if managed inappropriately. Even when horses have been returned to full pasture access, care should be taken to restrict grazing time when the grass is going through dynamic phases, such as rapid growth in the spring and late summer or at the onset of cold weather in the fall. Horses and ponies with EMS that fail to respond to management or develop laminitis again when permitted to graze must be held off pasture indefinitely.

MEDICAL TREATMENT

Veterinarians have a responsibility to recommend management changes and discourage horse owners from administering drugs as a substitute, but there are 2 indications for pharmacologic intervention: (1) short-term (3–6 months) treatment while management changes are taking effect, and (2) refractory cases.

Levothyroxine Sodium

When administered at high dosages levothyroxine induces weight loss in horses, and this is accompanied by an increase in insulin sensitivity.[62–64] In a recent study, pretreatment with levothyroxine for 14 days also prevented healthy horses from developing IR following endotoxin infusion.[65] Levothyroxine has been administered at an approximate dose of 0.1 mg/kg, which is rounded to 48 mg per day for horses weighing 450 to 525 kg. It is assumed that levothyroxine induces weight loss by raising circulating thyroxine concentrations and stimulating basal metabolic rate. Weight loss can be enhanced during treatment by restricting caloric intake and increasing exercise. Horses should not be permitted to graze on pasture because levothyroxine is likely to induce hyperphagia, which offsets its effects on body weight. Levothyroxine is primarily administered for the purpose of accelerating weight loss in obese horses, and can be prescribed for 3 to 6 months while other management practices are instituted.

Metformin Hydrochloride

Metformin is a biguanide drug that is administered to control hyperglycemia and increase tissue insulin sensitivity in humans with diabetes mellitus. This drug suppresses hepatic glucose production by activating AMP-activated protein kinase, which inhibits gluconeogenesis and lipogenesis while increasing fatty acid oxidation and lipolysis.[66] Two key gluconeogenesis enzymes, phosphoenolpyruvate carboxykinase and glucose-6-phosphatase, are inhibited by metformin through this mechanism. The insulin-sensitizing effects of metformin may also be mediated by skeletal muscle adenosine monophosphate kinase (AMPK), causing increased GLUT4 abundance within cell membranes and enhanced glucose uptake.[67] One study also describes AMPK-independent effects of metformin on cardiac muscle, with results indicating that p38 mitogen-activated protein kinase and protein kinase C pathways are activated.[68]

Only a small number of studies have been performed to examine the efficacy of metformin in horses. Durham and colleagues[69] reported that resting insulin concentrations and proxy measures of insulin sensitivity improved in insulin-resistant horses and ponies with metformin treatment (15 mg/kg every 12 hours orally). Administration of metformin at this dosage was associated with positive clinical outcomes, but a subsequent study revealed that the oral bioavailability of this drug is low in a horses.[70] A single dose of 3 g metformin has oral bioavailability of 7.1% $\pm$ 1.5% in fasted horses and 3.9% $\pm$ 1.0% in fed animals.[70] In a recent study, metformin was administered orally to 6 horses with EMS for 14 days after they were moved from stalls to grass paddocks, which was expected to exacerbate IR. All horses received metformin (15 mg/kg every 12 hours) for 2 weeks, followed by a washout period, and then treatment at a higher dosage (30 mg/kg every 12 hours) for 2 additional weeks.[71] Metformin treatment did not affect insulin sensitivity, but resting insulin concentrations decreased in response to treatment at the higher dosage. Of note, insulin sensitivity increased in response to turnout, which supports recommendations to provide horses with adequate space for exercise. At this point in time metformin is still recommended for the management of IR in horses, but further research is required to determine the appropriate dosage for horses.

Other Antidiabetic Drugs

Pioglitazone is the only other insulin-sensitizing drug that has been evaluated to date in horses. Healthy horses were treated with pioglitazone (1 mg/kg every 24 hours orally) for 14 days and then challenged with lipopolysaccharide.[72] Treatment with pioglitazone did not alter resting insulin sensitivity or prevent endotoxin-induced IR, but insulin receptor mRNA expression increased in skeletal muscle. Pioglitazone belongs to the thiazolidinedione class of antidiabetic drugs that includes rosiglitazone. These drugs stimulate peroxisome proliferator-activated receptor-γ (PPARγ), which is a nuclear receptor that regulates genes involved in glucose and lipid metabolism. Activation of PPARγ increases glucose uptake into adipose, muscle, and liver tissues, stimulates lipogenesis, and inhibits hepatic gluconeogenesis and glycogenolysis. Thiazolidinedione drugs improve glycemic control and increase insulin sensitivity in humans, but further research is required in horses.

SUMMARY

EMS is a clinical syndrome associated with laminitis that includes increased adiposity, hyperinsulinemia, and insulin resistance. This syndrome should be suspected in horses with generalized obesity and/or regional adiposity, and horses can be screened for insulin resistance by measuring resting glucose and insulin concentrations. Hyperinsulinemia is usually detected in insulin-resistant horses, while blood glucose concentrations are maintained within reference range. A simple oral sugar test can also be performed in the field to test for insulin resistance, and the CGIT is used to confirm the problem. Management focuses on diet and exercise interventions to address obesity, and most horses respond well to this approach. Horses that remain insulin resistant after weight loss and those with a leaner body condition are more challenging to diagnose and manage. Medical treatments are sometimes necessary in these cases, and more studies are required to assess insulin-sensitizing drugs in horses.

REFERENCES

1. Johnson PJ. The equine metabolic syndrome peripheral Cushing's syndrome. Vet Clin North Am Equine Pract 2002;18(2):271–93.
2. Frank N, Geor RJ, Bailey SR, et al. Equine metabolic syndrome. J Vet Intern Med 2010;24(3):467–75.
3. Bruce KD, Hanson MA. The developmental origins, mechanisms, and implications of metabolic syndrome. J Nutr 2010;140(3):648–52.
4. Treiber KH, Kronfeld DS, Hess TM, et al. Evaluation of genetic and metabolic predispositions and nutritional risk factors for pasture-associated laminitis in ponies. J Am Vet Med Assoc 2006;228(10):1538–45.
5. Carter RA, Treiber KH, Geor RJ, et al. Prediction of incipient pasture-associated laminitis from hyperinsulinaemia, hyperleptinaemia and generalised and localised obesity in a cohort of ponies. Equine Vet J 2009;41(2):171–8.
6. Frank N, Elliott SB, Brandt LE, et al. Physical characteristics, blood hormone concentrations, and plasma lipid concentrations in obese horses with insulin resistance. J Am Vet Med Assoc 2006;228(9):1383–90.
7. Cartmill JA, Thompson DL Jr, Storer WA, et al. Endocrine responses in mares and geldings with high body condition scores grouped by high vs. low resting leptin concentrations. J Anim Sci 2003;81(9):2311–21.
8. Kearns CF, McKeever KH, Roegner V, et al. Adiponectin and leptin are related to fat mass in horses. Vet J 2006;172(3):460–5.
9. Vick MM, Adams AA, Murphy BA, et al. Relationships among inflammatory cytokines, obesity, and insulin sensitivity in the horse. J Anim Sci 2007;85(5):1144–55.

10. Bailey SR, Habershon-Butcher JL, Ransom KJ, et al. Hypertension and insulin resistance in a mixed-breed population of ponies predisposed to laminitis. Am J Vet Res 2008;69(1):122–9.
11. Watson TD, Packard CJ, Shepherd J. Plasma lipid transport in the horse (*Equus caballus*). Comp Biochem Physiol B 1993;106(1):27–34.
12. Geor RJ. Current concepts on the pathophysiology of pasture-associated laminitis. Vet Clin North Am Equine Pract 2010;26(2):265–76.
13. Longland AC, Byrd BM. Pasture nonstructural carbohydrates and equine laminitis. J Nutr 2006;136(Suppl 7):2099S–102S.
14. Asplin KE, Sillence MN, Pollitt CC, et al. Induction of laminitis by prolonged hyperinsulinaemia in clinically normal ponies. Vet J 2007;174(3):530–5.
15. de Laat MA, McGowan CM, Sillence MN, et al. Equine laminitis: induced by 48 h hyperinsulinaemia in Standardbred horses. Equine Vet J 2010;42(2):129–35.
16. Elliott J, Bailey SR. Gastrointestinal derived factors are potential triggers for the development of acute equine laminitis. J Nutr 2006;136(Suppl 7):2103S–7S.
17. Bailey SR, Adair HS, Reinemeyer CR, et al. Plasma concentrations of endotoxin and platelet activation in the developmental stage of oligofructose-induced laminitis. Vet Immunol Immunopathol 2009;129(3–4):167–73.
18. van Eps AW, Pollitt CC. Equine laminitis induced with oligofructose. Equine Vet J 2006;38(3):203–8.
19. Kalck KA, Frank N, Elliott SB, et al. Effects of low-dose oligofructose treatment administered via nasogastric intubation on induction of laminitis and associated alterations in glucose and insulin dynamics in horses. Am J Vet Res 2009; 70(5):624–32.
20. Toth F, Frank N, Chameroy KA, et al. Effects of endotoxaemia and carbohydrate overload on glucose and insulin dynamics and the development of laminitis in horses. Equine Vet J 2009;41(9):852–8.
21. Henneke DR, Potter GD, Kreider JL, et al. Relationship between condition score, physical measurements and body fat percentage in mares. Equine Vet J 1983; 15(4):371–2.
22. Carter RA, Geor RJ, Burton SW, et al. Apparent adiposity assessed by standardised scoring systems and morphometric measurements in horses and ponies. Vet J 2009;179(2):204–10.
23. Prentice AM. Early influences on human energy regulation: thrifty genotypes and thrifty phenotypes. Physiol Behav 2005;86(5):640–5.
24. Armstrong C, Streeter C, Brooks S. Identification of SNPs within MCR4 as a candidate for obesity in the horse. J Equine Vet Sci 2009;29(5):322–3.
25. Ozanne SE, Hales CN. Early programming of glucose-insulin metabolism. Trends Endocrinol Metab 2002;13(9):368–73.
26. Ousey JC, Fowden AL, Wilsher S, et al. The effects of maternal health and body condition on the endocrine responses of neonatal foals. Equine Vet J 2008;40(7): 673–9.
27. George LA, Staniar WB, Treiber KH, et al. Insulin sensitivity and glucose dynamics during pre-weaning foal development and in response to maternal diet composition. Domest Anim Endocrinol 2009;37(1):23–9.
28. Treiber KH, Kronfeld DS, Geor RJ. Insulin resistance in equids: possible role in laminitis. J Nutr 2006;136(Suppl 7):2094S–8S.
29. Treiber KH, Kronfeld DS, Hess TM, et al. Use of proxies and reference quintiles obtained from minimal model analysis for determination of insulin sensitivity and pancreatic beta-cell responsiveness in horses. Am J Vet Res 2005;66(12): 2114–21.

30. Carter RA, McCutcheon LJ, George LA, et al. Effects of diet-induced weight gain on insulin sensitivity and plasma hormone and lipid concentrations in horses. Am J Vet Res 2009;70(10):1250–8.
31. Durham AE, Hughes KJ, Cottle HJ, et al. Type 2 diabetes mellitus with pancreatic b-cell dysfunction in 3 horses confirmed with minimal model analysis. Equine Vet J 2009;41(9):924–9.
32. Tóth F, Frank N, Martin-Jiménez T, et al. Measurement of C-peptide concentrations and responses to somatostatin, glucose infusion, and insulin resistance in horses. Equine Vet J 2010;42:149–55.
33. Samuel VT, Petersen KF, Shulman GI. Lipid-induced insulin resistance: unravelling the mechanism. Lancet 2010;375(9733):2267–77.
34. Stokes AM, Keowen ML, McGeachy M, et al. Potential role of the Toll-like receptor signaling pathway in equine laminitis [abstract]. J Equine Vet Sci 2010;30(2): 113–4.
35. Kahn CR. Insulin resistance, insulin insensitivity, and insulin unresponsiveness: a necessary distinction. Metabolism 1978;27(12 Suppl 2):1893–902.
36. Waller AP, Kohler K, Burns TA, et al. Regulation of glucose transport: novel insights into the pathogenesis of insulin resistance in horses. In: ACVIM forum proceedings. Anaheim (CA); 2010. p. 198.
37. Quinn RW, Burk AO, Hartsock TG, et al. Insulin sensitivity in Thoroughbred geldings: effect of weight gain, diet, and exercise on insulin sensitivity in Thoroughbred geldings. J Equine Vet Sci 2008;28(12):728–38.
38. Van Weyenberg S, Hesta M, Buyse J, et al. The effect of weight loss by energy restriction on metabolic profile and glucose tolerance in ponies. J Anim Physiol Anim Nutr (Berl) 2008;92(5):538–45.
39. Randle PJ, Garland PB, Newsholme EA, et al. The glucose fatty acid cycle in obesity and maturity onset diabetes mellitus. Ann N Y Acad Sci 1965;131(1): 324–33.
40. Shulman GI. Cellular mechanisms of insulin resistance. J Clin Invest 2000;106(2): 171–6.
41. Radin MJ, Sharkey LC, Holycross BJ. Adipokines: a review of biological and analytical principles and an update in dogs, cats, and horses. Vet Clin Pathol 2009;38(2):136–56.
42. Burns TA, Geor RJ, Mudge MC, et al. Proinflammatory cytokine and chemokine gene expression profiles in subcutaneous and visceral adipose tissue depots of insulin-resistant and insulin-sensitive light breed horses. J Vet Intern Med 2010;24(4):932–9.
43. Burns TA, Geor RJ, Mudge MC, et al. Characterization of adipose tissue macrophage infiltration in insulin-resistant and insulin-sensitive light breed horses [abstract]. J Vet Intern Med 2010;24(3):782.
44. Despres JP, Lemieux I, Bergeron J, et al. Abdominal obesity and the metabolic syndrome: contribution to global cardiometabolic risk. Arterioscler Thromb Vasc Biol 2008;28(6):1039–49.
45. Grundy SM. Metabolic syndrome pandemic. Arterioscler Thromb Vasc Biol 2008; 28(4):629–36.
46. De Sousa Peixoto RA, Turban S, Battle JH, et al. Preadipocyte 11beta-hydroxysteroid dehydrogenase type 1 is a keto-reductase and contributes to diet-induced visceral obesity in vivo. Endocrinology 2008;149(4):1861–8.
47. Santosa S, Jensen MD. Why are we shaped differently, and why does it matter? Am J Physiol Endocrinol Metab 2008;295(3):E531–5.

48. Schott HC, Graves EA, Refsal KR, et al. Diagnosis and treatment of pituitary pars intermedia dysfunction (classical Cushing's disease) and metabolic syndrome (peripheral Cushing's syndrome) in horses. Adv Vet Dermatol 2005; 5:159–69.
49. Houseknecht KL, Spurlock ME. Leptin regulation of lipid homeostasis: dietary and metabolic implications. Nutr Res Rev 2003;16(1):83–96.
50. Chen D, Garg A. Monogenic disorders of obesity and body fat distribution. J Lipid Res 1999;40(10):1735–46.
51. Gentry LR, Thompson DL Jr, Gentry GT Jr, et al. The relationship between body condition, leptin, and reproductive and hormonal characteristics of mares during the seasonal anovulatory period. J Anim Sci 2002;80(10):2695–703.
52. Caltabilota TJ, Earl LR, Thompson DL Jr, et al. Hyperleptinemia in mares and geldings: assessment of insulin sensitivity from glucose responses to insulin injection. J Anim Sci 2010;88(9):2940–9.
53. Wang Y, Zhou M, Lam KS, et al. Protective roles of adiponectin in obesity-related fatty liver diseases: mechanisms and therapeutic implications. Arq Bras Endocrinol Metabol 2009;53(2):201–12.
54. Wooldridge AA, Taylor DR, Zhong Q, et al. High molecular weight adiponectin is reduced in horses with obesity and inflammatory disease [abstract]. J Vet Intern Med 2010;24(3):781.
55. Wickham EP 3rd, Cheang KI, Clore JN, et al. Total and high-molecular weight adiponectin in women with the polycystic ovary syndrome. Metabolism 2010. [Epub ahead of print]. DOI:101016/j.metabol.2010.02.019.
56. Almeda-Valdes P, Cuevas-Ramos D, Mehta R, et al. Total and high molecular weight adiponectin have similar utility for the identification of insulin resistance. Cardiovasc Diabetol 2010;9:26.
57. Eiler H, Frank N, Andrews FM, et al. Physiologic assessment of blood glucose homeostasis via combined intravenous glucose and insulin testing in horses. Am J Vet Res 2005;66(9):1598–604.
58. Firshman AM, Valberg SJ. Factors affecting clinical assessment of insulin sensitivity in horses. Equine Vet J 2007;39(6):567–75.
59. Schuver A, Frank N, Chameroy K, et al. Use of an oral sugar test to assess insulin sensitivity in healthy and insulin-resistant horses [abstract]. J Vet Intern Med 2010;24(3):780.
60. Dugdale AH, Curtis GC, Cripps P, et al. Effect of dietary restriction on body condition, composition and welfare of overweight and obese pony mares. Equine Vet J 2010;42(7):600–10.
61. Geor RJ, Harris P. Dietary management of obesity and insulin resistance: countering risk for laminitis. Vet Clin North Am Equine Pract 2009;25(1):51–65, vi.
62. Frank N, Buchanan BR, Elliott SB. Effects of long-term oral administration of levothyroxine sodium on serum thyroid hormone concentrations, clinicopathologic variables, and echocardiographic measurements in healthy adult horses. Am J Vet Res 2008;69(1):68–75.
63. Frank N, Elliott SB, Boston RC. Effects of long-term oral administration of levothyroxine sodium on glucose dynamics in healthy adult horses. Am J Vet Res 2008; 69(1):76–81.
64. Sommardahl CS, Frank N, Elliott SB, et al. Effects of oral administration of levothyroxine sodium on serum concentrations of thyroid gland hormones and responses to injections of thyrotropin-releasing hormone in healthy adult mares. Am J Vet Res 2005;66(6):1025–31.

65. Tóth F, Frank N, Geor RJ, et al. Effects of pretreatment with dexamethasone or levothyroxine sodium on endotoxin-induced alterations in glucose and insulin dynamics in horses. Am J Vet Res 2010;71(1):60–8.
66. Kim YD, Park KG, Lee YS, et al. Metformin inhibits hepatic gluconeogenesis through AMP-activated protein kinase-dependent regulation of the orphan nuclear receptor SHP. Diabetes 2008;57(2):306–14.
67. Musi N, Hirshman MF, Nygren J, et al. Metformin increases AMP-activated protein kinase activity in skeletal muscle of subjects with type 2 diabetes. Diabetes 2002; 51(7):2074–81.
68. Saeedi R, Parsons HL, Wambolt RB, et al. Metabolic actions of metformin in the heart can occur by AMPK-independent mechanisms. Am J Physiol Heart Circ Physiol 2008;294(6):H2497–506.
69. Durham AE, Rendle DI, Newton JE. The effect of metformin on measurements of insulin sensitivity and beta cell response in 18 horses and ponies with insulin resistance. Equine Vet J 2008;40(5):493–500.
70. Hustace JL, Firshman AM, Mata JE. Pharmacokinetics and bioavailability of metformin in horses. Am J Vet Res 2009;70(5):665–8.
71. Chameroy K, Frank N, Elliott SB. Effects of metformin hydrochloride on glucose dynamics during transition to grass paddocks in insulin-resistant horses [abstract]. J Vet Intern Med 2010;24(3):690.
72. Wearn JG, Suagee JK, Crisman MV, et al. Effects of the insulin sensitizing drug pioglitazone on indices of insulin homeostasis in horses following endotoxin administration [abstract]. J Vet Intern Med 2010;24(3):709.

Equine Pituitary Pars Intermedia Dysfunction

Dianne McFarlane, DVM, PhD

KEYWORDS

• Cushing's • Horse • Pituitary • Laminitis
• Hypothalamus • Adrenal

Equine pituitary pars intermedia dysfunction (PPID), also known as equine Cushing's syndrome, is a widely recognized disease of aged horses. Over the past two decades the aged horse population has expanded significantly and in addition, client awareness of PPID has increased. As a result, there has been an increase in both diagnostic testing and treatment of the disease. This review focuses on the pathophysiology and clinical syndrome, as well as advances in diagnostic testing and treatment of PPID, with an emphasis on those findings that are new since the excellent comprehensive review by Schott in 2002.[1]

ANATOMY AND PHYSIOLOGY OF THE EQUINE PITUITARY PARS INTERMEDIA

Anatomy

The equine pituitary gland lies within the sella turcica, separated from the brain by a fold of dura mater known as the diaphragma sellae, suspended ventral to the hypothalamus by the infundibular stalk. The pituitary gland can be divided into 4 lobes: pars distalis, pars intermedia, pars tuberalis (collectively known as the adenohypophysis), and pars nervosa (neurohypophysis). The pars distalis is a collection of endocrine cells that synthesize, store, and release hormones in response to hypothalamic releasing and inhibiting factors. These factors reach the pars distalis by way of the hypophyseal portal system, which connects the capillaries of the median eminence to the capillaries of the pars distalis. The pars tuberalis is a thin band of endocrine cells enveloping the infundibular stalk. It is dense in the melatonin receptors through which it reads and decodes daily melatonin concentrations to coordinate the output of reproductive hormones with season.[2] The pars nervosa is a collection of axons and nerve terminals that originate in the paraventricular and superoptic nuclei of the hypothalamus. The pars nervosa stores and releases oxytocin and arginine vasopressin. The pars intermedia of the horse consists of a single endocrine type cell, the melanotrope, that

Department of Physiological Sciences, 264 McElroy Hall, Oklahoma State University, Stillwater, OK 74078, USA
E-mail address: diannem@okstate.edu

Vet Clin Equine 27 (2011) 93–113
doi:10.1016/j.cveq.2010.12.007 vetequine.theclinics.com

produces pro-opiomelanocortin (POMC) derived peptides. The pars intermedia is directly innervated by the dopaminergic neurons of the periventricular nucleus of the hypothalamus. It is unknown if neurons other than dopaminergic neurons directly innervate equine melanotropes.

Physiology

Melanotropes of the pars intermedia and corticotropes of the pars distalis both produce a hormone precursor protein, POMC. POMC undergoes extensive tissue-specific posttranslational processing to yield adrenocorticotropin (ACTH), melanocyte-stimulating hormones (MSHs), β-endorphin, corticotropin-like intermediate lobe peptide (CLIP), lipotropins, and several other small peptides. Prohormone convertases 1 and 2 (PC1 and PC2, respectively) are serine proteases that cleave the larger POMC into smaller peptides (**Fig. 1**). PC1 is expressed in both corticotropes and melanotropes, whereas PC2, which cleaves ACTH into α-MSH and CLIP, is only expressed in melanotropes. As a result, nearly all plasma ACTH in the healthy horse is produced in the pars distalis.[3] Prohormone convertase activity is inhibited by dopamine. In mice lacking the dopamine receptor, PC1 activity increases 4- to 5-fold and PC2 activity increases 2- to 3-fold.[4] This relative difference in the magnitude of increase in expression that the 2 enzymes display when dopamine is absent may explain why horses with PPID produce pars intermedia–derived ACTH; PC2 cannot keep pace with the relatively more abundant PC1.

Following cleavage by the prohormone convertases, POMC peptides are further processed by *N*-acetylation and carboxy terminal proteolysis yielding a population of peptides with altered bioactivity.[5–7] For example, initial cleavage of β-lipotropin by PC2 yields β-endorphin,[1–31] which is a highly potent opioid agonist. In the presence of dopamine, β-endorphin may be further modified to β-endorphin (1-27), acetylated

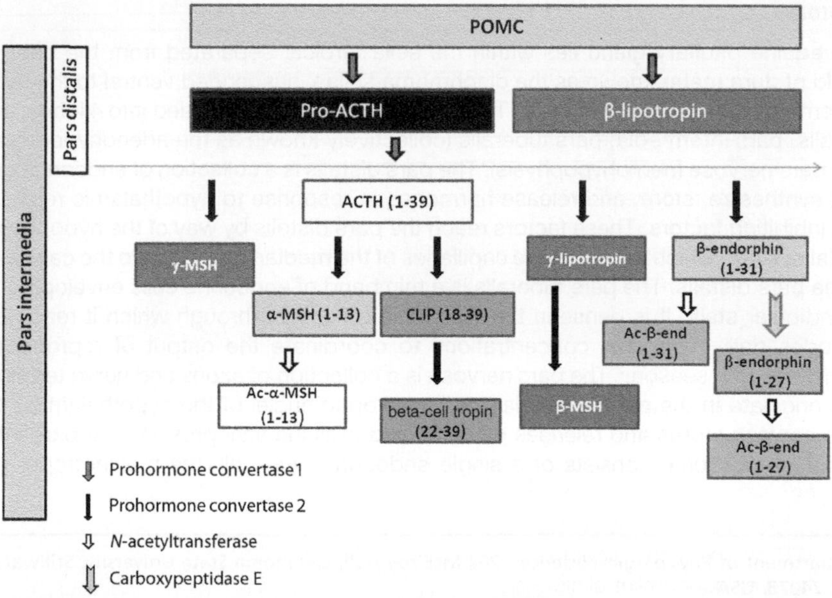

Fig. 1. POMC processing pathway. POMC is processed differently in the corticotropes of the pars distalis than in the melanotropes of the pars intermedia because of the differential expression of the enzymes involved in the posttranslational processing steps. Ac-α-MSH, acetyl-α-MSH; Ac-β-end, acetyl-β-end.

β-endorphin (1-27), and acetylated β-endorphin (1-31), all of which have minimal opioid agonist activity (see **Fig. 1**).[5–7]

The products of POMC are diverse and highly pleiotropic in function. Melanocortins exert a biologic effect through their interaction with a family of 5 G-protein coupled melanocortin receptors,[8,9] each with its own anatomic location and biologic activity. α-MSH is a primary product of POMC cleavage in the pars intermedia. It has a role in metabolism and obesity and is a potent antiinflammatory hormone. It is an antipyretic that is 25,000 times more potent than acetaminophen in reducing fever.[10,11] It has broad antiinflammatory effects that include decreasing the production of cytokines, costimulatory molecules, and other factors contributing to inflammation.[12] α-MSH also reduces neutrophilic oxidative burst, chemotaxis, and adhesion.[13,14] Little is known about the function of CLIP, the cleavage product generated from the C-terminal portion of ACTH. However, both CLIP and its cleavage product, beta-cell tropin, stimulate the release of insulin from rodent pancreatic beta cells.[15,16] β-Endorphin is a potent endogenous opioid agonist that functions in analgesia and in reduction of pain-associated inflammation.

Activity of the equine pars intermedia has been shown to be inhibited by dopamine and stimulated by thyrotropin-releasing hormone (TRH).[17,18] Both the dopamine D_2 receptor and the TRH receptor are expressed in the equine pars intermedia. Dopamine is released at the pars intermedia from the nerve terminals of the hypothalamic periventricular neurons that synapse directly to the melanotropes.[19] In the presence of dopamine, there is a decrease in POMC transcription and translation and secretion of POMC-derived peptide hormones. It is unknown whether TRH neurons directly innervate equine melanotropes as in amphibians[20,21] or TRH reaches the equine pars intermedia via the circulation. It is likely that in addition to dopamine and TRH, there are unidentified regulatory factors that modify equine pars intermedia function.

Similar to other species such as hamsters and sheep, activity of the pars intermedia in horses has a robust seasonal rhythm, with increased output as day length shortens (**Fig. 2**).[22–26] As a result, the plasma concentrations of α-MSH and ACTH are greatest in the autumn (August–October).[22–29] This adaptation helps animals to prepare for the metabolic and nutritional pressures of winter.[23–25] Because of the increase in pars intermedia activity, false-positive diagnostic test results are common when testing is performed in autumn and if reference ranges are not adjusted for season.[22,27] In addition, clinical signs of PPID may follow a seasonal pattern. Laminitis occurs most frequently in autumn.[30] Because pasture composition also changes significantly with season, studies are needed to determine the role of hormone level increase in seasonal development of laminitis.[31]

EPIDEMIOLOGY

PPID is a common endocrinopathy of aged horses and ponies. Recent epidemiologic investigations have suggested a disease prevalence of 15% to 30% in aged equids. According to data from owner surveys, hair coat abnormalities were present in 14% to 30% of aged horses.[32,33] Using the determination of plasma ACTH and α-MSH concentrations as a diagnostic test, 20% of aged horses showed positive test result for PPID by one or the other test, with 80% of the horses with positive test result having historical or concurrent clinical signs of disease.[33]

Similar to other neurodegenerative diseases, the most important risk factor for the development of PPID is age. Typically, recognition of clinical signs occurs in animals aged 18 to 20 years, with only rare reports in horses younger than 10 years.[1,17] Several breeds have been considered to be at greater risk for the development of PPID based

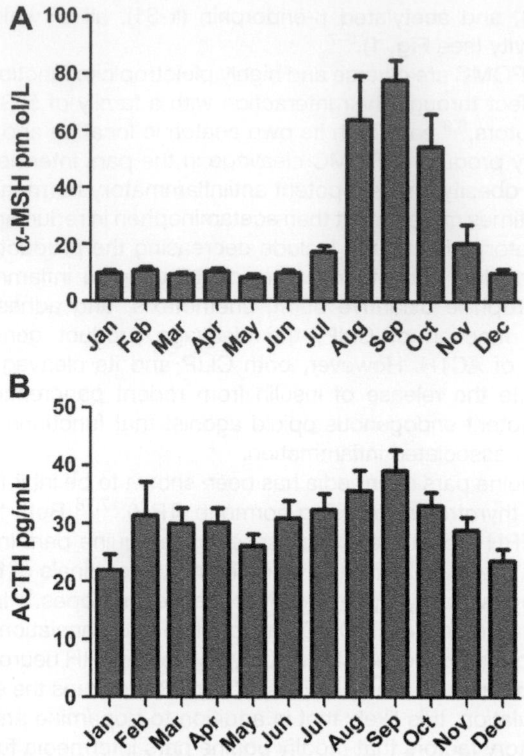

Fig. 2. Seasonal variability of POMC-derived hormones in horses. Mean (±SEM) monthly concentrations of plasma α-MSH (*A*) or ACTH (*B*) in 22 normal horses.

on clinical case reports, including ponies and Morgan horses. In the literature, 100 of 242 (42%) equids diagnosed with PPID were ponies.[34–44] However, in a recent study of 340 aged equids, neither breed nor height was associated with an increased risk for PPID, despite the ponies being significantly older than the horses.[33] Morgan horses were not part of the study population. One explanation for the conflicting results is that all pony breeds may not have a similar risk of PPID. Additional epidemiologic studies are needed to clarify the role of breed in the risk of PPID. Although early reports suggested that mares are at greater risk of developing PPID,[45] the current literature suggests that the distribution of PPID does not differ between males (n = 161) and females (n = 153).[34–44,46,47]

Geographic distribution of PPID has not been studied. Parkinson disease, a dopaminergic neurodegenerative disease of aged people, has been shown to have a regional distribution in the United States, with fewer cases in the south and more cases in agricultural areas.[48–50] It would be interesting to assess geographic data for PPID in the horse population. A shared pattern would suggest that similar environmental exposures may predispose to dopaminergic neurodegeneration in both diseases.

PATHOPHYSIOLOGY

Horses with PPID have hyperplasia of the pars intermedia with a single large adenoma or multiple small adenomas. PPID was previously characterized as a benign neoplasia of the equine pituitary gland. However, clinical, pharmacologic, biochemical, and histologic data indicate that PPID is a neurodegenerative disease with loss of dopaminergic inhibitory input to the melanotropes of the pars intermedia.[51] The clinical course of PPID is typical of a neurodegenerative disease; it is a slowly progressive disease that affects primarily aged animals. In response to administration of a dopamine agonist, plasma concentrations of POMC-derived peptides decrease in horses with PPID,[17] and treatment of horses with PPID with the dopamine agonist pergolide results in improvement of both the clinical signs and biochemical abnormalities associated with disease.[37–39] Furthermore, pars intermedia tissue from PPID horses was shown to have 8-fold less dopamine concentration than the tissue from age-matched controls,[52] and hypothalamic and pituitary tissues from horses with PPID were found to have a 6-fold reduction in levels of dopaminergic nerve terminals in the pars intermedia and a 50% reduction in levels of dopaminergic cell bodies in the periventricular nucleus.[53] An absence of dopamine is known to cause proliferation of melanotropes with increased production of POMC and POMC-derived peptides in culture,[54] dopamine receptor–deficient mice,[4] and surgically hypothalamic pituitary gland–disconnected animal models.[55,56] Considered collectively, these data strongly support the hypothesis that PPID is a dopaminergic neurodegenerative disease.

Although the precise cause of PPID is unknown, evidence suggests that oxidative stress may contribute to neuronal damage and cell death. Histologic examination of the pituitary gland of horses with PPID revealed a 16-fold increase in the levels of oxidative stress marker 3-nitrotyrosine in the nerve terminals of the periventricular dopaminergic neurons compared with healthy adult horses.[53] Lipofuscin pigment is also abundant in the pituitary neurons of horses with PPID.[57] Lipofuscin is an accumulation of oxidized cellular debris. Systemic oxidative stress or antioxidant failure does not seem to contribute to the development of PPID. The only indicator of systemic oxidative stress that has been shown in horses with PPID is a mild decrease in plasma thiol levels.[58] Peripheral total glutathione, malondialdehyde, glutathione peroxidase, and superoxide dismutase activities are unchanged in horses with PPID.[58,59] Although pituitary antioxidant capacity has not been shown to be impaired in horses with PPID, pituitary manganese superoxide dismutase activity has been found to decrease with age in horses.[59] Impairment of the activity of this mitochondrial antioxidant could contribute to the increased risk of PPID that occurs with age.[59] Further evaluation of the role of mitochondrial dysfunction and mitochondrial reactive oxygen species production in the pituitary gland of horses with PPID is warranted.

Neuronal accumulation and aggregation of misfolded proteins is a mechanism that contributes to the pathogenesis of most neurodegenerative diseases including Parkinson disease. In Parkinson disease, the protein that accumulates in the dopaminergic neurons is α-synuclein, a natively unfolded soluble monomeric protein that is expressed in nerve terminals and leukocytes. Under certain cellular conditions, α-synuclein can misfold and aggregate disrupting cellular function and triggering cell death.[60] Conditions that promote accumulation of α-synuclein include excessive concentration because of increased production or decreased clearance; posttranslational modifications, such as oxidation or nitration; and primary gene mutations.[61,62] Similar to what is observed in the brain of patients with Parkinson disease, α-synuclein was found to be more abundant in the pars intermedia of horses with PPID.[53] Increased gene expression of α-synuclein suggests that enhanced production has a role in α-synuclein accumulation in the horse with PPID (Dianne McFarlane, unpublished data, 2010). In addition to being more abundant, pars intermedia α-synuclein seems to be excessively nitrated, a modification known to promote α-synuclein aggregation.[53,63] It is unknown if failure of protein clearance also contributes to α-synuclein accumulation in horses with PPID. Misfolded proteins are removed primarily through autophagy, the process by which damaged proteins or organelles are recycled by the lysosome. Impaired autophagy has been suggested to play a critical role in the pathogenesis of protein-misfolding diseases, including Parkinson disease.[64] Assessment of autophagy in the periventricular neurons of horses with PPID is needed.

CLINICAL SIGNS OF PPID

The clinical signs of PPID have been discussed in detail in previous reviews.[1] However, the mechanistic cause of these signs remains largely unknown. In addition, the interrelationship of the clinical signs present in individual animals is not well described. For example, it is not clear in the literature if the horses with PPID with abnormal fat deposits also have insulin resistance, hyperglycemia, polyuria/polydipsia (PU/PD), and laminitis. It is conceivable that PPID is a collection of syndromes each with a unique set of clinical signs and hormone profiles. Knowing how the clinical signs are related to each other and to an array of hormones would improve the understanding of the pathologic mechanisms of PPID.

Hirsutism

The most unique and specific clinical sign associated with PPID is the development of an abnormal hair coat, including hirsutism, delayed shedding, incomplete shedding, and lightening of coat color in aged horses.[46] Aged horses with hirsutism or with a history of hirsutism and those that fail to shed completely have been shown to be 5 times more likely to have a positive PPID test result than aged horses with normal coats,[33] and hirsutism was found to have a positive predictive value of 90% for PPID using postmortem examination as the gold standard.[46] The pathologic mechanisms responsible for hair coat abnormalities in PPID have not been studied.

Muscle Atrophy

A common sign of PPID is muscle wasting or sarcopenia, affecting most prominently the epaxial and gluteal musculature. Sarcopenia is also a characteristic of aging in horses and people in the absence of disease.[33,65,66] Characterization of muscle changes in horses with PPID revealed atrophy of type 2 fibers, sarcoplasmic lipid accumulation, increased myofiber size variation, and subsarcolemmal accumulation of swollen mitochondria.[67] These findings are consistent with those of glucocorticoid excess in other species.[68,69] However, other hormone derangements, including insulin resistance, and chronic inflammation can also cause sarcopenia.[65,70] Further studies are needed to clarify the mechanism underlying muscle wasting in PPID.

Laminitis

Endocrinopathy is the most common cause of laminitis in the horse. Both equine metabolic syndrome and PPID are associated with an increased risk of laminitis.[30,71,72] Although the cause of laminitis remains elusive, recent work has suggested that high serum insulin concentration both predicts and provokes laminitis. Studies have documented that horses and ponies with high fasting insulin concentrations are more likely to founder.[40,72,73] Recently, induction of clinical, radiographic, and histologic signs of laminitis in normal horses and ponies was achieved using a model that creates hyperinsulinemia while maintaining normal insulin sensitivity and blood glucose concentration.[74,75] High nonphysiologic doses of insulin were used in the model. Alterations in cortisol metabolism may also have a role in the development of laminitis. Preliminary data suggest that tissue-specific variation in 11β-hydroxysteroid dehydrogenase activity occurs in the neck adipose tissue of horses with acute laminitis and equine metabolic syndrome.[76,77] Tissue activity of 11β-hydroxysteroid dehydrogenase has not been evaluated in horses with PPID.

PU/PD

PU/PD occurs in approximately 30% (80 of 260) of horses with PPID.[30,34,36–42,45,47,72] Proposed mechanisms for the development of PU/PD include loss of antidiuretic hormone because of compression of the pars nervosa, increased thirst because of central actions of hypercortisolemia, and osmotic diuresis because of hyperglycemia and glucosuria. The observation that horses can have marked hyperglycemia without an increase in voluntary water intake suggests that a mechanism other than osmotic diuresis is responsible in at least some cases of PPID.[35]

Hyperhidrosis

Excessive sweating has been reported to occur more frequently in horses with PPID.[1] Using a quantitative intradermal terbutaline sweat test,[78] 4 of 8 horses with PPID were observed to sweat excessively (Dianne McFarlane, unpublished data, 2010). Although some horses with PPID may sweat only because of a long hair coat, other horses with PPID-associated hyperhidrosis continue to sweat excessively even in a cool environment or when body clipped.

Abnormal Fat Distribution and Insulin Resistance

Abnormal fat distribution is present in 15% to 30% of horses with PPID,[34–38,40,47] and insulin resistance, defined by increased fasting insulin level, is present in 60% (61 of 103) of horses with PPID.[1,33,58,79] Fat pads are typically located above the eyes in the supraorbital fossa, along the crest of the neck, over the tail head, and in the sheath or mammary region.[80,81] It is unclear whether fat deposition occurs as a result of PPID or abnormal fat accumulation is a predisposing condition for the development of PPID. Adiposity and insulin resistance cause chronic inflammation and mitochondrial impairment resulting in oxidative stress, which may have a role in the development of PPID. Longitudinal population studies are needed to determine how frequently horses with obesity and its related conditions progress to develop PPID.

Opportunistic Infections and Immunosuppression

Opportunistic or secondary infections occur in approximately 35% (63 of 180) of horses with PPID compared with 11% (4 of 33) of healthy aged horses (Dianne McFarlane, unpublished data, 2010).[34,36,38,40–42,45,47,57] Common infections include dermatophilosis, sinus infection, pneumonia, and abscesses. Horses with PPID are also likely to have occult infections presumably because of the absence of a significant inflammatory response to pathogens. Horses with PPID often have a pathologic evidence of chronic pneumonia at necropsy without a history of clinical disease.[57] Horses with PPID also have been shown to have higher fecal strongyle egg counts, suggesting that they are more susceptible to endoparasitism.[82]

Previous literature has suggested that high serum cortisol concentration is responsible for immunosuppression in PPID; however, this view is likely oversimplified. As discussed earlier, blood concentrations of several immunosuppressive hormones are increased in horses with PPID, including α-MSH, β-endorphin, and ACTH. These hormones may function in concert to alter the immune response and create a pathogen permissive environment. Aging, in the absence of disease, is associated with changes in immune function characterized by a loss in the ability to respond appropriately to challenges and an increased baseline inflammatory state. Horses with PPID have a leukocyte proinflammatory cytokine profile typical of adult rather than aged horses.[44] In contrast, cytokine response to endotoxin stimulation is greater in peripheral blood mononuclear cells from horses with PPID than from adult horses. Neutrophil function also seems to be impaired with PPID; chemotaxis and oxidative burst are decreased compared with age-matched controls.[83] Equine neutrophilic oxidative burst activity was found to be strongly correlated to α-MSH/insulin ratio but not correlated to serum cortisol concentration from the same sample.[83]

Behavioral Abnormalities

Horses are often described as becoming more lethargic or docile with the development of PPID. Lethargy may result due to metabolic abnormalities, such as insulin resistance; concurrent disease; or high plasma β-endorphin concentrations. Occasionally, a horse is perceived as lethargic because of reluctance to move secondary to laminitis. Clinical signs of laminitis secondary to PPID can be subtle, possibly because of high pain tolerance secondary to increased β-endorphin concentration.

Reproductive Infertility

PPID should be considered in the differential diagnosis of aged mares that fail to conceive or have abnormal estrous cycles. Decreased dopaminergic regulation of reproductive hormonal output and chronic uterine infections may contribute to infertility in mares with PPID. Treatment of infertile mares with PPID with pergolide may restore reproductive function and normal cycling.[38,42] Administration of pergolide to pregnant mares does not seem to be associated with adverse effects. Discontinuing pergolide administration a month before foaling to avoid periparturient complications such as agalactia is recommended.

Neurologic Disease

Neurologic impairment, including ataxia, blindness, seizures, and narcolepsy, has been suggested to occur in 6% to 50% of PPID cases. In a herd of 37 aged horses, neurologic impairment was observed more commonly in horses with PPID (27%) than in aged horses without PPID (5%) (Dianne McFarlane, unpublished data, 2010); however, larger studies are needed.

Clinical Pathology

Routine hematologic and serum biochemical analyses should be part of a complete health examination of an aged horse with or without PPID. In most horses with PPID, routine blood analysis is nondiagnostic but it may provide information regarding general health and PPID-associated secondary diseases. The most common abnormality identified by serum biochemical evaluation in the laboratory in a horse with PPID is hyperglycemia. Although nonspecific, when hyperglycemia is present in routine blood analysis of an aged horse, PPID should be considered. Other abnormalities in horses with PPID may include increased liver enzyme activities, which may be an indication of steroid-induced hepatopathy. Histologic findings consistent with steroid-induced hepatopathy, specifically swollen vacuolated hepatocytes, were reported in 73% of horses with PPID, and 71% of the horses with hepatocellular swelling also had adrenocortical hyperplasia.[57]

DIAGNOSTIC TESTS FOR PPID

With the past decade has come the realization that diagnosis of PPID is not straightforward. Rather, it is complicated by the slow progressive nature of PPID, seasonal variation in hormone output, and overlapping endocrine response to various diseases and pathologic events. In addition, the lack of a true gold standard has impeded the ability to adequately validate traditional or novel diagnostic tests. Hence, there is confusion regarding the best way to diagnose PPID, and many equine clinicians have been frustrated trying to arrive at an accurate diagnosis in patients. Testing for PPID in the autumn is associated with false-positive test results regardless of the diagnostic method used. Studies that were conducted before 2004 validating diagnostic tests must be interpreted cautiously because the investigators would have not accounted for the potential influence of season in either the study design or the data interpretation.[31,37] In all methods of testing, false-negative test results are common early in disease. As with other neurodegenerative diseases, the slow progressive nature of PPID makes it likely that significant pathologic effects have already occurred before diagnostic testing can identify the animal as having PPID. Repeated testing of horses with negative test results but with clinical signs compatible with PPID is recommended.

Dexamethasone Suppression Test

Dexamethasone suppression test has long been considered the gold standard antemortem test, although its superiority over other diagnostic methods remains unproven.[84] In the normal horse, inhibition of ACTH release from the pars distalis by dexamethasone results in suppression of cortisol release from the adrenal gland (**Table 1**). Horses with PPID cannot suppress cortisol release because of ACTH secretion from the pars intermedia, which is not subject to glucocorticoid feedback. The dexamethasone suppression test was originally reported to have 100% sensitivity and specificity using postmortem examination as the gold standard.[84] However, horses in this study were selected based on the presence or absence of overt signs of PPID, which would have favorably biased test performance. There are at present no unbiased studies that compare the overnight dexamethasone suppression test directly with other diagnostic tests using clinical signs and postmortem examination as the gold standard. In the author's experience, some patients with confirmed PPID have an abnormal plasma ACTH concentration before an abnormal dexamethasone suppression test result, whereas in others the converse is observed. At present, data are insufficient to say which diagnostic method is the best at different stages of disease. It is the author's opinion that PPID is a clinical syndrome of different causes, all culminating in dysfunction of the pars intermedia. Therefore, it is unlikely that 1 testing strategy will be optimal in all cases.

Endogenous Plasma ACTH or α-MSH Concentration

Measurement of plasma concentrations of ACTH and α-MSH has also been shown to be useful in the diagnosis of PPID.[22,36] In the healthy horse, α-MSH is primarily a product of the pars intermedia, whereas ACTH is produced by the corticotropes of the pars distalis. In PPID, ACTH is also released from the pars intermedia. Measurement of plasma ACTH concentration for diagnosis of the disease may be confounded by many factors. ACTH levels have been shown to increase in response to stress, competition, and exercise.[85,86] The effect of disease, debilitation, inflammation, or trauma on ACTH concentration in horses has not been extensively investigated. It is

Table 1
Diagnostic testing methods for PPID

Diagnostic Test	Procedure	Sample	Interpretation	Comments (Also See Text)
Overnight DEX Suppression	Collect serum between 4–6 PM. Administer DEX at 40 μg/kg BW IM. Collect serum 19–20 h later	2 serum samples, 1 mL each: 1 preDEX administration and 1 post-DEX administration	Serum cortisol of >1 μg/dL at 19 h post-DEX administration suggests PPID	A mildly decreased resting cortisol (pre-DEX administration) is typical of a PPID-affected horse. A resting cortisol of <1.8 μg/dL is suggestive of iatrogenic adrenal insufficiency
Endogenous Plasma ACTH Concentration	Collect EDTA plasma, preferably in plastic blood collection tube. Separate plasma by centrifugation, and freeze for submission to laboratory. Avoid hemolysis and heat. Process sample within 8 h of collection	EDTA plasma sample, 1 mL	Normal reference range depends on methodology and laboratory. Typically an ACTH concentration <35 pg/mL (chemiluminescent immunoassay) or <45–50 pg/mL (radioimmunoassay) is considered normal	ACTH is likely affected by many biologic events, all of which are not well documented at present. Seasons can have a profound effect, with higher concentrations seen in autumn
Endogenous Plasma α-MSH Concentration	Collect EDTA plasma, preferably in plastic blood collection tube. Separate plasma by centrifugation, and freeze for submission to laboratory. Avoid hemolysis and heat. Process sample within 8 h of collection	1 EDTA plasma sample, 1 mL	Nonautumn reference range: >35 pmol/L suggests PPID	Plasma α-MSH concentration is extremely seasonal. High concentrations are observed in autumn

TRH Stimulation Assay	Collect serum. Administer TRH, 1 mg IV. Collect serum 30–60 min after TRH	2 serum samples, 1 mL each: pre-TRH administration and 30–60 min post-TRH administration	30%–50% increase in serum cortisol 30 min after TRH administration suggests PPID	Pharmaceutical TRH is expensive, TRH compounded for this use may be difficult to obtain. False-positive results may be common
Combined DEX Suppression/ TRH Stimulation Test	Collect plasma between 8 and 10 AM Administer DEX at 40 μg/kg BW IM. Administer TRH, 1 mg IV, 3 h after DEX administration. Collect serum 30 min after TRH and 24 h after DEX administration	3 plasma samples, 1 mL each: pre-DEX administration, 30 min post-TRH administration, and 24 h post-DEX administration	Plasma cortisol >1 μg/dL at 24 h post-DEX administration or ≥66% increase in cortisol levels 3 h after TRH administration suggests PPID	Some diagnostic laboratories prefer to use serum for measurement of cortisol levels. The effect of season on the combined test has not been assessed but would likely result in false-positive results as each of the component tests do
Domperidone Response Test	Collect EDTA plasma at 8 AM. Administer domperidone at 3.3 mg/kg BW po. Collect EDTA plasma at 2 and 4 h after domperidone administration	3 EDTA plasma samples, 1 mL each	A 2-fold increase in plasma ACTH concentration suggests PPID	Higher doses (5 mg/kg po) may improve response. The 2-h sample is more diagnostic in the summer and autumn, and the 4-h sample is best in the winter and spring

Abbreviations: BW, body weight; DEX, dexamethasone; IM, intramuscularly; IV, intravenously.

likely other diseases or events may confound interpretation of plasma ACTH concentration for the diagnosis of PPID.

Plasma α-MSH concentration is a direct product of the pars intermedia, and an increased plasma α-MSH concentration is highly suggestive of PPID. α-MSH has been shown to be strongly influenced by season, and seasonal reference ranges are needed to maximize the discriminatory ability of this test. Measuring α-MSH concentration has been shown to have improved diagnostic accuracy than measuring ACTH concentration.[28] Although not offered as a commercial test at present, measurement of plasma α-MSH concentration may provide a slight improvement as a single sample test for PPID compared with tests available at present.

TRH Stimulation Test

The TRH stimulation test is based on the observation that horses with PPID have a 30% to 50% increase in serum cortisol concentration following administration of TRH, whereas normal horses do not respond.[87] TRH directly stimulates equine melanotropes; plasma α-MSH concentration increased more than 400% in healthy horses following TRH administration.[20] The TRH stimulation test has the advantage of being both a safe and expedient (30 minutes) test. However, false-positive test results are common, with 1 of 3 healthy horses being falsely identified as having PPID in one study.[20] Adrenal gland release of cortisol may be modulated by several poorly defined physiologic and pathologic events. In addition, the disparity between plasma ACTH and cortisol concentrations in horses with PPID suggests that the excessive ACTH produced in horses with PPID may be immunologically active but biologically inert.[88] To circumvent this problem, Beech and colleagues[89] investigated the measurement of ACTH following TRH administration and suggested that this measurement may be a more discriminating test for PPID than the measurement of cortisol release.

Combined Dexamethasone Suppression/TRH Stimulation Test

The combination of the 2 provocative tests described earlier improves the sensitivity and specificity compared with either test considered alone.[46] The disadvantage of this approach is the need for multiple samples within 24 hours.

Domperidone Response Test

The domperidone response test measures ACTH release in response to administration of domperidone, a dopamine receptor antagonist. Because healthy horses are thought to have minimal ACTH production from the pars intermedia and because their corticotropes are not regulated by dopamine, only horses with PPID should produce ACTH when relieved of dopaminergic inhibition.[90,91]

Serum Insulin Concentration

Fasting serum insulin concentration is increased in approximately 60% of horses with PPID.[1,33,58,79] Conditions other than PPID may also increase fasting insulin levels, most notably, equine metabolic syndrome. A high percentage of false-positive and false-negative test results provides limited value to this test for the diagnosis or screening of PPID. However, monitoring fasting insulin concentration is recommended in all horses suspected of having PPID because it has been shown to be predictive for the development of laminitis.[72,73]

Cortisol Circadian Rhythm Loss

Loss of cortisol circadian rhythm occurs in horses with PPID.[84] It has been suggested that monitoring the circadian rhythm of cortisol may be useful for the diagnosis of

PPID.[92] However, loss of circadian rhythm is a common manifestation of a generalized disease and it also occurs as part of normal aging. In a study of 50 healthy horses, 64% had a difference of less than 30% in morning and evening serum cortisol levels, which is the suggested cutoff for the diagnosis of PPID (Dianne McFarlane, unpublished data, 2010).[92] This very low specificity makes this test unsuitable as a diagnostic test.

Urinary Cortisol/Creatinine Ratio

The utility of the measurement of cortisol/creatinine concentration in a single urine sample to diagnose PPID has been evaluated[43] in healthy horses, horses with PPID, and horses with non-PPID illness (grass sickness). Although urinary cortisol/creatinine ratio was higher in horses with PPID than in healthy controls, there was not a significant difference in the ratio among the 3 groups, and the diagnostic sensitivity (85%) and specificity (55%) for PPID was poor. This poor performance was likely the result of the nonspecific cortisol response that occurs as part of a general sickness syndrome.

ACTH Stimulation Test

Administration of ACTH results in release of cortisol from the adrenal gland. The magnitude of the cortisol response is correlated to the adrenal gland size. Therefore, an equal dose of ACTH elicits a greater cortisol response in animals with hyperadrenocorticism than in normal animals. The performance of this test for diagnosing PPID has been assessed in 3 small studies that used postmortem examination as the gold standard. Although the test had 75% sensitivity for the diagnosis of PPID in 2 of the studies,[34,79] the third study found no difference in ACTH-stimulated cortisol response between PPID-affected and healthy aged horses.[84] Adrenal gland hyperplasia is observed in only 20% to 30% of horses with PPID; therefore, an exaggerated response to ACTH in horses with PPID is unlikely to be a consistent finding.[45,47,57]

Advanced Imaging Modalities

The use of advanced diagnostic imaging may not ever prove practical for the diagnosis of PPID because of the expense and the need for general anesthesia. However, recent studies have demonstrated that contrast-enhanced magnetic resonance imaging has the capability to image the equine pituitary gland in enough detail such that the pars intermedia can be differentiated from the adjacent lobes.[93] This advancement will enable the monitoring of dynamic changes of the pituitary with season, with disease, and in response to treatment and therefore has a strong potential to enhance the understanding of the development and progression of PPID.

Necropsy

Postmortem examination of the horse with PPID reveals a grossly enlarged pituitary, often 2 to 5 times the normal size. This enlargement is caused by hypertrophy and hyperplasia of the pars intermedia with microadenomas (<1 cm) or macroadenomas (>1 cm). Large adenomas may contain areas of hemorrhage and necrosis. Affected melanotropes are pleomorphic (polyhedral or spindle shaped) with eosinophilic granular cytoplasm. Cells are organized into nodules or follicular structures separated by fine septal tissue.[35,47,57,90,94] Lipofuscin deposition is common and often severe in the region of the pars nervosa adjacent to the pars intermedia. Other lesions include compression of the adjacent structures, including the pars distalis, pars nervosa, pars tuberalis, or in rare cases, the optic chiasm or hypothalamus. Other, nonpituitary lesions related to disease complications such as laminitis or pneumonia are commonly present.[35,47,57] Evidence of inflammation and oxidative damage may be observed in multiple organs, including the heart, liver, kidney, and lungs.[57]

TREATMENT

Horses with PPID benefit from the provision of an optimized geriatric health management program and the pharmaceutical treatment of the disease. Similar to other aged horses, PPID-affected animals require aggressive preventative health care. The importance of excellent dental care, hoof care, nutrition, and parasite control cannot be overemphasized. PPID-affected horses typically benefit from a processed senior-type concentrate that is easy to masticate and digest. In theory, feeds high in antioxidants could slow the neurodegenerative process associated with PPID, although evidence for this action is lacking. The specific amount and type of feed needs to be individualized to the horse's weight and hormone profile. In horses with insulin resistance, a highly soluble carbohydrate feed should be avoided. However, unlike the horses with equine metabolic syndrome, the PPID-affected insulin-resistant horses often also have concurrent muscle wasting, complicating their nutritional requirements. Fortunately, many commercial feeds are now available designed specifically for the aged or endocrine-impaired horse. Fecal egg counts should be routinely performed in horses with PPID because of their predisposition to strongyle infections.[82] Horses with PPID may have difficulty with thermoregulation, so ample fresh water, shelter, and shade should be provided, with body clipping and blanketing as needed. Medical conditions are more frequent in aged horses, especially in those with PPID; therefore, careful and frequent observation for the evidence of secondary illness is important. When well cared for, horses with PPID can live into their 30s and even 40s.

The drug of choice in the treatment of PPID is pergolide mesylate. Pergolide is an ergot-derived dopamine D_2 receptor agonist, which downregulates POMC peptide production. The efficacy of pergolide at improving clinical signs of disease and diagnostic test response has been documented in several studies.[37–39,41,42] Pergolide, which was used to treat Parkinson disease, was voluntarily withdrawn from the market in 2007 for use in humans because of the reports of cardiac regurgitation and vegetative valvular lesions.[95,96] Heart lesions have not been reported in horses receiving pergolide. After its removal from market, the Food and Drug Administration's Center for Veterinary Medicine issued a limited exemption from the Animal Medicinal Drug Use Clarification Act regulations, allowing pergolide to be compounded for veterinary use from bulk sources until a new animal drug application for the product is approved. Care must be taken, however, when using compounded pergolide because it is unstable in aqueous vehicles and needs to be stored refrigerated in the dark.[97] Aqueous drug form should not be used more than 30 days after formulation.[97]

Most clinicians start with a dose of 1 mg per horse then titrate to effect in increments of 0.5 to 1.0 mg units. Clinical and diagnostic test improvement is typically not apparent for several months, so recheck examinations with recommendations for dose adjustments every 6 to 12 months are appropriate. Adverse effects are uncommon at this dose; however, anorexia can occur. Anorexia usually can be resolved by abruptly decreasing the dose, then slowly increasing the dose over time until the desired dose is achieved. Some horses improve if the total dose is split and administered twice daily. Lifelong treatment with pergolide is recommended. There are reports of horses that have been maintained on pergolide treatment for more than 10 years (Schott, personal communication, 2010). Anecdotal reports suggest that dose requirements increase slowly over time in treated animals, likely because of a continued progression of disease or the development of drug tolerance. Because of the seasonal fluctuation in hormone production by the pars intermedia, it may be possible to strategically treat mild cases of PPID for only 6 months of the year (eg, June–December); however, this therapeutic approach has not yet been critically assessed. In vitro studies have suggested that pergolide may also have antioxidant activity and may provide neuroprotective benefits.[98,99] These properties could be beneficial in slowing the progression of PPID. Further work is needed to determine the benefit of early therapeutic intervention in the time course and ultimate outcome of the disease.

Recent improvements in the methodology to measure serum pergolide levels have allowed pharmacokinetic studies to be performed in humans and horses.[100,101] Preliminary work has shown that pergolide is rapidly absorbed following oral administration in horses. Exact bioavailability was not determined.[101] As expected, the pharmacodynamic effects of pergolide (change in hormone concentration) were not predicted by the pharmacokinetic parameters of the drug.[101]

Cyproheptadine has been suggested as a second-line drug used in combination with pergolide when maximal doses of pergolide alone are insufficient to achieve resolution of clinical signs. As a monotherapeutic agent, cyproheptadine has limited efficacy.[38,39] Cyproheptadine is a mixed-action drug, with serotonin antagonist, antihistamine, and antimuscarinic effects. Cyproheptadine lowers seizure threshold in mice, so it should be used cautiously in horses with a history of seizures or central neurologic disease.[102]

Trilostane is a competitive inhibitor of 3β-hydroxysteroid dehydrogenase, the enzyme responsible for production of cortisol from cholesterol. Trilostane was reported to improve clinical signs of PPID but not the dexamethasone suppression test results.[40] Trilostane may be beneficial to those horses with PPID with adrenal gland hyperplasia and hypercortisolemia; however, it would have no effect on the excessive production of pituitary-derived hormones.

Many nutraceuticals, botanicals, and natural remedies are available for the treatment of PPID. To date, only 1 such product has been tested in horses with PPID. In this study, a commercial *Vitex agnus castus* (chasteberry, Vitex) extract failed to resolve clinical signs or improve diagnostic test results in 14 horses.[103] In fact, several animals' condition worsened, and use of the extract was discontinued early. In contrast, 8 of 9 horses subsequently treated with pergolide improved. The lack of efficacy and safety evidence makes these remedies contraindicated in horses with PPID.

SUMMARY

Much has been learned about equine PPID over the past decade; however, far more remains to be accomplished. There is a critical need for accurate and early testing methods with season-specific reference ranges. Disease risk factors need to be clarified and preventative strategies developed. Understanding the complexity of the hormonal derangements in PPID and using this knowledge to formulate more individualized and targeted therapy plans may help avoid the life-threatening complications that occur with PPID.

REFERENCES

1. Schott HC. Pituitary pars intermedia dysfunction: equine Cushing's disease. Vet Clin North Am Equine Pract 2002;18:237–70.
2. Masson-Pevet M, Gauer F. Seasonality and melatonin receptors in the pars tuberalis in some long day breeders. Biol Signals 1994;3:63–70.
3. Wilson MG, Nicholson WE, Holscher MA, et al. Proopiolipomelanocortin peptides in normal pituitary, pituitary tumor, and plasma of normal and Cushing's horses. Endocrinology 1982;110:941–54.

4. Saiardi A, Borrelli E. Absence of dopaminergic control on melanotrophs leads to Cushing's-like syndrome in mice. Mol Endocrinol 1998;12:1133–9.
5. Ham J, Smyth DG. Regulation of bioactive beta-endorphin processing in rat pars intermedia. FEBS Lett 1984;175:407–11.
6. Millington WR, Dybdal NO, Mueller GP, et al. N-acetylation and C-terminal proteolysis of beta-endorphin in the anterior lobe of the horse pituitary. Gen Comp Endocrinol 1992;85:297–307.
7. Wilkinson CW. Roles of acetylation and other post-translational modifications in melanocortin function and interactions with endorphins. Peptides 2006;27:453–71.
8. Getting SJ. Targeting melanocortin receptors as potential novel therapeutics. Pharmacol Ther 2006;111:1–15.
9. Cummings DE, Schwartz MW. Melanocortins and body weight: a tale of two receptors. Nat Genet 2000;26:8–9.
10. Lipton JM, Glyn JR, Zimmer JA. ACTH and alpha-melanotropin in central temperature control. Fed Proc 1981;40:2760–4.
11. Murphy MT, Richards DB, Lipton JM. Antipyretic potency of centrally administered alpha-melanocyte stimulating hormone. Science 1983;221:192–3.
12. Lipton JM, Catania A. Anti-inflammatory actions of the neuroimmunomodulator alpha-MSH. Immunol Today 1997;18:140–5.
13. Catania A, Rajora N, Capsoni F, et al. The neuropeptide alpha-MSH has specific receptors on neutrophils and reduces chemotaxis in vitro. Peptides 1996;17:675–9.
14. Oktar BK, Yuksel M, Alican I. The role of cyclooxygenase inhibition in the effect of alpha-melanocyte-stimulating hormone on reactive oxygen species production by rat peritoneal neutrophils. Prostaglandins Leukot Essent Fatty Acids 2004;71:1–5.
15. Beloff-Chain A, Morton J, Dunmore S, et al. Evidence that the insulin secretagogue, beta-cell-tropin, is ACTH 22-39. Nature 1983;301:255–8.
16. Marshall JB, Kapcala LP, Manning LD, et al. Effect of corticotropin-like intermediate lobe peptide on pancreatic exocrine function in isolated rat pancreatic lobules. J Clin Invest 1984;74:1886–9.
17. Orth DN, Holscher MA, Wilson MG, et al. Equine Cushing's disease: plasma immunoreactive proopiolipomelanocortin peptide and cortisol levels basally and in response to diagnostic tests. Endocrinology 1982;110:1430–41.
18. McFarlane D, Beech J, Cribb A. Alpha-melanocyte stimulating hormone release in response to thyrotropin releasing hormone in healthy horses, horses with pituitary pars intermedia dysfunction and equine pars intermedia explants. Domest Anim Endocrinol 2006;30:276–88.
19. Saland LC. The mammalian pituitary intermediate lobe: an update on innervation and regulation. Brain Res Bull 2001;54:587–93.
20. Danger JM, Perroteau I, Franzoni MF, et al. Innervation of the pars intermedia and control of alpha-melanotropin secretion in the newt. Neuroendocrinology 1989;50:543–9.
21. Shioda S, Nakai Y, Hori T, et al. Innervation of thyrotropin-releasing hormone-containing neurons in the bullfrog pars intermedia. Neurosci Lett 1987;81:53–6.
22. McFarlane D, Donaldson MT, McDonnell SM, et al. Effects of season and sample handling on measurement of plasma alpha-melanocyte-stimulating hormone concentrations in horses and ponies. Am J Vet Res 2004;65:1463–8.
23. Logan A, Weatherhead B. Photoperiodic dependence of seasonal changes in pituitary content of melanocyte-stimulating hormone. Neuroendocrinology 1980;30:309–12.

24. Lincoln GA, Rhind SM, Pompolo S, et al. Hypothalamic control of photoperiod-induced cycles in food intake, body weight, and metabolic hormones in rams. Am J Physiol Regul Integr Comp Physiol 2001;281:R76–90.
25. Schuhler S, Ebling FJ. Role of melanocortin in the long-term regulation of energy balance: lessons from a seasonal model. Peptides 2006;27:301–9.
26. Place NJ, McGowan CM, Lamb SV, et al. Seasonal variation in serum concentrations of selected metabolic hormones in horses. J Vet Intern Med 2010;24:650–4.
27. Donaldson MT, McDonnell SM, Schanbacher BJ, et al. Variation in plasma adrenocorticotropic hormone concentration and dexamethasone suppression test results with season, age, and sex in healthy ponies and horses. J Vet Intern Med 2005;19:217–22.
28. McFarlane D, Paradis MR, Zimmel D, et al. The effect of latitude of residence, breed and pituitary dysfunction on seasonal plasma ACTH and MSH concentration [abstract]. J Vet Intern Med 2010;24:689.
29. Frank N, Elliott SB, Chameroy KA, et al. Association of season and pasture grazing with blood hormone and metabolite concentrations in horses with presumed pituitary pars intermedia dysfunction. J Vet Intern Med 2010;24(5):1167–75.
30. Donaldson MT, Jorgensen AJ, Beech J. Evaluation of suspected pituitary pars intermedia dysfunction in horses with laminitis. J Am Vet Med Assoc 2004;224:1123–7.
31. Hoffman RM, Wilson JA, Kronfeld DS, et al. Hydrolyzable carbohydrates in pasture, hay, and horse feeds: direct assay and seasonal variation. J Anim Sci 2001;79:500–6.
32. Brosnahan MM, Paradis MR. Assessment of clinical characteristics, management practices, and activities of geriatric horses. J Am Vet Med Assoc 2003;223:99–103.
33. McGowan TW. Aged horse health, management and welfare [doctoral thesis]. St Lucia, Australia: University of Queensland; 2008.
34. Hillyer MH, Taylor FR, Mair TS, et al. Diagnosis of hyperadrenocorticism in the horse. Equine Vet Educ 1992;4:131–4.
35. van der Kolk JH, Kalsbeek HC, van Garderen E, et al. Equine pituitary neoplasia: a clinical report of 21 cases (1990–1992). Vet Rec 1993;133:594–7.
36. Couetil L, Paradis MR, Knoll J. Plasma adrenocorticotropin concentration in healthy horses and in horses with clinical signs of hyperadrenocorticism. J Vet Intern Med 1996;10:1–6.
37. Schott HC, Coursen CL, Eberhart SW, et al. The Michigan Cushing's project. In: Proceedings of the 47th Annual Convention of the American Association of Equine Practitioners. 2001. p. 22–4.
38. Donaldson MT, LaMonte BH, Morresey P, et al. Treatment with pergolide or cyproheptadine of pituitary pars intermedia dysfunction (equine Cushing's disease). J Vet Intern Med 2002;16:742–6.
39. Perkins GA, Lamb S, Erb HN, et al. Plasma adrenocorticotropin (ACTH) concentrations and clinical response in horses treated for equine Cushing's disease with cyproheptadine or pergolide. Equine Vet J 2002;34:679–85.
40. McGowan CM, Neiger R. Efficacy of trilostane for the treatment of equine Cushing's syndrome. Equine Vet J 2003;35:414–8.
41. Munoz MC, Doreste F, Ferrer O, et al. Pergolide treatment for Cushing's syndrome in a horse. Vet Rec 1996;139:41–3.
42. Sgorbini M, Panzani D, Maccheroni M, et al. Equine Cushing-like syndrome: diagnosis and therapy in two cases. Vet Res Commun 2004;28(Suppl 1):377–80.

43. Chandler KJ, Dixon RM. Urinary cortisol:creatinine ratios in healthy horses and horses with hyperadrenocorticism and non-adrenal disease. Vet Rec 2002;150: 773–6.
44. McFarlane D, Holbrook TC. Cytokine dysregulation in aged horses and horses with pituitary pars intermedia dysfunction. J Vet Intern Med 2008;22:436–42.
45. Heinrichs M, Baumgartner W, Capen CC. Immunocytochemical demonstration of proopiomelanocortin-derived peptides in pituitary adenomas of the pars intermedia in horses. Vet Pathol 1990;27:419–25.
46. Frank N, Andrews FM, Sommardahl CS, et al. Evaluation of the combined dexamethasone suppression/thyrotropin-releasing hormone stimulation test for detection of pars intermedia pituitary adenomas in horses. J Vet Intern Med 2006;20:987–93.
47. Boujon CE, Bestetti GE, Meier HP, et al. Equine pituitary adenoma: a functional and morphological study. J Comp Pathol 1993;109:163–78.
48. Wright WA, Evanoff BA, Lian M, et al. Geographic and ethnic variation in Parkinson disease: a population-based study of US Medicare beneficiaries. Neuroepidemiology 2010;34:143–51.
49. Lanska DJ. The geographic distribution of Parkinson's disease mortality in the United States. J Neurol Sci 1997;150:63–70.
50. Priyadarshi A, Khuder SA, Schaub EA, et al. Environmental risk factors and Parkinson's disease: a metaanalysis. Environ Res 2001;86:122–7.
51. McFarlane D. Advantages and limitations of the equine disease, pituitary pars intermedia dysfunction as a model of spontaneous dopaminergic neurodegenerative disease. Ageing Res Rev 2007;6:54–63.
52. Millington WR, Dybdal NO, Dawson R Jr, et al. Equine Cushing's disease: differential regulation of beta-endorphin processing in tumors of the intermediate pituitary. Endocrinology 1988;123:1598–604.
53. McFarlane D, Dybdal N, Donaldson MT, et al. Nitration and increased alpha-synuclein expression associated with dopaminergic neurodegeneration in equine pituitary pars intermedia dysfunction. J Neuroendocrinol 2005;17: 73–80.
54. Gehlert DR, Bishop JF, Schafer MP, et al. Rat intermediate lobe in culture: dopaminergic regulation of POMC biosynthesis and cell proliferation. Peptides 1988;9(Suppl 1):161–8.
55. Goudreau JL, Lindley SE, Lookingland KJ, et al. Evidence that hypothalamic periventricular dopamine neurons innervate the intermediate lobe of the rat pituitary. Neuroendocrinology 1992;56:100–5.
56. Engler D, Pham T, Liu JP, et al. Studies of the regulation of the hypothalamic-pituitary-adrenal axis in sheep with hypothalamic-pituitary disconnection. II. Evidence for in vivo ultradian hypersecretion of proopiomelanocortin peptides by the isolated anterior and intermediate pituitary. Endocrinology 1990;127: 1956–66.
57. Glover CM, Miller LM, Dybdal NO, et al. Extrapituitary and pituitary pathological findings in horses with pituitary pars intermedia dysfunction: a retrospective study. J Equine Vet Sci 2009;29:146–53.
58. Keen JA, McLaren M, Chandler KJ, et al. Biochemical indices of vascular function, glucose metabolism and oxidative stress in horses with equine Cushing's disease. Equine Vet J 2004;36:226–9.
59. McFarlane D, Cribb AE. Systemic and pituitary pars intermedia antioxidant capacity associated with pars intermedia oxidative stress and dysfunction in horses. Am J Vet Res 2005;66:2065–72.

60. Conway KA, Lee SJ, Rochet JC, et al. Acceleration of oligomerization, not fibrillization, is a shared property of both alpha-synuclein mutations linked to early-onset Parkinson's disease: implications for pathogenesis and therapy. Proc Natl Acad Sci U S A 2000;97:571–6.
61. Betarbet R, Canet-Aviles RM, Sherer TB, et al. Intersecting pathways to neurodegeneration in Parkinson's disease: effects of the pesticide rotenone on DJ-1, alpha-synuclein, and the ubiquitin-proteasome system. Neurobiol Dis 2006;22: 404–20.
62. Kirik D, Rosenblad C, Burger C, et al. Parkinson-like neurodegeneration induced by targeted overexpression of alpha-synuclein in the nigrostriatal system. J Neurosci 2002;22:2780–91.
63. Good PF, Hsu A, Werner P, et al. Protein nitration in Parkinson's disease. J Neuropathol Exp Neurol 1998;57:338–42.
64. Cuervo AM, Stefanis L, Fredenburg R, et al. Impaired degradation of mutant alpha-synuclein by chaperone-mediated autophagy. Science 2004;305:1292–5.
65. Narici MV, Maffulli N. Sarcopenia: characteristics, mechanisms and functional significance. Br Med Bull 2010;95:139–59.
66. Sakuma K, Yamaguchi A. Molecular mechanisms in aging and current strategies to counteract sarcopenia. Curr Aging Sci 2010;3:90–101.
67. Aleman M, Nieto JE. Gene expression of proteolytic systems and growth regulators of skeletal muscle in horses with myopathy associated with pituitary pars intermedia dysfunction. Am J Vet Res 2010;71:664–70.
68. Pleasure DE, Walsh GO, Engel WK. Atrophy of skeletal muscle in patients with Cushing's syndrome. Arch Neurol 1970;22:118–25.
69. Tice LW, Engel AG. The effects of glucocorticoids on red and white muscles in the rat. Am J Pathol 1967;50:311–33.
70. Lim S, Kim JH, Yoon JW, et al. Sarcopenic obesity: prevalence and association with metabolic syndrome in the Korean Longitudinal Study on Health and Aging (KLoSHA). Diabetes Care 2010;33:1652–4.
71. Geor RJ. Pasture-associated laminitis. Vet Clin North Am Equine Pract 2009;25: 39–50, vi.
72. Carter RA, Treiber KH, Geor RJ, et al. Prediction of incipient pasture-associated laminitis from hyperinsulinaemia, hyperleptinaemia and generalised and localised obesity in a cohort of ponies. Equine Vet J 2009;41:171–8.
73. McGowan CM, Frost R, Pfeiffer DU, et al. Serum insulin concentrations in horses with equine Cushing's syndrome: response to a cortisol inhibitor and prognostic value. Equine Vet J 2004;36:295–8.
74. de Laat MA, McGowan CM, Sillence MN, et al. Equine laminitis: induced by 48 h hyperinsulinaemia in Standardbred horses. Equine Vet J 2010;42: 129–35.
75. Asplin KE, Sillence MN, Pollitt CC, et al. Induction of laminitis by prolonged hyperinsulinaemia in clinically normal ponies. Vet J 2007;174:530–5.
76. Johnson PJ, Ganjam VK, Slight SH, et al. Tissue-specific dysregulation of cortisol metabolism in equine laminitis. Equine Vet J 2004;36:41–5.
77. Schott H, Graves E, Refsal KR, et al. Diagnosis and treatment of pituitary pars intermedia dysfunction (classical Cushing's disease) and metabolic syndrome (peripheral Cushing's syndrome) in horses. In: Hillier A, Foster AP, Kwochka KW, editors. Advances in veterinary dermatology. Oxford (UK): Blackwell Publisher; 2004. p. 159–69 [Conference Proceedings].
78. MacKay RJ. Quantitative intradermal terbutaline sweat test in horses. Equine Vet J 2008;40:518–20.

79. van der Kolk JH, Wensing T, Kalsbeek HC, et al. Laboratory diagnosis of equine pituitary pars intermedia adenoma. Domest Anim Endocrinol 1995;12:35–9.
80. Carter RA, Geor RJ, Burton SW, et al. Apparent adiposity assessed by standardised scoring systems and morphometric measurements in horses and ponies. Vet J 2009;179:204–10.
81. Frank N, Elliott SB, Brandt LE, et al. Physical characteristics, blood hormone concentrations, and plasma lipid concentrations in obese horses with insulin resistance. J Am Vet Med Assoc 2006;228:1383–90.
82. McFarlane D, Hale GM, Johnson EM, et al. Fecal egg counts after anthelmintic administration to aged horses and horses with pituitary pars intermedia dysfunction. J Am Vet Med Assoc 2010;236:330–4.
83. McFarlane D, McDaniel K. Neutrophil function in healthy aged horses and horses with pituitary dysfunction [abstract]. J Vet Intern Med 2010;24:688–9.
84. Dybdal NO, Hargreaves KM, Madigan JE, et al. Diagnostic testing for pituitary pars intermedia dysfunction in horses. J Am Vet Med Assoc 1994;204:627–32.
85. Fazio E, Medica P, Aronica V, et al. Circulating beta-endorphin, adrenocorticotrophic hormone and cortisol levels of stallions before and after short road transport: stress effect of different distances. Acta Vet Scand 2008;50:6.
86. Nagata S, Takeda F, Kurosawa M, et al. Plasma adrenocorticotropin, cortisol and catecholamines response to various exercises. Equine Vet J Suppl 1999;30: 570–4.
87. Beech J, Garcia M. Hormonal response to thyrotropin-releasing hormone in healthy horses and in horses with pituitary adenoma. Am J Vet Res 1985;46: 1941–3.
88. Orth DN, Nicholson WE. Bioactive and immunoreactive adrenocorticotropin in normal equine pituitary and in pituitary tumors of horses with Cushing's disease. Endocrinology 1982;111:559–63.
89. Beech J, Boston R, Lindborg S, et al. Adrenocorticotropin concentration following administration of thyrotropin-releasing hormone in healthy horses and those with pituitary pars intermedia dysfunction and pituitary gland hyperplasia. J Am Vet Med Assoc 2007;231:417–26.
90. Miller MA, Pardo ID, Jackson LP, et al. Correlation of pituitary histomorphometry with adrenocorticotrophic hormone response to domperidone administration in the diagnosis of equine pituitary pars intermedia dysfunction. Vet Pathol 2008; 45:26–38.
91. Sojka JE, Jackson LP, Moore G, et al. Domperidone causes an increase in endogenous ACTH concentration in horses with pituitary pars intermedia dysfunction (equine Cushing's disease). In: Proceedings of the 52nd Annual Convention of the American Association of Equine Practitioners. 2006. p. 320–3.
92. Douglas R. Circadian cortisol rhythmicity and equine Cushing's-like disease. J Equine Vet Sci 1999;19:684–753.
93. Schott H, Pease A, Patterson J, et al. CT and MR imaging of equine pituitary glands. In: Proceedings of the 28th Annual Forum of the American College of Veterinary Internal Medicine. 2010. p. 196.
94. van der Kolk JH, Heinrichs M, van Amerongen JD, et al. Evaluation of pituitary gland anatomy and histopathologic findings in clinically normal horses and horses and ponies with pituitary pars intermedia adenoma. Am J Vet Res 2004;65:1701–7.
95. Baseman DG, O'Suilleabhain PE, Reimold SC, et al. Pergolide use in Parkinson disease is associated with cardiac valve regurgitation. Neurology 2004;63: 301–4.

96. Available at: http://www.fda.gov/NewsEvents/Newsroom/PressAnnouncements/2007/ucm108877.htm. Accessed July, 2010.
97. Davis JL, Kirk LM, Davidson GS, et al. Effects of compounding and storage conditions on stability of pergolide mesylate. J Am Vet Med Assoc 2009;234:385–9.
98. Gille G, Rausch WD, Hung ST, et al. Pergolide protects dopaminergic neurons in primary culture under stress conditions. J Neural Transm 2002;109:633–43.
99. Uberti D, Piccioni L, Colzi A, et al. Pergolide protects SH-SY5Y cells against neurodegeneration induced by H(2)O(2). Eur J Pharmacol 2002;434:17–20.
100. Thalamas C, Rajman I, Kulisevsky J, et al. Pergolide: multiple-dose pharmacokinetics in patients with mild to moderate Parkinson disease. Clin Neuropharmacol 2005;28:120–5.
101. Wright AM. Pharmacokinetics of pergolide in normal mares [master's thesis]. Manhattan (NY): Kansas State University; 2009.
102. Singh D, Goel RK. Proconvulsant potential of cyproheptadine in experimental animal models. Fundam Clin Pharmacol 2010;24:451–5.
103. Beech J. Comparison of *Vitex agnus castus* extract and pergolide in treatment of equine Cushing's syndrome. In: Proceedings of the 48th Annual Convention of the American Association of Equine Practitioners. 2002. p. 175–7.

Disorders of the Equine Thyroid Gland

Babetta A. Breuhaus, DVM, PhD

KEYWORDS

- Horse • Hypothyroidism • Hyperthyroidism
- Nonthyroidal illness syndrome • Thyroid hormone
- Thyrotropin • Goiter

THYROID GLAND ANATOMY AND FUNCTION

The thyroid gland, found dorsal to the trachea just distal to the larynx, is a smooth, firm, bilobed organ, approximately 2.5 cm × 2.5 cm × 5 cm,[1] weighing approximately 0.04 g/kg body weight.[2] This gland is not readily seen or palpated in normal horses, although it may become visible as horses age. Histologically, this gland is composed of cuboidal to low columnar epithelial cells arranged in follicles. The epithelial cells produce thyroglobulin, a glycoprotein containing multiple tyrosine residues. Iodine is concentrated in the gland, oxidized, and bound to tyrosine to form monoiodotyrosine (MIT) and diiodotyrosine (DIT). These iodotyrosine residues are then coupled to form thyroxine (T_4) and triiodothyronine (T_3), which remain bound to thyroglobulin and are stored within the follicles in an approximate ratio (in humans) of 23% MIT, 33% DIT, 35% T_4, and 7% T_3.[3] In humans, there is enough thyroid hormone stored within the thyroid gland to maintain euthyroidism for approximately 2 to 3 months if iodine ingestion were to cease completely.

Thyroid hormone secretion is stimulated by thyrotropin (thyroid-stimulating hormone [TSH]) from the anterior pituitary gland, which in turn is regulated by thyrotropin-releasing hormone (TRH) from the hypothalamus. TSH also has trophic effects on the thyroid gland, increasing epithelial (follicular) cell size and activity; increasing iodide uptake; increasing secretion of thyroglobulin into the colloid; increasing the synthesis of MIT, DIT, T_4, and T_3, and reuptake of colloid by follicular cells by endocytosis.[3] Once secreted, thyroid hormones travel in the blood, primarily bound to proteins, including thyroid hormone–binding globulin, transthyretin, and albumin. Although only the unbound free fractions are metabolically active, this protein binding helps maintain a pool of readily available hormone and prevents the circulating hormones from being rapidly excreted by the kidneys, which only excrete free T_4 and T_3. T_4 binds more tightly to binding proteins than does T_3, resulting in a lower metabolic clearance rate and a longer half-life (7 days for T_4 vs 1 day for T_3 in

Department of Clinical Sciences, North Carolina State University, 4700 Hillsborough Street, Raleigh, NC 27606, USA
E-mail address: Betta_breuhaus@ncsu.edu

Vet Clin Equine 27 (2011) 115–128
doi:10.1016/j.cveq.2010.12.002
vetequine.theclinics.com

humans).[3] In addition to this tighter protein binding, T_4 does not bind with thyroid hormone receptors as avidly as does T_3. Together, these properties result in T_3 being more metabolically active than T_4. Because the thyroid gland releases a much larger amount of T_4 compared with T_3, the majority of T_3 is derived from deiodination of T_4 in the peripheral tissues by type 1 (D1) and type 2 (D2) deiodinases, which contain selenium as the iodine acceptor in the catalytic unit (selenocysteine). Type 3 (D3) deiodinase, which is also a selenoprotein, is the main T_4 and T_3 inactivating enzyme. The conversion of T_4 to reverse T_3 by D1 and D3 deiodinases is important to regulate thyroid hormone function.

The primary action of thyroid hormones is to stimulate oxygen consumption. Thyroid hormones stimulate protein synthesis and catabolism, help regulate lipid metabolism, and stimulate basal metabolic rate and body heat production. These hormones are not essential for life but play important roles in growth and organ maturation. The actions of thyroid hormones are divided into genomic and nongenomic actions. Genomic actions are mediated by thyroid hormone receptors that are nuclear transcription factors that increase or decrease the expression of genes that regulate cell function. Nongenomic actions can be initiated by receptors at the plasma membrane, within the cytoplasm, or at the mitochondrion. Nongenomic actions include roles in cell division, angiogenesis, protein trafficking, cell migration, platelet aggregation, nitric oxide synthase and Na^+/K^+-ATPase activation, modulation of Ca^{2+}-ATPase and Na^+/H^+ exchanger (Na^+/H^+ antiporter) activity, modulation of neurons and myocyte Na^+ currents, and epidermal growth factor receptor activity. For a detailed review on thyroid hormone actions, see elsewhere.[4]

The thyroid gland also contains parafollicular cells, commonly referred to as C cells. These cells secrete factors that help regulate follicular cell activity. They also secrete calcitonin, which is important in the regulation of extracellular calcium concentration. Calcitonin decreases osteoclastic bone activity and serum calcium concentration. Calcium regulation and calcitonin are discussed in more detail elsewhere in this issue by Ramiro Toribio.

DIAGNOSTIC TESTS OF THYROID GLAND FUNCTION IN HORSES

Measurement of Thyroid Hormone Levels

Single point-in-time measurements of thyroid hormone concentrations, although simple to perform, are not always considered to be the most reliable indicators of thyroid function. A variety of drugs, as well as physiologic or pathophysiologic states, can cause the measured values to be low, even when the thyroid gland itself is normal. In the horse, some of these causes include fasting; phenylbutazone or corticosteroid administration; strenuous exercise; diets high in energy, protein, zinc or copper; and nonthyroidal illnesses.[5–15] Thus, it is important that thyroid hormone measurements be performed in horses that have not received any medications for at least 2, and preferably, 4 weeks before testing. If a horse has been receiving thyroid hormone supplementation without prior documentation of hypothyroidism, it is best to wean the horse off the supplementation and then test thyroid function once the horse has not received any supplementation for at least 4 weeks.

If only single thyroid hormone measurements are available, it is also important to measure the free fractions of T_4 and T_3 because certain states (such as liver and other diseases), drugs (such as salicylates and phenylbutazone), or hormones (such as estrogen), can alter protein binding.[16] During illness in humans, measurement of serum-free T_4 concentration by direct methods often underestimates values when compared with measurements of free T_4 concentration after dialysis or ultrafiltration.[17–21]

This situation also seems to be the case in dogs[22] and horses.[15] Thus, serum concentrations of free T_4 measured by equilibrium dialysis are more likely to reflect the true thyroid status in ill horses compared with other methods of free T_4 concentration measurement. Measuring free T_4 concentrations by dialysis instead of directly may help prevent equine clinicians from misdiagnosing ill horses as being hypothyroid. Resting thyroid hormone and TSH concentrations from 71 healthy adult horses are given in **Table 1**.

Stimulation Tests

Stimulation tests provide a better indication of thyroid status than single measurements of thyroid hormone concentrations. These tests involve measuring thyroid hormone concentrations before and after giving TRH or TSH to stimulate thyroid hormone release. Various techniques and results have been described.[7–9,23–27] These tests are usually not performed by ambulatory clinicians because multiple blood samples are required to be taken over several hours and sterile TRH and TSH are not readily available and can be expensive.

To perform a stimulation test, a control blood sample is obtained, TRH (1 mg to the average 450–500-kg horse) or TSH (5 IU) is given intravenously, and subsequent blood samples are obtained. According to most references, T_3 concentrations should double at 2 hours and T_4 concentrations should double at 4 hours. In 36 normal horses that participated in various studies conducted by the author, the mean (and range) increase in total T_4 concentration was 2.2 (1.3–3.8) times the control value at 4 hours. Increases in concentrations of free T_4 and free T_4 by dialysis (mean and range) were 1.7 (1.1–2.1) times and 1.8 (1.1–2.8) times the control values at 4 hours, respectively. Increases in concentrations of total and free T_3 (mean and range) were 3 (1.1–10.3) times and 4.2 (1–53) times the control values at 2 hours, respectively. The seemingly lower T_4 responses to TRH injection are in agreement with findings by others.[23,28–30] Closer examination of the data by the author revealed that, in general, the few horses with smaller increases in concentrations of T_4 or T_3 either started with higher resting values or their peaks occurred later (T_4) or earlier (T_3) than 4 or 2 hours. Horses with lower T_4 responses, in general, did not have lower T_3 responses. Horses with high responses tended to have very low resting thyroid hormone concentrations. Thus, one must be careful when interpreting the results of a TRH stimulation test.

Suppression Test

A T_3 suppression test has been described to confirm the diagnosis of hyperthyroidism.[31,32] A control blood sample is obtained before the intramuscular administration of 2.5 mg T_3 diluted in 5 mL of sterile saline, given twice daily for 7 doses (4 days). Additional blood samples are drawn 5 minutes before each dose of T_3,

Table 1
Normal baseline concentrations of thyroid hormones in adult horses (n = 71)

	Total T_4 nmol/L	Free T_4 pmol/L	Free T_4 by Dialysis pmol/L	Total T_3 nmol/L	Free T_3 pmol/L	TSH ng/mL
Range	6–46	6–21	7–47	0.3–2.9	0.1–5.9	0.02–0.97
Median	19	11	22	0.9	1.7	0.23
95% CI	18–22	10–12	21–25	0.9–1.1	1.8–2.4	0.21–0.37
Mean	20	11	23	1.0	2.1	0.29
SD	9.4	2.8	8.9	0.5	1.3	0.23

Abbreviation: CI, confidence interval.

then twice daily on days 5 and 7, and in the morning of day 10. In normal horses, T_4 and T_3 measurements are within the reference range in the control blood sample. Administration of T_3 should result in a 10- to 20-fold increase in serum T_3 concentration, whereas serum T_4 concentration should gradually decrease, remaining suppressed for at least 5 days after the last dose of T_3. In hyperthyroid horses, control (pre-T_3) blood samples have increased concentrations of T_4 and T_3. The increase in serum T_3 concentration after T_3 administration is not as pronounced as in normal horses, but serum T_3 concentration does remain increased throughout the administration period. Serum concentration of T_4 is not suppressed.

Imaging

Ultrasonographic examination of the thyroid gland reveals whether enlargement is because of solid tissue or is cystic. It also allows measurement of the gland, comparison to the contralateral gland, and provides guidance for biopsy. Nuclear scintigraphy is a well-established tool for the evaluation of thyroid function, detection of metastatic disease, and measurement of metabolic tumor volume in humans and small animals.[33,34] Nuclear scintigraphy of the thyroid gland has been described in the horse.[31,32,35,36] This technique is especially useful to determine thyroid gland function and whether there are differences in function between lobes. Such information is important if one is considering performing hemithyroidectomy to control hyperthyroidism.

THYROID DISORDERS IN ADULT HORSES

Neoplasia

Probably the oldest described and documented abnormalities of the thyroid gland in the horse are hyperplasia and neoplasia. It is not uncommon to find mildly enlarged or neoplastic thyroid glands at necropsy of older horses that showed no outward evidence while the horse was alive. Schlotthauer[2] examined the thyroid glands of 100 consecutive horses at necropsy. He divided the gross and histologic evaluation of the glands into 4 groups: normal (34%), hyperplastic (20%), colloid goiter (9%), and adenomatous (37%). Since then, multiple reports of thyroid tumors have been published, describing hyperplastic nodules, adenomas, adenocarcinomas, carcinomas, and C-cell tumors.[31,32,35–50] It has been suggested that thyroid tumors are more common in horses older than 17 years.[46] Although it has been suggested that thyroid tumors occur more often in domestic animals living in iodine-deficient areas,[51] there have been no studies to show this to be true in horses. Most thyroid tumors in horses are benign and do not seem to metastasize.

In most reports, serum concentrations of thyroid hormones remained normal in horses with thyroid tumors, although occasionally, thyroid tumors have been associated with hypothyroidism[36,52,53] or hyperthyroidism.[31,32,49] Reported clinical signs of hypothyroidism include lethargy, exercise intolerance, and poor hair coat. Clinical signs of hyperthyroidism include weight loss, tachycardia, tachypnea, hyperactive behavior, ravenous appetite, alopecia, and cachexia.

Serum thyroid hormone concentrations should be measured in horses with enlarged thyroid glands. Additional diagnostics should include ultrasonography and biopsy and, depending on those results, a T_3 suppression test and/or nuclear scintigraphy may be indicated. The diet should be examined to make certain that iodine intake is appropriate because too little can result in goiter. The recommended daily iodine ingestion in adult horses is 0.007 mg/kg or 0.35 mg/kg dry matter diet, assuming consumption of 2% of body weight. Iodine should be increased to 0.4 mg/kg dry matter diet for the last trimester of pregnancy.[54]

If thyroid neoplasia is diagnosed, it is not necessary to remove the thyroid glands immediately if serum thyroid hormone concentrations are normal and the glands are not enlarged enough to compromise breathing or eating. If serum thyroid hormone concentrations are low, the horse can be supplemented with one of several products, described in more detail in the following sections. If the horse is hyperthyroid or if the glands begin enlarging rapidly, they should be surgically removed[55] and the horse placed on replacement therapy. If surgery is contemplated, it should be performed before the glands get large enough to complicate their removal. If the size of the gland is not a problem but the horse is hyperthyroid, propylthiouracil (PTU) can be administered orally to decrease concentrations of circulating thyroid hormones. PTU inhibits thyroid hormone synthesis by antagonizing thyroid peroxidase (catalyzes oxidation of iodide to iodine), inhibiting thyroglobulin synthesis, inhibiting thyroid follicular cell growth, and inhibiting the conversion of T_4 to T_3 (inhibits D1 deiodinase).[56] Use of PTU in horses was first described in an equine experimental model of hypothyroidism.[57–59] With a daily oral dose of 4 mg/kg it took approximately 4 weeks for horses to become hypothyroid. More recently, PTU (8 mg/kg/d) was administered orally to treat a hyperthyroid horse.[32] Once the serum concentrations of thyroid hormones decreased, this dose was given every other day. The dose of PTU should be titrated to keep thyroid hormones concentrations in the normal range. When administering PTU, gloves and mask should be worn.

Hypothyroidism

Disorders of thyroid function can result from alterations in TRH, TSH, or thyroid hormone synthesis or release, alterations in conversion to T_3 in peripheral tissues, and alterations in thyroid hormone receptor sensitivity. The prevalence of primary hypothyroidism in adult horses is very low. Autoimmune thyroid disease is common in humans and dogs, but, with the exception of one report, has not been described in horses. In the one study that is available,[60] 156 of 622 slaughtered horses from Eastern Europe were found to have grossly abnormal thyroid glands. In 80% of these 156 horses, histologic appearance was consistent with a Hashimoto thyroiditis–like disease, including variation in follicle size and shape, rarefaction of colloid, and lymphocytic infiltration and fibrosis. Serum obtained from 9 of these horses revealed higher thyroglobulin, antithyroglobulin, and antithyroid peroxidase autoantibody titers than in 9 healthy horses. Neither did the report indicate how the serum was obtained from the affected horses nor did it indicate what the time frame was in relation to the time of death. Thyroid hormone concentrations were not measured. There was no information on whether the horses exhibited any signs of hypothyroidism.

Extrapolating from humans and dogs, one might expect hypothyroidism in horses to be manifested as lethargy, cold intolerance, and weight gain or obesity. Traditionally, horses that were thought of as easy keepers, those that gained weight on little feed and tended to accumulate fat in the crest of the neck and over the rump, were considered to be hypothyroid. These horses were also thought to be prone to developing laminitis as well as various other problems, including infertility in mares, anhidrosis, and exertional rhabdomyolysis. Horses with these problems often were administered long-term supplemental thyroid hormones, either without actual thyroid hormone measurement or despite measurement of normal circulating concentrations. Evidence that has accumulated over the past 10 years suggests that many of the clinical signs traditionally associated with hypothyroidism in horses are more appropriately signs of equine metabolic syndrome or insulin resistance. Studies have also been unable to substantiate hypothyroidism as a cause for infertility in mares[61,62] or anhidrosis.[63] In reports of horses made hypothyroid by surgical thyroidectomy[64–71] or by PTU administration,[56–59] neither obesity nor laminitis occurred. In studies of young growing horses, thyroidectomy resulted in decreased growth rate, delayed physeal closure and tooth eruption, cold insensitivity, lethargy, a coarse hair coat, a coarse and thickened face, decreased rectal temperature, decreased serum phosphorus concentration, and increased serum cholesterol concentration.[64] However, in subsequent studies in adult horses, there were very few, if any, clinical signs associated with experimentally produced hypothyroidism. In addition, semen from thyroidectomized stallions is fertile,[66] and thyroidectomized mares are capable of conceiving and carrying foals to term.[64,66] Thyroidectomy also did not alter the response of blood lipids to feed deprivation.[68] Thyroidectomy has been shown to result in decreased resting heart rate, cardiac output, respiratory rate, and rectal temperature[71] and increased serum concentrations of triglycerides, cholesterol, and very-low-density lipoproteins.[67] However, despite statistical differences, all these measurements in adult horses remained within normal range, making it impossible to use them to help identify a hypothyroid horse clinically. To date, in a few published case reports of horses that were actually documented to be hypothyroid, clinical signs were primarily lethargy, exercise intolerance, and poor hair coat.[37,53,54] There is one report of keratoconjunctivitis sicca in a hypothyroid horse.[72] Overall, the number of horses documented to have naturally occurring primary hypothyroidism remains low.

Nonthyroidal Illness Syndrome (Euthyroid Sick Syndrome)

Nonthyroidal illness results in central hypothyroidism. Release of hypothalamic TRH is decreased by several mechanisms. Decreased leptin concentration (eg, from fasting or poor appetite) reduces the set point for thyroid hormone feedback inhibition of TRH release. At the same time, local concentrations of T_3 are increased, both by increased iodothyronine deiodinase D2 (eg, from sepsis or trauma), leading to increased conversion of T_4 to T_3 in the hypothalamus, and by decreased iodothyronine deiodinase D3 leading to decreased conversion of T_3 to diiodothyronine (T_2) (deactivation).[73] TSH release is also inhibited, partly because of the decreased TRH and secondarily to negative feedback from stress, glucocorticoids, and locally produced cytokines, including interleukin 6, tumor necrosis factor α, and interferon γ.[73] In addition, nonthyroidal illness can result in decreased thyroid hormone–binding proteins and decreased binding protein affinity and capacity.[73] This effect of illness decreases the serum concentrations of total T_4 or T_3, but has less of an effect on serum concentrations of the free fractions. In fact, if free fractions are measured by equilibrium dialysis or ultrafiltration, the free T_4 concentration is often normal or increased and there is only a modest decrease in concentration of free T_3.[73]

Nonthyroidal illness syndrome has been well described in humans and dogs. Most assume that the syndrome exists in horses, but few studies have documented it, much less characterized it in horses. Preliminary evidence suggests that nonthyroidal illness in horses and foals is similar to that in other species.[15,74] This is important because horses with nonthyroidal illness syndrome will have low thyroid hormone concentrations, especially total T_3 and T_4, which may lead to the misdiagnosis of primary hypothyroidism. In such cases, treatment of the underlying disease rather than thyroid hormone supplementation is indicated.

THYROID HORMONE SUPPLEMENTATION

Horses that have undergone thyroidectomy or that have been properly diagnosed as hypothyroid can be supplemented with T_4 or a combination of T_4 and T_3. T_4 is available in several forms. Iodinated casein contains approximately 1% T_4 and is given at 5 to 15 g/horse/d orally.[64] The recommended starting dosage of levothyroxine has been

20 μg/kg/d orally,[75,76] but more recent studies suggest that doses as high as 50 to 100 μg/kg/d may be well tolerated, at least for a short period.[29,30,77,78] It should be noted that horses in those studies were administered T_4 in a small meal of grain, which may have affected absorption, because fiber or bran cereal can decrease the oral absorption of thyroid hormones in humans.[79] Thus, the required dose of T_4 may vary, depending on whether it is given to fasted horses or if it is fed with a meal. Serum thyroid hormone concentrations should be monitored during supplementation so that dosages can be adjusted to maintain thyroid hormone levels in the normal range. If a sensitive TSH assay becomes commercially available, dosages should be adjusted to normalize TSH. In people receiving levothyroxine, it takes 4 weeks for thyroid hormone and TSH concentrations to stabilize.[79]

The controversial practice of administering thyroid hormones to obese euthyroid horses in an attempt to promote weight loss and decrease episodes of laminitis has received attention in the past 5 to 10 years. Anecdotally, many practitioners report that horses remain overweight despite thyroid hormone supplementation and that there is no evidence that the incidence of laminitis is altered. In fact, it would be difficult to design a study to test whether or not thyroid hormone supplementation alters the onset or severity of laminitis. However, the common practice has been to adjust the thyroid hormone dose to maintain serum thyroid hormone concentrations within the normal range. If this procedure is followed in a euthyroid horse, one is simply exchanging the horse's own thyroid hormones for a supplement. In addition, in many cases there has been no attempt to control or alter the diet. In order to lose weight, it is recommended that the feed intake be controlled at 1.5% to 2% of the desired body weight per day, preferably as grass hay or other feed that is low in soluble carbohydrates. If this diet is achieved, a horse is likely to lose weight, with or without thyroid hormone supplementation.

There is some evidence that thyroid hormone supplementation might be useful in accelerating weight loss and improving insulin sensitivity, which might decrease bouts of laminitis. Administration of increasing doses of levothyroxine at 2-week intervals (50–200 μg/kg/d) to 8 euthyroid horses increased serum total and free T_4 concentrations and blunted thyroid hormone and TSH responses to TRH. Serum concentrations of free T_3 were increased and TSH concentrations were decreased only at the highest dose. The horses showed no adverse clinical signs except agitation (also only at the highest dose) and lost weight.[29] Plasma concentrations of triglycerides, cholesterol, and very-low-density lipoproteins decreased, and insulin sensitivity increased.[77] It would be difficult to design a study to test whether or not thyroid hormone supplementation alters the onset or severity of laminitis.

Untreated hyperthyroidism or long-term T_4 administration in people can have undesirable effects, including loss of bone density,[80] tachycardia, increased heart rate variability, atrial premature contractions or atrial fibrillation,[81–83] left ventricular hypertrophy,[84] and increased risk of myocardial infarction and congestive heart failure.[80] To explore the potential effects of long-term thyroid hormone administration to euthyroid horses, Frank and colleagues[30,78] administered 48 mg (100 μg/kg/d) levothyroxine per day to 6 euthyroid mares for 48 weeks. Every 4 weeks they performed physical examinations, complete blood cell counts, and serum chemistry panels and measured serum concentrations of cardiac isoenzymes. They performed cardiac ultrasonographic examinations, TRH stimulation tests, and intravenous glucose tolerance tests at weeks 16, 32, and 48. This dose of levothyroxine increased the serum total T_4 concentrations 4 to 5 times the presupplementation concentrations. Serum total T_3 concentrations were decreased at week 32 but returned to the presupplementation concentrations by week 48. However, free fractions were not measured. At this level of supplementation, total T_4 and T_3 concentrations no longer responded to TRH. The horses lost weight, even though intake was not controlled or measured (horses spent time at pasture). Heart rate was variable, with no consistent pattern. Results of evaluation of blood remained within the reference range. Echocardiographic measurements remained fairly stable, except that the left ventricular free wall thickness appeared to be steadily increasing, ultimately becoming statistically significantly increased at 48 weeks. Fractional shortening was decreased at 16 and 32 weeks but remained within normal range; the clinical significance of this data is unclear. Resting serum insulin concentration and acute insulin response to glucose decreased, whereas insulin sensitivity increased. These changes were correlated to body weight, and it is impossible to determine whether they were caused directly by the thyroid hormone administration or indirectly by the weight loss. The investigators concluded that thyroid hormone supplementation may be useful in the treatment of obesity and insulin resistance.

THYROID HORMONES IN FOALS

When considering thyroid function in foals, it is important to know that serum thyroid hormone concentrations are much higher in neonates, slowly decreasing to adult concentrations over the first weeks of life.[74,85,86] For this reason, it is important to use age-matched reference ranges. Thyroid hormone and TSH concentrations from 18 normal foals aged less than 12 hours are given in **Table 2**.

Thyroid hormones are essential for normal organ development and growth, and, as might be expected, deficiencies result in more significant clinical problems in foals than adults. Thyroid disorders known to occur in foals include nonthyroidal illness syndrome,[74] congenital goiter, and a syndrome of musculoskeletal abnormalities associated with thyroid gland hyperplasia. Little more is known about these disorders since they were reviewed in a previous volume in the Veterinary Clinics of North America.[76]

Congenital Goiter

Enlarged thyroid glands at birth are associated with low serum thyroid hormone concentrations and can be caused by either too little[87,88] or too much[89–91] iodine in the mare's diet during gestation or by ingestion of goitrogenic plants. Clinical signs in these foals can be mild, with the foal exhibiting little more than the goiter, to a more severe presentation, with the foal born weak, with poor sucking and righting reflexes, hypothermia, and developmental abnormalities of the musculoskeletal system, including tendon contracture or rupture and delayed bone development,

Table 2
Normal baseline concentrations of thyroid hormones in equine neonates aged less than 12 hours (n = 18)

	Total T_4 nmol/L	Free T_4 pmol/L	Free T_4 by Dialysis pmol/L	Total T_3 nmol/L	Free T_3 pmol/L	TSH ng/mL
Range	238–337	46–118	78–184	3.4–10.8	2.4–20.3	0.12–0.72
Median	277	78	106	8.2	7.8	0.22
95% CI	268–296	70–90	96–125	6.3–8.5	6.6–11.6	0.21–0.41
Mean	282	80	110	7.4	9.1	0.31
SD	28.2	20.3	29.5	2.3	5.0	0.20

Abbreviation: CI, confidence interval.

particularly of the small cuboidal bones of the carpus and tarsus. The hair coat may also be sparse. Mustard has been suggested as a potential dietary goitrogen in the horse, and selenium deficiency may contribute. One of the most commonly identified causes of excessive iodine ingestion is kelp, a seaweed product. Mares supplemented with kelp remain euthyroid because the adult thyroid gland can increase iodine excretion to balance absorption. However, the fetal thyroid gland cannot autoregulate until very close to term. Excessive iodine ingestion by the mare crosses the placenta and inhibits the fetal thyroid gland, resulting in congenital goiter and hypothyroidism.

Treatment of these foals includes supportive care, correcting the mare's diet if necessary, and, if the foal is actually hypothyroid at the time of birth, thyroid hormone supplementation. Because T_3 has higher and more rapid biologic activity than T_4, a combination of T_3 and T_4 administration may be indicated in an extremely weak foal. However, dosage recommendations for foals are not well established. An attempt should be made to increase thyroid hormone concentrations to an appropriate level for the age of the foal. The current dosage recommendation for levothyroxine (T_4) for foals is 20 to 50 μg/kg/d orally, and for T_3 is 1 μg/kg/d orally.[92] Irvine[93] suggested that T_4 be given at 0.176 × body weight in kg × desired T_4 in μg/L/d and that the dose of T_3 would be one-third of the T_4 dose. Exercise should be restricted in foals born with incompletely ossified cuboidal bones and/or ruptured extensor tendons. Lightweight splints may be necessary to prevent foals from knuckling or to prevent collapse of the cuboidal bones. If used, splints must be applied carefully and monitored closely.

Thyroid Gland Hyperplasia and Musculoskeletal Deformity

A syndrome characterized by thyroid gland hyperplasia, increased gestational length, and musculoskeletal abnormalities (including mandibular prognathia, flexural limb deformities of the front legs, ruptured digital extensor tendons, and incomplete ossification of the carpal and tarsal bones) has been described, primarily in the Pacific Northwest region of the United States and Canada, but it has sporadically been reported elsewhere as well.[94–101] Despite prolonged gestation, foals are born dysmature and often have a silky hair coat. The cause is unknown, but nitrate, low iodine, low selenium, or goitrogenic plant ingestion by the mare during gestation has been proposed.[99,100] At the time of birth, baseline serum concentrations of T_4 and T_3 are usually within the normal neonatal ranges, but the response to TSH administration is decreased.[100] Because thyroid hormone concentrations are normal at the time of birth and because thyroid hormone supplementation often does not reverse the musculoskeletal changes in these foals, they are usually not administered.

REFERENCES

1. Sojka JE. Hypothyroidism in horses. Comp Cont Educ Pract Vet 1995;17:845–52.
2. Schlotthauer CF. The incidence and types of disease of the thyroid gland of adult horses. J Am Vet Med Assoc 1931;78:211–8.
3. Barrett KE, Barman SM, Boitano S, et al. The thyroid gland. In: Ganong's review of medical physiology. New York: McGraw-Hill; 2010. p. 301–14.
4. Cheng SY, Leonard JL, Davis PJ. Molecular aspects of thyroid hormone actions. Endocr Rev 2010;31:130 70.
5. Messer NT, Johnson PJ, Refsal KR, et al. Effect of food deprivation on baseline iodothyronine and cortisol concentrations in healthy, adult horses. Am J Vet Res 1995;56:116–21.

6. Messer NT, Ganjam VK, Nachreiner RF, et al. Effects of dexamethasone administration on serum thyroid hormone concentrations in clinically normal horses. J Am Vet Med Assoc 1995;206:63–6.
7. Morris DD, Garcia M. Thyroid-stimulating hormone: response test in healthy horses, and effect of phenylbutazone on equine thyroid hormones. Am J Vet Res 1983;44:503–7.
8. Morris DD, Garcia M. Effects of phenylbutazone and anabolic steroids on adrenal and thyroid gland function tests in healthy horses. Am J Vet Res 1985;46:359–64.
9. Sojka JE, Johnson MA, Bottoms GD. Serum triiodothyronine, total thyroxine, and free thyroxine concentrations in horses. Am J Vet Res 1993;54:52–5.
10. Ramirez S, Wolfsheimer KJ, Moore RM, et al. Duration of effects of phenylbutazone on serum total thyroxine and free thyroxine concentrations in horses. J Vet Intern Med 1997;11:371–4.
11. Schott HC, Marteniuk J, Refsal KR, et al. Thyroid hormone responses to endurance exercise [abstract]. J Vet Intern Med 1997;11:105.
12. Graves EA, Schott HC 2nd, Marteniuk JV, et al. Thyroid hormone responses to endurance exercise. Equine Vet J Suppl 2006;36:32–6.
13. Glade MJ, Reimers TJ. Effects of dietary energy supply on serum thyroxine, triiodothyronine and insulin concentrations in young horses. J Endocrinol 1985;104:93–8.
14. Swinker AM, McCurley JR, Jordan ER, et al. Effects of dietary excesses on equine serum thyroid hormone levels. J Anim Sci 1989;65(Suppl 1):255–6.
15. Breuhaus BA, Refsal KR, Beyerlein SL. Measurement of free thyroxine concentration in horses by equilibrium dialysis. J Vet Intern Med 2006;20:371–6.
16. Molina PE, Ashman R. Thyroid gland. In: Endocrine physiology. New York: McGraw-Hill; 2010. p. 75–100.
17. Kaptein EM, MacIntyre SS, Weiner JM, et al. Free thyroxine estimate in nonthyroidal illness: comparison of eight methods. J Clin Endocrinol Metab 1981;52:1073–7.
18. Ekins RP. Principles of measuring free thyroid hormone concentrations in serum. NuCompact 1985;16:305–13.
19. Alexander NM. Free thyroxin in serum: labeled thyroxin-analog methods fall short of their mark. Clin Chem 1986;32:417.
20. Nelson JC, Tomei RT. Direct determination of free thyroxin in undiluted serum by equilibrium dialysis/radioimmunoassay. Clin Chem 1988;34:1737–44.
21. Herbomez M, Forzy G, Gasser F, et al. Clinical evaluation of nine free thyroxine assays: persistent problems in particular populations. Clin Chem Lab Med 2003;41:942–7.
22. Schachter S, Nelson RW, Scott-Moncrieff C, et al. Comparison of serum-free thyroxine concentrations determined by standard equilibrium dialysis, modified equilibrium dialysis, and 5 radioimmunoassays in dogs. J Vet Intern Med 2004;18:259–64.
23. Beech J, Garcia M. Hormonal response to thyrotropin-releasing hormone in healthy horses and in horses with pituitary adenoma. Am J Vet Res 1985;46:1941–3.
24. Chen CL, Li WI. Effect of thyrotropin releasing hormone (TRH) on serum levels of thyroid hormones in Thoroughbred mares. J Equine Vet Sci 1986;6:58–61.
25. Held JP, Oliver JW. A sampling protocol for the thyrotropin-stimulating test in the horse. J Am Vet Med Assoc 1984;184:326–7.
26. Lothrup CD, Nolan HL. Equine thyroid function assessment with the thyrotropin-releasing hormone response test. Am J Vet Res 1986;47:942–4.

27. Harris P, Marlin D, Gray J. Equine thyroid function tests: a preliminary investigation. Br Vet J 1992;148:71–80.
28. Rothschild CM, Hines MT, Breuhaus BA, et al. Effects of trimethoprim-sulfadiazine on thyroid function of horses. J Vet Intern Med 2004;18:370–3.
29. Sommardahl CS, Frank N, Elliott SB, et al. Effects of oral administration of levothyroxine sodium on serum concentrations of thyroid gland hormones and responses to injections of thyrotropin-releasing hormone in healthy adult mares. Am J Vet Res 2005;66:1025–31.
30. Frank N, Buchanan BR, Elliott SB. Effects of long-term oral administration of levothyroxine sodium on serum thyroid hormone concentrations, clinicopathologic variables, and echocardiographic measurements in healthy adult horses. Am J Vet Res 2008;69:68–75.
31. Alberts MK, McCann JP, Woods PR. Hemithyroidectomy in a horse with confirmed hyperthyroidism. J Am Vet Med Assoc 2000;217:1051–4.
32. Tan RH, Davies SE, Crisman MV, et al. Propylthiouracil for treatment of hyperthyroidism in a horse. J Vet Intern Med 2008;22:1253–8.
33. Sarkar S. Benign thyroid disease: what is the role of nuclear medicine? Semin Nucl Med 2006;36:185–93.
34. Feeney DA, Anderson KL. Nuclear imaging and radiation therapy in canine and feline thyroid disease. Vet Clin North Am Small Anim Pract 2007;37:799–821.
35. Hillidge CJ, Sanecki RK, Theodorakis MC. Thyroid carcinoma in a horse. J Am Vet Med Assoc 1982;181:711–4.
36. Held JP, Patton CS, Toal RL, et al. Work intolerance in a horse with thyroid carcinoma. J Am Vet Med Assoc 1985;187:1044–5.
37. Joyce JR, Thompson RB, Kyzar JR, et al. Thyroid carcinoma in a horse. J Am Vet Med Assoc 1976;168:610–2.
38. Hani H, von Tscharner C, Straub R. Thyroid carcinoma with bone metastases in the horse. Schweiz Arch Tierheilkd 1979;121:413–20.
39. Turk JR, Nakata YJ, Leathers CW, et al. Ultimobranchial adenoma of the thyroid gland in a horse. Vet Pathol 1983;20:114–7.
40. Lucke VM, Lane JG. C-cell tumours of the thyroid in the horse. Equine Vet J 1984;16:28–30.
41. Yoshikawa T, Yoshikawa H, Oyamada T, et al. A follicular adenoma with C-cell hyperplasia in the equine thyroid. Nippon Juigaku Zasshi 1984;46:615–23.
42. van der Velden MA, Meulenaar H. Medullary thyroid carcinoma in a horse. Vet Pathol 1986;23:622–4.
43. Chiba S, Okada K, Numakunai S, et al. A case of equine thyroid follicular carcinoma accompanied with adenohypophysial adenoma. Nippon Juigaku Zasshi 1987;49:551–4.
44. Tateyama S, Tanimura N, Moritomo Y, et al. The ultimobranchial remnant and its hyperplasia or adenoma in equine thyroid gland. Nippon Juigaku Zasshi 1988; 50:714–22.
45. Hovda LR, Shaftoe S, Rose ML, et al. Mediastinal squamous cell carcinoma and thyroid carcinoma in an aged horse. J Am Vet Med Assoc 1990;197:1187–9.
46. Dalefield RR, Palmer DN. The frequent occurrence of thyroid tumours in aged horses. J Comp Pathol 1994;110:57–64.
47. Kuwamura M, Shirota A, Yamate J, et al. C-cell adenoma containing variously sized thyroid follicles in a horse. J Vet Med Sci 1998;60:387–9.
48. Ramirez S, McClure JJ, Moore RM, et al. Hyperthyroidism associated with a thyroid adenocarcinoma in a 21-year-old gelding. J Vet Intern Med 1998;12: 475–7.

49. De Cock HE, MacLachlan NJ. Simultaneous occurrence of multiple neoplasms and hyperplasias in the adrenal and thyroid gland of the horse resembling multiple endocrine neoplasia syndrome: case report and retrospective identification of additional cases. Vet Pathol 1999;36:633–6.
50. Ueki H, Kowatari Y, Oyamada T, et al. Non-functional C-cell adenoma in aged horses. J Comp Pathol 2004;131:157–65.
51. Capen CC. The endocrine glands. In: Jubb KV, Kennedy PC, Palmer N, editors. Pathology of domestic animals. 3rd edition. New York: Academic Press; 1985. p. 266–82.
52. Stanley O, Hillidge CJ. Alopecia associated with hypothyroidism in a horse. Equine Vet J 1982;14:165–7.
53. Hillyer MN, Taylor FG. Cutaneous manifestations of suspected hypothroidism in a horse. Equine Vet Educ 1992;4:116–8.
54. National Research Council. Nutrient requirements of horses. 6th edition. Washington, DC: National Academy of Sciences; 2007.
55. El Sheikh M, McGregor AM. Antithyroid drugs: their mechanism of action and clinical use. In: Weetman AP, Grossman A, editors. Pharmacotherapeutics of the thyroid gland. New York: Springer-Verlag; 1997. p. 188–206.
56. Elce YA, Ross MW, Davidson EJ, et al. Unilateral thyroidectomy in 6 horses. Vet Surg 2003;32:187–90.
57. Breuhaus BA. Thyroid-stimulating hormone in adult euthyroid and hypothyroid horses. J Vet Intern Med 2002;16:109–15.
58. Johnson PJ, Messer NT, Ganjam VK, et al. Effects of propylthiouracil and bromocryptine on serum concentrations of thyrotrophin and thyroid hormones in normal female horses. Equine Vet J 2003;35:296–301.
59. Cartmill JA, Thompson DLJ, Gentry LR, et al. Effects of dexamethasone, glucose infusion, adrenocorticotropin, and propylthiouracil on plasma leptin concentrations in horses. Domest Anim Endocrinol 2003;24:1–14.
60. Perillo A, Passantino G, Passantino L, et al. First observation of an Hashimoto thyroiditis-like disease in horses from eastern Europe: histopathological and immunological findings. Immunopharmacol Immunotoxicol 2005;27:241–53.
61. Gutierrez CV, Riddle WT, Bramlage LR. Serum thyroxine concentrations and pregnancy rates 15 to 16 days after ovulation in broodmares. J Am Vet Med Assoc 2002;220:64–6.
62. Meredith TB, Dobrinski I. Thyroid function and pregnancy status in broodmares. J Am Vet Med Assoc 2004;224:892–4.
63. Breuhaus BA. Thyroid function in anhidrotic horses. J Vet Intern Med 2009;23: 168–73.
64. Lowe JE, Baldwin BH, Foote RH, et al. Equine hypothyroidism: the long term effects of thyroidectomy on metabolism and growth in mares and stallions. Cornell Vet 1974;64:276–95.
65. Lowe JE, Baldwin BH, Foote RH, et al. Semen characteristics in thyroidectomized stallions. J Reprod Fertil Suppl 1975;23:81–6.
66. Lowe JE, Foote RH, Baldwin BH, et al. Reproductive patterns in cyclic and pregnant thyroidectomized mares. J Reprod Fertil Suppl 1987;35:281–8.
67. Frank N, Sojka JE, Latour MA, et al. Effect of hypothyroidism on blood lipid concentrations in horses. Am J Vet Res 1999;60:730–3.
68. Frank N, Sojka JE, Latour MA. Effects of hypothyroidism and withholding of feed on plasma lipid concentrations, concentration and composition of very-low-density lipoprotein, and plasma lipase activity in horses. Am J Vet Res 2003;64:823–8.

69. Frank N, Sojka JE, Patterson BW, et al. Effect of hypothyroidism on kinetics of metabolism of very-low-density lipoprotein in mares. Am J Vet Res 2003;64: 1052–8.
70. Frank N, Sojka JE, Latour MA. Effect of hypothyroidism on the blood lipid response to higher dietary fat intake in mares. J Anim Sci 2004;82:2640–6.
71. Vischer CM, Foreman JH, Constable PD, et al. Hemodynamic effects of thyroidectomy in sedentary horses. Am J Vet Res 1999;60:14–21.
72. Schwarz BC, Sallmutter T, Nell B. Keratoconjunctivitis sicca attributable to parasympathetic facial nerve dysfunction associated with hypothyroidism in a horse. J Am Vet Med Assoc 2008;233:1761–6.
73. Warner MH, Beckett GJ. Mechanisms behind the non-thyroidal illness syndrome: an update. J Endocrinol 2010;205:1–13.
74. Breuhaus BA, LaFevers DH. Thyroid function in normal, sick and premature foals. J Vet Intern Med 2005;19:445.
75. Chen CL, McNulty ME, McNulty BA, et al. Serum levels of thyroxine and triiodothyronine in mature horses following oral administration of synthetic thyroxine (Synthroid R). J Equine Vet Sci 1984;4:5–6.
76. Frank N, Sojka J, Messer NT. Equine thyroid dysfunction. Vet Clin North Am Equine Pract 2002;18:305–19.
77. Frank N, Sommardahl CS, Eiler H, et al. Effects of oral administration of levothyroxine sodium on concentrations of plasma lipids, concentration and composition of very-low-density lipoproteins, and glucose dynamics in healthy adult mares. Am J Vet Res 2005;66:1032–8.
78. Frank N, Elliott SB, Boston RC. Effects of long-term oral administration of levothyroxine sodium on glucose dynamics in healthy adult horses. Am J Vet Res 2008;69:76–81.
79. Woeber KA. Update on the management of hyperthyroidism and hypothyroidism. Arch Fam Med 2000;9:743–7.
80. Sawin CT. Thyroid disease in older persons. In: Braverman LE, editor. Diseases of the thyroid. 2nd edition. Totowa (NJ): Humana Press; 2003. p. 85–105.
81. Biondi B, Fazio S, Carella C, et al. Cardiac effects of long term thyrotropin-suppressive therapy with levothyroxine. J Clin Endocrinol Metab 1993;77: 334–8.
82. Sawin CT, Geller A, Wolf PA, et al. Low serum thyrotropin concentrations as a risk factor for atrial fibrillation in older persons. N Engl J Med 1994;331: 1249–52.
83. Casu M, Cappi C, Patrone V, et al. Sympatho-vagal control of heart rate variability in patients treated with suppressive doses of l-thyroxine for thyroid cancer. Eur J Endocrinol 2005;152:819–24.
84. Shapiro LE, Sievert R, Ong L, et al. Minimal cardiac effects in asymptomatic athyreotic patients chronically treated with thyrotropin-suppressive doses of l-thyroxine. J Clin Endocrinol Metab 1997;82:2592–5.
85. Irvine CH, Evans MJ. Post-natal changes in total and free thyroxine and triiodothyronine in foal serum. J Reprod Fertil 1975;23(Suppl):709–15.
86. Chen CL, Riley AM. Serum thyroxine and triiodothyronine concentrations in neonatal foals and mature horses. Am J Vet Res 1981;42:1415–7.
87. Hintz HF, Ralston SL. The horse industry and feeding horses for optional reproduction and growth. In: Naylor JM, Ralston SL, editors. Large animal clinical nutrition. St Louis (MO): Mosby; 1991. p. 407–16.
88. Osame S, Ichajo S. Clinicopathological observations on thoroughbred foals with enlarged thyroid gland. J Vet Med Sci 1994;56:771–2.

89. Baker HJ, Lindsey JR. Equine goiter due to excess dietary iodine. J Am Vet Med Assoc 1968;153:1618–30.
90. Drew B, Barber WP, Williams DG. The effect of excess dietary iodine on pregnant mares and foals. Vet Rec 1975;97:93–5.
91. Durham AE. Congenital goitre in two colt foals born to mares fed excess iodine during pregnancy. Equine Vet Educ 1995;7:239–41.
92. Madigan JE. Endocrine problems. In: Madigan JE, editor. Manual of equine neonatal medicine. Woodland (CA): Live Oak Publishing; 1994. p. 206–9.
93. Irvine CH. Hypothyroidism in the foal. Equine Vet J 1984;16:302–5.
94. Shaver JR, Fretz PB, Doige CE, et al. Skeletal manifestations of suspected hypothyroidism in two foals. J Equine Med Surg 1979;3:269–75.
95. McLaughlin BG, Doige CE. A study of ossification of carpal and tarsal bones in normal and hypothyroid foals. Can Vet J 1982;23:164–8.
96. McLaughlin BG, Doige CE, McLaughlin PS. Thyroid hormone levels in foals with congenital musculoskeletal lesions. Can Vet J 1986;27:264–7.
97. Allen AL, Doige CE, Fretz PB, et al. Hyperplasia of the thyroid gland and concurrent musculoskeletal deformities in western Canadian foals: reexamination of a previously described syndrome. Can Vet J 1994;35:31–8.
98. Fretz PB. Congenital hypothyroidism-dysmaturity syndrome in western Canadian foals: clinical manifestations, management, treatment, prognosis, and follow-up. In: Proceedings of the 40th Convention of the American Association of Equine Practitioners. Lexington (KY): The American Association of Equine Practitioners; 1994. p. 63.
99. Allen AL, Townsend HG, Doige CE, et al. A case–control study of the congenital hypothyroidism and dysmaturity syndrome of foals. Can Vet J 1996;37:349–58.
100. Hines MT, Gay C, Talcott T. Congenital hypothyroidism and dysmaturity syndrome of foals: diagnosis and possible risk factors. In: Proceedings 15th American College of Veterinary Internal Medicine, Lake Buena Vista. Lakewood (CO): ACVIM; 1997. p. 363–4.
101. Allen AL, Fretz PB, Card CE, et al. The effects of partial thyroidectomy on the development of the equine fetus. Equine Vet J 1998;30:53–9.

Disorders of Calcium and Phosphate Metabolism in Horses

Ramiro E. Toribio, DVM, MS, PhD

KEYWORDS

- Hypocalcemia • Hypercalcemia • Parathyroid • Horse • Foal
- Hyperphosphatemia

CALCIUM

Several cellular processes (intracellular, extracellular, physiologic, and pathologic) depend on calcium as a regulatory ion. Calcium is necessary for blood coagulation, neuromuscular excitability, muscle contraction, enzymatic activation, hormone secretion, cell division, and cell membrane stability.[1] Calcium is also central to cell death by participating in free radical production, cytokine release, protease activation, and apoptosis. Because of its physiologic and pathologic functions, keeping extracellular calcium concentrations within a narrow range is important.[1] Calcium is found in 3 main compartments: *the skeleton, soft tissues*, *and the extracellular fluid* where it has structural and nonstructural functions. Approximately 99% of the total body calcium is in the skeleton as hydroxyapatite crystals, providing support against gravity, protecting internal organs (brain, spinal cord, lungs, heart), acting as a niche for blood-forming elements, and serving as a reservoir for calcium. The rest of the calcium is in the cell membrane, mitochondria, endoplasmic reticulum (0.9%), and in the extracellular fluid (0.1%).[2] Cytosolic free calcium concentrations are low. In equine blood, calcium is found in free or ionized form (50%–58%); bound to proteins (40%–45%); and complexed to anions, such as citrate, bicarbonate, phosphate, and lactate (5%–10%) (**Fig. 1**).[1–6] Free or ionized calcium (Ca^{2+}) is the biologically active form of calcium. Albumin is the main calcium-binding protein and its affinity for Ca^{2+} is pH-dependent. In acidosis there is decreased Ca^{2+} binding to albumin (higher blood Ca^{2+}); whereas, in alkalosis blood Ca^{2+} concentrations are lower. Total calcium concentrations remain unchanged. Hypoalbuminemia results in total hypocalcemia (pseudohypocalcemia) with Ca^{2+} concentrations within the normal range. Plasma and serum calcium concentrations are lower in foals than in adult horses.[7]

1 mg/dL $\times$ 0.25 = mmol/L; 1 mmol/L = 4 mg/dL of calcium.

Department of Veterinary Clinical Sciences, College of Veterinary Medicine, The Ohio State University, 601 Vernon Tharp Street, Columbus, OH 43210, USA
E-mail address: toribio.1@osu.edu

Vet Clin Equine 27 (2011) 129–147
doi:10.1016/j.cveq.2010.12.010 vetequine.theclinics.com

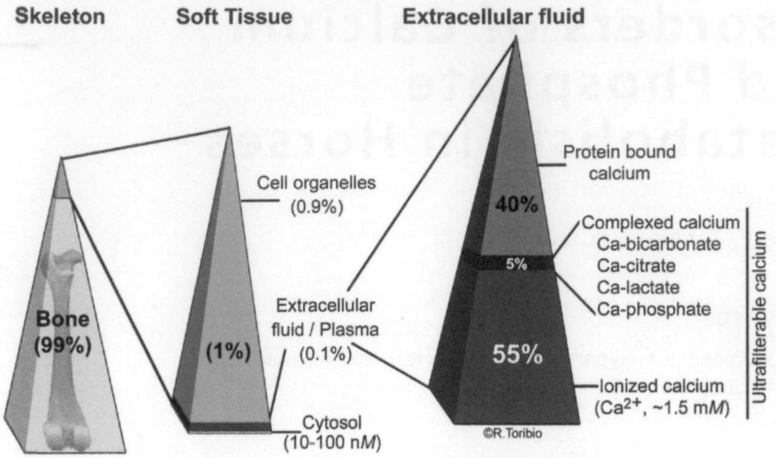

Fig. 1. Calcium distribution in the body. Around 99% of the total calcium in the body is in bone with the remaining 1% present in the extracellular fluid (0.1%) and cellular organelles (0.9%). In the extracellular compartment, calcium exists as a free, ionized or active form (Ca^{2+}), bound to proteins, and complexed to anions, such as bicarbonate, phosphate, citrate, and lactate. In horses, serum ionized calcium represents 50% to 58% of the total extracellular calcium.[4–6] Ionized and complex calcium are filtered through the glomerulus (ultrafilterable) but are rapidly reabsorbed by the nephron. (*Courtesy of* Ramiro E. Toribio, DVM, MS, PhD, Columbus, OH.)

As for calcium, total magnesium in blood is bound to proteins, complexed to anions and free or ionized (Mg^{2+}; active). See the article by Stewart elsewhere in this issue for further exploration of this topic.

PHOSPHORUS

Phosphorus represents approximately 1.0% of the body weight, with most (85%) located in the bone matrix as hydroxyapatite, 15.0% in blood and soft tissues, and less than 0.1% in the extracellular fluid. In blood and soft tissue, phosphorus is the major intracellular anion existing in organic (phospholipids, nucleic acids, phosphoproteins, creatine phosphate, adenosine triphosphate, cyclic adenosine monophosphate, nicotinamide adenine dinucleotide phosphate, 2,3-diphosphoglycerate) and inorganic forms. Similar to free cytosolic calcium, free cytosolic phosphate concentration is low. In blood, phosphorus exists as organic and inorganic phosphates. Organic phosphate consists of phosphate esters (phospholipids) bound to proteins and blood cells, representing most of the phosphorus in circulation (70%); however, only inorganic phosphate (P_i) is measured by routine methods. P_i is found as ionized phosphate (approximately 50%), complexed with cations (Na^+, Ca^{2+}, Mg^{2+}; approximately 35%), and bound to proteins (approximately 15%). Four forms of P_i exist in biologic fluids: H_3PO_4, $H_2PO_4^-$, HPO_4^{2-}, PO_3^{2-}; however, at physiologic pH only divalent (HPO_4^{2-}) and monovalent ($H_2PO_4^-$) are present at significant concentrations. The average valence of serum P_i of −1.8, giving a milliequivalency of 1.8 mEq per 1 mmol of P_i. 1 mmol/L = 3.1 mg/dL; mg/dl × 0.323 = mmol/L.

Phosphate plays essential roles in muscle contraction; neurologic function; enzyme activity; electrolyte transport; oxygen transport; gene transcription; and in the metabolism of proteins, carbohydrates, and fats.[8] Unlike Ca^{2+}, serum P_i has more fluctuations that are influenced by diet, age, physiologic status, activity, diseases, glycemia, hormones, and quality of sample (pH, hemolysis, hyperlipemia, hyperproteinemia, gammopathies). Serum P_i ranges from 2.5 to 5.0 mg/dL (0.8–1.6 mmol/L) in adult horses and is higher (up to 8.0 mg/dL) in foals. Serum P_i is not a reliable marker of body stores but is considered a better indicator of dietary intake and body status when compared with serum Ca^{2+} because P_i homeostasis is not precise.

REQUIREMENTS, ABSORPTION, AND ELIMINATION

The requirements of calcium and phosphorus depend on age, physiologic status, and physical activity. Although there is no nutritional drive for calcium, there appears to be a drive for phosphorus because horses with phosphorus deficiency will eat or lick materials, such as dirt, rocks, and bones (pica). A balanced equine diet must have 0.15% to 1.5% of calcium and 0.15% to 0.6% of phosphorus in feed dry matter. Calcium/phosphorus ratios less than 1:1 can have negative effects on skeletal development; however, ratios as high as 6:1 may not be detrimental in growing animals as long as phosphorus intake is adequate.[9] Adult horses should receive around 40 mg of calcium/kg/day. Pregnant mares require 50 to 60 g of calcium/d; whereas, lactating mares and growing horses require 50 to 75 g of calcium/d. Average horses should absorb 20 to 25 mg of calcium and 10 to 12 mg of phosphorus/kg/d to balance losses.[10–12]

Compared with other species, horses absorb a larger proportion (up to 75%) of dietary calcium,[13] which primarily takes place in the proximal small intestine (**Fig. 2**).[12,14] Calcium absorption is inhibited by dietary phosphate (phytate) and oxalates.[15,16] Plants containing high amounts of oxalates are associated with pathologies of calcium deficiency. The dietary cation-anion balance (DCAB) affects intestinal calcium absorption; diets with a low DCAB (anionic, acid) increase calcium absorption.[17] In horses, glucocorticoids decrease intestinal calcium absorption, decrease bone resorption, and increase the urinary excretion of calcium.[18,19] Calcium elimination depends on physiologic status, amount of calcium ingested, substances that interfere with calcium

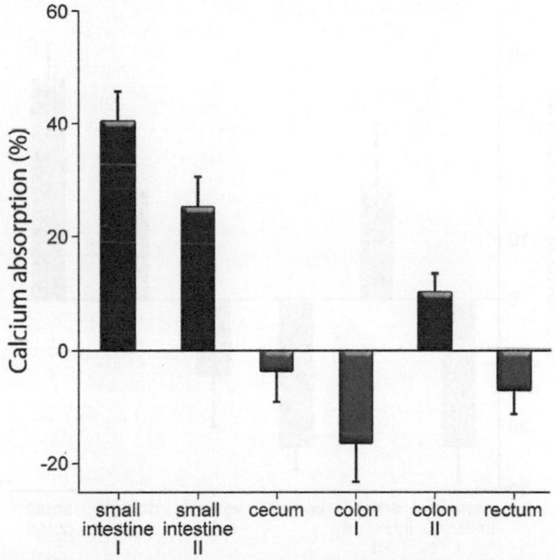

Fig. 2. Intestinal absorption of calcium in horses. As shown, most calcium absorption takes place in the small intestine and absorption in the large intestine is minimal. (*Adapted from* Schryver HF, Craig PH, Hintz HF, et al. The site of calcium absorption in the horse. J Nutr 1970;100:1127–31; with permission.)

absorption, and diseases. Calcium is eliminated through the kidneys, milk, sweat, feces, and the fetus. Most renal reabsorption of Ca^{2+} (>70%) takes place in the proximal tubules and the fractional excretion of Ca^{2+} in horses is high (5%–10%).[20,21] Endogenous losses of calcium are around 20 to 25 mg/kg/BW/d.[10] With a 50% calcium digestibility, a 500 kg horse requires 20 g of calcium to replace losses, or 40 mg/kg/d; these requirements are higher in growing and lactating animals.

Phosphorus absorption in horses ranges from 30% to 55% and occurs in the small and large intestines (**Fig. 3**).[12,22,23] Dietary aluminum and phytate reduce P_i absorption. Most renal P_i reabsorption (>80%) occurs in the proximal tubules and the urinary fractional excretion of P_i in horses is low (<0.5%). Serum P_i is a better indicator of dietary phosphorus intake and status than serum calcium concentrations. The urinary fractional clearance of calcium and phosphorus have been proposed as a tool to estimate intake.[24] However, interpretation of calcium clearance is difficult because of the large and variable amounts of calcium eliminated in the equine urine.[25] Chronic excess of phosphorus is associated with signs of calcium deficiency, including abnormal cartilage and bone development, lameness, fractures, and osteodystrophia fibrosa (nutritional secondary hyperparathyroidism). Chronic phosphorus deficiency is manifested as weight loss, weakness, depraved appetite (pica), lameness, and developmental orthopedic diseases (DOD). Calcium and phosphorus content and availability in some mineral supplements are presented in **Tables 1** and **2**.

CALCIUM AND PHOSPHORUS HOMEOSTASIS

Extracellular Ca^{2+} concentrations are controlled by a homeostatic system that includes 3 body systems (kidney, intestine, and bone) and 3 hormones (parathyroid hormone [PTH], calcitonin [CT], and 1,25-dihydroxyvitamin D_3 [$1,25(OH)_2D_3$] or calcitriol).[3,5,26] Mg^{2+} is also involved in Ca^{2+} homeostasis; PTH release, PTH action, and $1,25(OH)_2D_3$ synthesis are Mg^{2+}-dependent processes. A decrease in extracellular Ca^{2+}

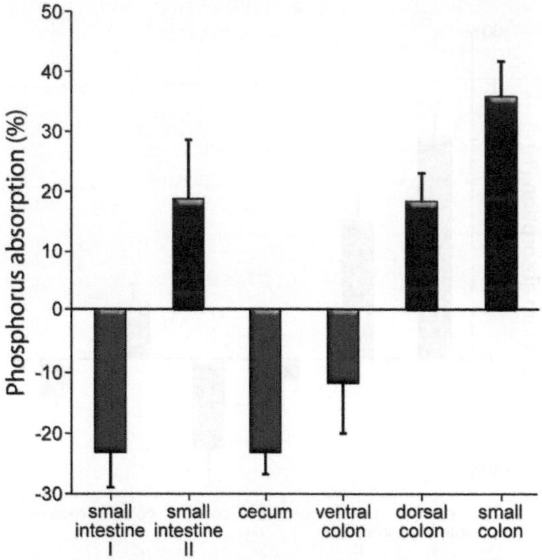

Fig. 3. Intestinal absorption of phosphorus in horses. Although some absorption takes place in the small intestine, most phosphorus absorption occurs in the large intestine. (*Adapted from* Schryver HF, Hintz HF, Craig PH, et al. Site of phosphorus absorption from the intestine of the horse. J Nutr 1972;102:143–7; with permission.)

Table 1
Calcium and phosphorus content in some mineral supplements

Supplement	Ca (%)	P (%)
Calcium carbonate	34.0	0
Defluorinated phosphate	32.0	15
Bone meal	30.0	14
Dicalcium phosphate	27.0	21
Monocalcium phosphate	17.0	21
Monosodium phosphate	0.0	22
Calcium gluconate 23%	2.14	0

Data from Toribio RE. Disorders of calcium and phosphorus. In: Reed SM, Bayly WM, Sellon DC, editors. Equine internal medicine. St Louis (MO): Saunders/Elsevier; 2010. p. 1277–91.

concentrations increase PTH secretion by the parathyroid gland, which in turn acts in the kidney to increase calcium reabsorption and $1,25(OH)_2D_3$ synthesis and in bone to increase osteoclastic bone resorption (**Fig. 4**).[1,21] PTH also increases the urinary excretion of phosphorus (phosphaturic hormone). The hormone $1,25(OH)_2D_3$ increases intestinal absorption and renal reabsorption of Ca^{2+} and P_i. An increase in Ca^{2+} leads to CT secretion by the C cells of the thyroid gland to inhibit osteoclastic activity. Parathyroid hormone-related protein (PTHrP) is an autocrine/paracrine factor that activates the PTH receptor and is important for Ca^{2+} homeostasis in the fetus but not in adults.[27,28] PTHrP concentrations are elevated in various equine malignancies (see later discussion).

Serum P_i concentrations are regulated by intestinal absorption and renal reabsorption. Rapid translocations of P_i can occur between the intracellular and extracellular P_i pools. The kidney is the major regulator of P_i concentrations.[1] PTH, vitamin D, and phosphatonins are critical hormones in P_i homeostasis.[1,8,29] Phosphatonins represent a series of endocrine factors (fibroblast growth factor-23[FGF-23], secreted frizzled related protein-4 [sFRP-4]) that increase urinary P_i excretion.[29] As previously mentioned, P_i homeostasis is not as precise as that of Ca^{2+}.

CALCIUM DISORDERS

Disorders of calcium regulation include hypocalcemia and hypercalcemia, which can be acute or chronic, and often associated with abnormal phosphate and magnesium

Table 2
Availability of calcium and phosphorus in feeds and supplements for horses

Source	Ca (%)	P (%)
Corn	—	38
Timothy hay	70	42
Alfalfa hay	77	38
Wheat bran	—	34
Limestone	67	—
Dicalcium phosphate	73	44
Bone meal	71	46
Monosodium phosphate	—	47
Calcium gluconate 23%	100[a]	0

[a] From intravenous administration.

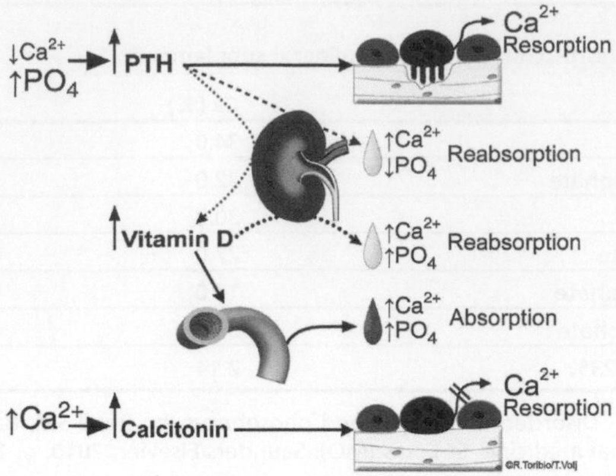

Fig. 4. Calcium and phosphate homeostasis. A decrease in extracellular Ca^{2+} concentrations or an increase in phosphate (PO4) concentrations leads to a PTH release from the parathyroid gland, which in turn increases renal reabsorption of Ca^{2+}, renal activation of vitamin D, urinary PO4 excretion, and bone resorption. In turn, vitamin D increases intestinal absorption and renal reabsorption of Ca^{2+} and PO_4. An increase in Ca^{2+} concentration stimulates the thyroid gland to secrete calcitonin to inhibit osteoclastic bone resorption. (*Courtesy of* Ramiro E. Toribio, DVM, MS, PhD, and Tim Vojt, Columbus, OH.)

metabolism. Clinical signs depend on how severe hypocalcemia or hypercalcemia is and how rapid it develops. Specific pathologic conditions of calcium dysregulation include hypoparathyroidism,[30,31] primary hyperparathyroidism,[32] nutritional secondary hyperparathyroidism,[33] renal failure,[34] humoral hypercalcemia of malignancy,[35–37] vitamin D toxicity,[38] exercise-induced hypocalcemia,[39] idiopathic hypocalcemia of foals,[40] cantharidiasis,[41] and sepsis.[5,42,43]

Hypocalcemic Disorders

Equine conditions associated with acute hypocalcemia are listed in **Box 1**. Signs of acute hypocalcemia result from increased neuromuscular excitability and decreased smooth muscle cell contractility; whereas, chronic calcium deficiency presents as abnormal cartilage and bone development, aberrant mineralization, DOD, and lameness. Extracellular Ca^{2+} concentrations affect the voltage at which Na^{+} channels are activated; Ca^{2+} acts as a Na^{+} channel antagonists by decreasing Na^{+} permeability and increasing the depolarization threshold. Thus, a decrease in Ca^{2+} concentrations leads to hyperactivation of Na^{+} channels: hyperexcitability that manifests as muscle fasciculations, tremors, tetany, and seizures. Tachycardia and cardiac arrhythmias may be present; however, bradycardia may occur in severe hypocalcemia. As Ca^{2+} and Mg^{2+} homeostasis are linked, it is not unusual for horses with hypocalcemia to also have low Mg^{2+} concentrations.

Horses with acute hypocalcemia may develop sustained skeletal muscular contractions or tetany. Any horse with severe hypocalcemia can develop tetany, although it is more frequent in lactating mares and horses transported for long distances. In mares, tetany may occur immediately before foaling up to the end of the lactation period. Mares producing large amounts of milk and eating diets low in calcium, in lush pastures, or performing physical work are at a higher risk. Clinical signs include depression, ataxia, anxiety, muscle fasciculations and tremors, spasticity, tachypnea, dysphagia, hypersalivation, hyperhidrosis, and colic.[44]

Box 1
Equine conditions associated with acute hypocalcemia

Colic
Enterocolitis
Sepsis and endotoxemia
Endurance exercise
Lactation and transport
Acute renal failure
Rhabdomyolysis
Pleuropneumonia
Pancreatitis
Furosemide administration
Hypoparathyroidism
Hypomagnesemia
Cantharidin toxicosis
Dystocia and retained placenta
Hypocalcemic tetany

Hypocalcemic seizures

Similar to hypocalcemic tetany, a decrease of Ca^{2+} concentration in the central nervous system increases neuroexcitability. Hypocalcemic seizures have been reported in foals and horses with hypocalcemia, sepsis, and hypoparathyroidism.[40] In general, horses and foals with hypocalcemic seizures have hypomagnesemia. Clinical signs usually improve with calcium treatment, although some animals may require repeated treatments with calcium and magnesium salts to improve. Antiseizure therapy or sedation may be required. The prognosis for these animals is guarded because repeated treatments are required to control clinical signs and some horses remain refractory to medical therapy.

Synchronous diaphragmatic flutter

Horses and foals with severe hypocalcemia may develop a rhythmic movement on the flank from diaphragmatic contractions that are synchronous with the heartbeat. This condition is known as synchronous diaphragmatic flutter (SDF) or *thumps*, and has been reported in horses with gastrointestinal disease, sepsis, lactation tetany, blister beetle toxicosis, endurance exercise, hypoparathyroidism, and alkalosis.[5,31,45–49] SDF can also be present in hypocalcemic foals. Hypomagnesemia is a frequent finding in animals with SDF. Depolarization of the right atrium stimulates action potentials in the hyperexcitable phrenic nerve as it crosses over the heart. SDF is frequent in horses after prolonged exercise in which there are major electrolytes losses (Ca^{2+}, Na^{+}, K^{+}, Mg^{2+}, Cl^{-}) from excessive sweating.[50,51] Exercising horses often develop alkalosis from hyperventilation (respiratory alkalosis) and chloride loss in the sweat (metabolic hypoohloromic alkalosis).[52] Alkalosis results in increased binding of Ca^{2+} and Mg^{2+} to albumin, leading to ionized hypocalcemia and hypomagnesemia. Hypomagnesemia should always be included in the differential diagnosis of hypocalcemia and SDF (see the article by Stewart elsewhere in this issue for further exploration of this topic).

Ileus and retained placenta

The development of ileus and retained placenta during hypocalcemia is in part a consequence of decreased smooth muscle tone and contractility. Although the Ca^{2+} required for skeletal muscle contraction comes from the sarcoplasmic reticulum, the source of Ca^{2+} for smooth muscle contraction is the extracellular space. In addition, smooth muscle cells have less Na^{+} and more Ca^{2+} voltage-gated channels than skeletal muscle fibers, and therefore, Na^{+} is less important for the action potential and muscle contraction. For these reasons, any condition associated with hypocalcemia can impair smooth muscle contractility that clinically manifests as ileus, poor uterine tone, or retained placenta. The administration of calcium salts should be considered in horses with ileus or retained placenta.

Hypoparathyroidism

Although rare, hypoparathyroidism has been documented in horses and foals.[31,46,53] Primary hypoparathyroidism results from decreased secretion of PTH; whereas, secondary hypoparathyroidism results from magnesium depletion or inflammatory cytokines (sepsis). In humans, various genetic mutations are linked to primary hypoparathyroidism; however, this has not been proven in any domestic animal. Hypoparathyroidism should be suspected in any horse or foal with refractory hypocalcemia. Clinical signs are those of hypocalcemia, including hyperexcitability, SDF, ataxia, seizures, tachycardia, tachypnea, muscle fasciculations, bruxism, stiff gait, recumbency, ileus, and colic.[31,44,46] Laboratory findings include hypocalcemia, hyperphosphatemia, hypercalciuria, hypophosphaturia, and low or normal serum PTH concentrations. Hypomagnesemia may be present.[31,46] Secondary (functional or acquired) hypoparathyroidism per se has not been documented in horses or foals; however, hypocalcemia and impaired parathyroid gland function occur in critically ill foals and horses, and the author thinks this is a form of secondary hypoparathyroidism.[40,54] In foals, this condition is known as *neonatal idiopathic hypocalcemia*.[40] Prognosis for survival in foals with refractory hypocalcemia is poor.

Hypocalcemia in critically ill horses and foals

Sepsis and endotoxemia are the most common cause of hypocalcemia in critically ill equine patients. Hypocalcemia is common in horses with severe gastrointestinal disease[5] and in septic foals.[54] The pathogenesis of hypocalcemia in patients with sepsis is multifactorial, including parathyroid gland dysfunction, intracellular calcium sequestration, and intestinal losses.[5,44] Inflammatory mediators known to be increased in horses with gastrointestinal disease, sepsis, and endotoxemia impair equine parathyroid cell function[20] and likely are involved in the pathogenesis of hypocalcemia in critically ill horses and foals.

Exercise-induced hypocalcemia

Horses under intense physical activity develop electrolyte and acid-base abnormalities. Hypocalcemia and hypomagnesemia are consistent findings in exercising horses. Hypocalcemia may result from Ca^{2+} losses in the sweat; increased Ca^{2+} binding to albumin, lactate, phosphate, and bicarbonate during alkalosis; and parathyroid gland dysfunction.[39]

Equine cantharidiasis

Blister beetle toxicosis (cantharidiasis) is primarily reported in the Southwestern and Midwestern United States and results from the ingestion of alfalfa contaminated with blister beetles (*Epicauta spp.*) that produce cantharidin (cantharidic acid), an irritant of intestinal and urinary mucosal surfaces. Consistent laboratory abnormalities with cantharidiasis are acute hypocalcemia and hypomagnesemia. The pathogenesis of hypocalcemia is unclear but severe gastrointestinal disease and acute renal failure/tubular necrosis are the most likely reasons. Clinical signs are those of acute hypocalcemia.

Oxalate toxicity

The ingestion of oxalates may cause chronic hypocalcemia or a negative calcium balance by reducing calcium absorption; a diet with greater than 1% of oxalates can reduce most intestinal calcium absorption.[16] Clinical signs associated with oxalate excess are those of phosphate excess, chronic calcium deficiency, and nutritional secondary hyperparathyroidism.

Treatment of Hypocalcemia

To treat hypocalcemia it is important to consider calcium deficit, maintenance, losses, and sequestration. The protein status should also be taken into consideration. Ionized calcium (Ca^{2+}) gives a better assessment of the calcium status than total calcium because plasma proteins do not affect it; however, few laboratories measure Ca^{2+} and most treatment decisions are based on total calcium concentrations. Parenteral calcium therapy is more critical in horses that develop hypocalcemia rapidly, in horses that cannot restore normocalcemia, or in horses at risk of ileus than in horses with chronic hypocalcemia. Although most horses with low Ca^{2+} concentrations do not show signs of hypocalcemia, delaying therapy may result in complications, such as ileus and arrhythmias. Calcium therapy should be considered in horses with mild hypocalcemia because horses with functional kidneys can eliminate large amounts of calcium; hypercalcemia from excessive calcium administration is rare, in particular if the horse is receiving fluid therapy; and calcium therapy is inexpensive.

As routine therapy, adding 50 mL of 23% calcium gluconate per 5 L of lactated Ringer's solution (twice the maintenance rate) is sufficient to restore normocalcemia in horses with mild hypocalcemia. Higher doses (100–150 mL) may be required in animals with severe hypocalcemia. In animals with chronic or refractory hypocalcemia, oral supplementation with calcium carbonate (limestone; 100–300 g/horse/d) or dicalcium phosphate (100–200 g/horse/d) should be considered. The value of adding vitamin D treatment is questionable and some horses may develop toxicity (hypervitaminosis D). However, low doses of vitamin D might be of benefit to horses with decreased calcium absorption and reabsorption. Hypocalcemia may not resolve in several animals until they receive magnesium supplementation.

Hypercalcemic Disorders

Equine disorders associated with hypercalcemia include primary and secondary hyperparathyroidism, chronic renal failure, humoral hypercalcemia of malignancy, and hypervitaminosis D. Calcinosis and idiopathic systemic granulomatous disease are rare and often not associated with hypercalcemia. Unlike hypocalcemia in which treatment is often successful, the prognosis for hypercalcemia in horses in general is poor.

Primary hyperparathyroidism

This condition results from the excessive and autonomous secretion of PTH by a parathyroid gland that is not responsive to the negative feedback of Ca^{2+}.[1] Primary hyperparathyroidism has been reported in horses with parathyroid adenomas or parathyroid hyperplasia.[32,55–59] High PTH concentrations lead to increased renal Ca^{2+} reabsorption, decreased renal P_i reabsorption (↑renal elimination), and increased renal $1,25(OH)_2D_3$ synthesis; whereas, bone resorption is enhanced (osteodystrophia fibrosa).

Laboratory abnormalities include hypercalcemia, hypophosphatemia, hypocalciuria, and hyperphosphaturia. PTHrP concentrations are within normal limits. Clinical findings include lameness, fractures, poor body condition, and enlargement of facial bones. On radiographs there is decreased bone density, fibrous proliferation of the maxilla and mandible, and loss of the lamina dura surrounding the molars.[32] Nasal passages may be narrow. Although not documented in horses, in theory treatment will consist of surgical removal of the affected parathyroid gland. However, a major challenge would be to find the affected parathyroid gland. Scintigraphy failed to identify hyperactive parathyroid tissue in a horse and a mule.[59]

Secondary hyperparathyroidism

In the case of secondary hyperparathyroidism, the excessive secretion of PTH is a response of the parathyroid gland to hyperphosphatemia and hypovitaminosis D from chronic renal failure (renal secondary hyperparathyroidism), hyperphosphatemia, or hypocalcemia from nutritional imbalances (nutritional secondary hyperparathyroidism). *Renal secondary hyperparathyroidism* is not well recognized in horses. Although in other species chronic renal failure (CRF) is associated with hyperphosphatemia, horses with CRF usually have hypophosphatemia. Further, the hypercalcemia of horses with CRF likely results from the inability of the diseased kidneys to eliminate Ca^{2+} (Ca^{2+} retention) rather than increased PTH concentrations. As a consequence of the high extracellular Ca^{2+} concentrations, and unlike other species, PTH concentrations in horses with CRF are often normal or low.[30,60] *Nutritional secondary hyperparathyroidism* is a well-documented disease of horses.

Nutritional secondary hyperparathyroidism

Horses fed diets low in calcium, high in phosphorus, high in oxalates, or with a phosphorus/calcium ratio of greater than or equal to 3:1 may develop *nutritional secondary hyperparathyroidism* (NSH), also known as bran disease, miller's disease, big head, osteodystrophia fibrosa, osteitis fibrosa, and equine osteoporosis.[56] Excessive dietary phosphorus reduces intestinal calcium absorption and results in hyperphosphatemia. Plants with high oxalate content predispose to NSH because oxalates interfere with calcium absorption. High-phosphorus and low-calcium diets stimulate PTH secretion in the horse.[56] Hyperphosphatemia inhibits renal synthesis of $1,25(OH)_2D_3$. Because $1,25(OH)_2D_3$ inhibits parathyroid cell function, hypovitaminosis D contributes to parathyroid cell hyperplasia and excessive PTH secretion. PTH increases osteoclastic activity, bone resorption and bone loss,[61] accumulation of unmineralized connective tissue (osteodystrophia fibrosa), and facial enlargement (big head). Horses with NSH preserve normocalcemia at the expense of the skeletal reserves and do not develop signs of acute hypocalcemia.

Clinical signs of NSH include physeal enlargement, limb deformities, lameness, stiff gait, and unthriftiness. There is facial bone enlargement that may not be evident in old horses. The increased bone resorption around molars may result in masticatory problems. Upper airway obstruction and stridor, dyspnea, and epiphora may be present.[62,63] Laboratory findings include hyperphosphatemia, hypocalcemia or normocalcemia, and increased PTH concentrations. The urinary fractional excretion of calcium is low (hypocalciuria); whereas, the excretion of phosphate is high (hyperphosphaturia). Serum alkaline phosphatase activity and collagen degradation products may be increased. Laboratory findings may be within normal limits if the animal is eating a balanced diet. On radiographs there is decreased bone density; however, bone density must be decreased by 30% before differences can be observed radiographically.[64] Resorption of alveolar sockets and loss of the dental lamina dura may be present before other radiographic changes are detected. Soft-tissue mineralization was reported in a foal.[65]

Regarding prevention and treatment, diet evaluation is indicated. Eliminate or reduce any grain-based diet and avoid plants with high oxalate content. The addition of alfalfa to the diet may be helpful. Supplementation with calcium carbonate (limestone; $CaCO_3$) or dicalcium phosphate should be considered. An affected animal may require a total of 100 to 300 g/d. The diet should have a Ca/P ratio of 3 to 4:1. Supplementation with vitamin D has been proposed. Horses may require 9 to 12 months for complete recovery, although some bone changes may not regress. Horses with severe signs should be confined to a stall or small paddock. The use of nonsteroidal antiinflammatory drugs may be indicated in animals with severe pain.

Hypervitaminosis D

The ingestion or administration of vitamin D_2 (ergocalciferol) or vitamin D_3 (cholecalciferol) results in hypervitaminosis D, a life-threatening disease of horses and other domestic animals.[38,66–68] Several plants contain $1,25(OH)_2D$-like compounds. The ingestion of *Solanum glaucophyllum (S. malacoxylon)* results in a condition known as *enteque seco* in Argentina and *espichamento* in Brazil.[66,69] In Hawaii, hypervitaminosis D may be caused by *Solanum sodomaeum* and by Jessamine (*Cestrum diurnum*) in the southern United States.[67] In Europe, the ingestion of golden oat (*Trisetum flavescens*) causes enzootic calcinosis. Hypervitaminosis D increases the intestinal absorption and renal reabsorption of calcium and phosphorus. Hyperphosphatemia is the most consistent laboratory finding in horses with vitamin D intoxication[70]; whereas, serum calcium concentrations are variable.[38,67,68] High vitamin D concentrations lead to parathyroid cell atrophy and decreased PTH secretion. Azotemia and hyposthenuria may be present.[38]

These horses have weight loss, poor appetite, lameness, painful stiffness, and are reluctant to move. Mineral deposition in the kidneys leads to renal failure, polyuria, and polydipsia. Sudden death from cardiovascular mineralization has been reported.[38] Lameness may occur from calcification of ligaments and tendons. On radiographs, there is increased bone density, decreased size of the medullary cavity, and calcification of soft tissues.

Therapeutic measures are based on reducing dietary calcium and phosphate intake. Glucocorticoids are used in humans with hypervitaminosis D to inhibit intestinal calcium absorption. In horses, glucocorticoids decrease intestinal absorption of calcium, increase urinary excretion of calcium, and decrease bone resorption.[44] Dexamethasone has been administered to horses with hypervitaminosis D with questionable results.[68]

The prognosis for horses with hypervitaminosis D is poor. On necropsy there is mineralization of soft tissues, large vessels, and endocardium. Mineralization may be found in the kidney, liver, lymph nodes, lungs, ligaments, and tendons. Osteopetrosis of long bones can be present. The parathyroid glands are often atrophied.[71]

Hypercalcemia of malignancy

Humoral hypercalcemia of malignancy (HHM, pseudohyperparathyroidism) refers to a paraneoplastic condition of horses with different types of cancer. In horses, HHM has been associated with squamous cell carcinomas, adrenocortical carcinoma, lymphoma, multiple myeloma, and ameloblastoma (**Fig. 5**).[1] These malignancies secrete (PTHrP), which interacts with PTH receptors to increase bone resorption, renal Ca^{2+} reabsorption, and renal P_i elimination.[27] Laboratory abnormalities include hypercalcemia, hypophosphatemia, hypocalciuria, hyperphosphaturia, normal or low PTH

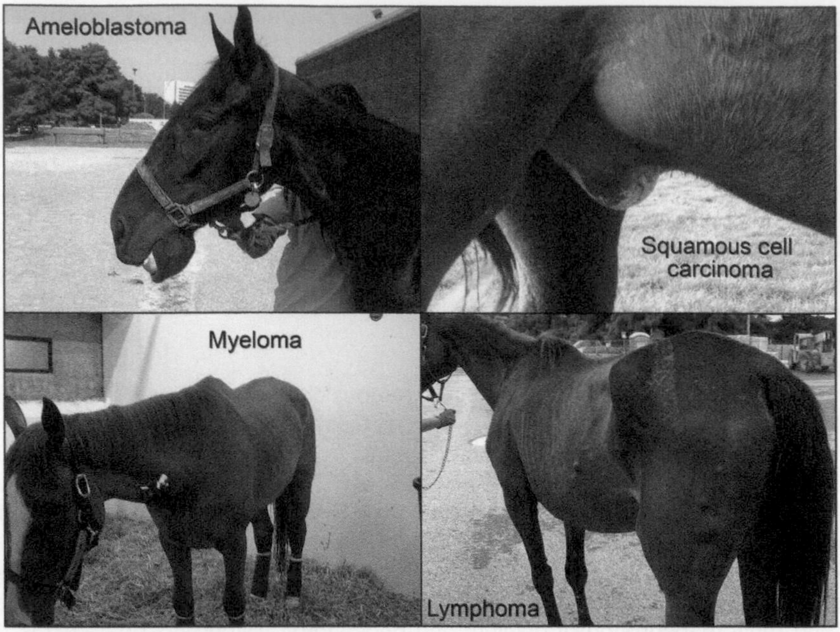

Fig. 5. Horses with various types of cancer (ameloblastoma, multiple myeloma, squamous cell carcinoma in the prepuce, and cutaneous lymphoma) and humoral hypercalcemia of malignancy from increased blood concentrations of PTHrP. (*Courtesy of* Ramiro E. Toribio, DVM, MS, PhD, Columbus, OH, USA.)

concentrations, and increased concentrations of PTHrP. Soft-tissue mineralization may be present. HHM should be suspected in any horse with hypercalcemia, no evidence of renal disease, and normal or low concentrations of PTH. The prognosis for horses with HHM is poor.

Idiopathic systemic granulomatous disease

Idiopathic systemic granulomatous disease is a rare immune disease of horses and ponies, characterized by weight loss, crusting skin lesions often affecting mucocutaneous junctions and coronary bands (**Fig. 6**). There is granuloma formation in several organs and the skin.[72–74] Although most of these animals have serum calcium within the normal range, hypercalcemia has also been documented.[72] Increased expression of PTHrP by the macrophages of granulomas was found in a pony with this pathology.[72] In the equivalent condition of humans, sarcoidosis, hypercalcemia is attributed to excessive and unregulated production of $1,25(OH)_2D_3$ by macrophages.[75] In distribution, this disease may resemble the multisystemic eosinophilic epitheliotropic disease of horses.

Calcinosis

Systemic calcinosis, characterized by hyperphosphatemia and calcification of soft tissues (liver, heart, kidney, lungs, vessels, muscle), has been documented in horses with various diseases (colitis, respiratory distress, laminitis, and muscle fiber necrosis).[76] The exact cause of the calcinosis remains unclear, although it is speculated to result from hyperphosphatemia or hyperparathyroidism.

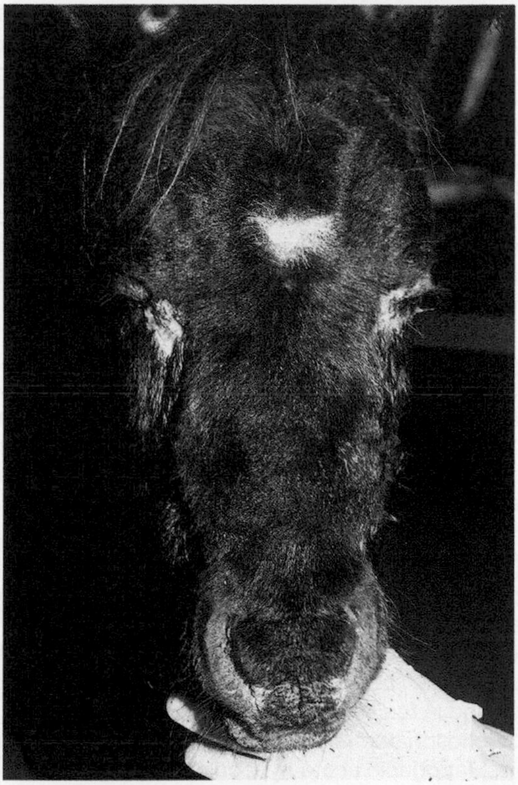

Fig. 6. Miniature pony diagnosed with idiopathic systemic granulomatous disease. The animal had a history of weight loss, fever, crusting lesions on the skin, mucocutaneous junctions, and coronary bands. Blood tests revealed anemia and hypercalcemia. On histology, granulomata that were immunopositive for PTHrP were present in the skin, lungs, liver, and kidney. There was no evidence of eosinophilic infiltration. (*Courtesy of* Ramiro E. Toribio, DVM, MS, PhD, Columbus, OH.)

Neonatal hypercalcemia and asphyxia

Clinical observations by several clinicians indicate that some critically ill newborn foals develop hypercalcemia with no evidence of renal disease, hyperparathyroidism, or excessive calcium administration. A consistent feature in these foals is peripartum asphyxia. Although the cause of this condition remains unknown, the author speculates that it is associated with placental insufficiency and excessive production of PTHrP.

Treatment of Hypercalcemia

In general, hypercalcemia is not considered an equine emergency; however, the differential diagnosis of hypercalcemia is important for its subsequent treatment and prognosis. Few disorders are associated with equine hypercalcemia (hyperparathyroidism, CRF, HHM, hypervitaminosis D). Mild hypercalcemia is not life threatening and therapy should be directed to the primary cause. Parathyroidectomy would be the treatment of choice for primary hyperparathyroidism, although this is impractical for several reasons (eg, localizing the pathologic gland, cost). Surgical removal of epithelial tumors or irradiation can be a successful treatment for HHM. Some horses with lymphoma may improve with chemotherapy. When severe hypercalcemia requires medical treatment, initial therapy should include the administration of 0.9% saline solution and loop diuretics. Furosemide is the diuretic of choice because it inhibits the $Na^+/K^+/2Cl^-$ cotransporter in the distal tubules, increasing the urinary excretion of calcium. Thiazide diuretics are contraindicated because they stimulate calcium reabsorption. Glucocorticoid administration should be considered, in particular for horses with hypervitaminosis D. For horses with CRF, dietary management based on low calcium diets (no alfalfa) and free access to water, electrolytes, and carbohydrates may improve their quality of life, in particular if the azotemia is mild. Regardless of the cause, the prognosis for horses with hypercalcemia is guarded.

PHOSPHATE DISORDERS

Phosphate disorders are closely linked to disorders of the calcium metabolism. It would be unusual for horses receiving diets with low or high phosphorus content to develop hypophosphatemia or hyperphosphatemia, although the clinical signs of either one can be evident.

Hyperphosphatemia

Excessive dietary phosphate and hyperphosphatemia are associated with nutritional secondary hyperparathyroidism (described in the calcium section). Hyperphosphatemia occurs in horses with acute renal failure, massive tissue necrosis (eg, tumor lysis syndrome, rhabdomyolysis, hemolysis, intestinal infarction), hypervitaminosis D, hypoparathyroidism, and in foals treated with phosphate-containing enemas. Horses with prolonged hyperphosphatemia are also at risk of developing soft-tissue mineralization and calcinosis. Iatrogenic acute hypocalcemia may occur in animals receiving excessive amounts of oral or parenteral phosphate salts (eg, enemas).

Hypophosphatemia

Hypophosphatemia occurs with renal failure, malignancies secreting phosphatonins or PTHrP (HHM), hyperparathyroidism, parenteral nutrition, and hyperinsulinism. Hypophosphatemia usually results from the intracellular shift of P_i in patients with severe sepsis, malnourishment (refeeding syndrome), alkalosis, or hyperglycemia (hyperinsulinemia).[77] It is not unusual for animals under partial or total parenteral to develop hypophosphatemia (often associated with hypokalemia and hypomagnesemia), which suggests that this is an insulin-mediated phenomenon. Insulin increases the activity of the Na^+/K^+ ATPase and Na^+-P_i cotransporter, shifting K^+ and P_i to the intracellular compartment. Although in other species osteomalacia (old animals) and rickets (young animals) are consequences of phosphorus deficiency, these conditions are not well recognized in horses. Horses with chronic phosphorus deficiency may develop an aberrant appetite for dirt and inanimate objects (pica). Increased cell fragility and hemolysis from hypophosphatemia, although suspected in many cases, remain to be documented in the equine literature.

Treatment

Therapy to hyperphosphatemia should be directed at reducing dietary intake of phosphate and addressing the primary problem. Information on phosphate binders (eg, aluminum hydroxide) is lacking in horses. Calcium carbonate can have a dual effect by acting as a phosphate binder and by increasing calcium availability. The value and practicality of dialysis as a therapy for hyperphosphatemia in horses remains to be shown. The use of diuretics that increase urinary phosphate excretion (eg, acetazolamide) should be considered in some instances.

For the treatment of acute hypophosphatemia, the extracellular deficit should be overestimated because P_i is a major intracellular anion and cell depletion is likely to be present when extracellular P_i concentrations are low. The author prefers to use parenteral potassium phosphate, although sodium phosphate is a good alternative. Oral administration of potassium phosphate or monosodium phosphate can also be used. Oral supplementation with dicalcium phosphate should be considered in chronic hypophosphatemia (see **Table 2**). Hypokalemia and hypomagnesemia are frequent findings in horses and foals with hypophosphatemia, particularly those with energy dysregulation and parenteral nutrition. Because the regulation of these ions is linked, in addition to phosphate administration, treatment with magnesium and potassium salts may be required.

SUMMARY

Although most attention in the clinical setting is given to electrolytes, such as sodium and potassium, disorders of calcium and phosphate homeostasis can be fatal, impair the future of the animal, or lead to problems that can be expensive to treat (eg, ileus, developmental orthopedic diseases). Most horses with gastrointestinal disease develop hypocalcemia (and hypomagnesemia), and supplementing their fluids with calcium gluconate is generally a safe measure because the equine kidney can handle large amounts of calcium. Although phosphate treatment in intensive care units is rare, careful assessment of serum phosphate concentrations, particularly in animals under parenteral nutrition, should be given. An important aspect of serum calcium and phosphate concentrations is that their values can have prognostic significance in conditions such as cancer and chronic renal failure (hypercalcemia), or tissue necrosis (hyperphosphatemia). Thus, integrating and not overlooking these minerals can assist in a better management of equine patients.

REFERENCES

1. Toribio RE. Disorders of calcium and phosphorus. In: Reed SM, Bayly WM, Sellon DC, editors. Equine internal medicine. St Louis (MO): Saunders/Elsevier; 2010. p. 1277–91.
2. Rosol TJ, Capen CC. Calcium-regulating hormones and diseases of abnormal mineral (calcium, phosphorus, magnesium) metabolism. In: Kaneko JJ, Harvey JW, Bruss ML, editors. Clinical biochemistry of domestic animals. San Diego (CA): Academic Press; 1997. p. 619–702.
3. Hurwitz S. Homeostatic control of plasma calcium concentration. Crit Rev Biochem Mol Biol 1996;31:41–100.
4. Kohn CW, Brooks CL. Failure of pH to predict ionized calcium percentage in healthy horses. Am J Vet Res 1990;51:1206–10.
5. Toribio RE, Kohn CW, Chew DJ, et al. Comparison of serum parathyroid hormone and ionized calcium and magnesium concentrations and fractional urinary clearance of calcium and phosphorus in healthy horses and horses with enterocolitis. Am J Vet Res 2001;62:938–47.
6. Lopez I, Estepa JC, Mendoza FJ, et al. Fractionation of calcium and magnesium in equine serum. Am J Vet Res 2006;67:463–6.
7. Berlin D, Aroch I. Concentrations of ionized and total magnesium and calcium in healthy horses: Effects of age, pregnancy, lactation, pH and sample type. Vet J 2009;181:305–11.

8. Endres DB, Rude RK. Mineral and bone metabolism. In: Burtis CA, Ashwood ER, Bruns DE, editors. Tietz textbook of clinical chemistry and molecular diagnostics. St Louis (MO): Elsevier Saunders; 2006. p. 1891–963.
9. Jordan RM, Meyers VS, Yoho B, et al. Effect of calcium and phosphorus levels on growth, reproduction, and bone development of ponies. J Anim Sci 1975;40:78.
10. Schryver HF, Craig PH, Hintz HF. Calcium metabolism in ponies fed varying levels of calcium. J Nutr 1970;100:955–64.
11. Schryver HF, Hintz HF, Craig PH. Phosphorus metabolism in ponies fed varying levels of phosphorus. J Nutr 1971;101:1257–63.
12. Schryver HF, Hintz HF, Lowe JE. Calcium and phosphorus in the nutrition of the horse. Cornell Vet 1974;64:493–515.
13. Schryver HF, Foose TJ, Williams J, et al. Calcium excretion in feces of ungulates. Comp Biochem Physiol A 1983;74:375–9.
14. Schryver HF, Craig PH, Hintz HF, et al. The site of calcium absorption in the horse. J Nutr 1970;100:1127–31.
15. Schryver HF, Hintz HF, Craig PH. Calcium metabolism in ponies fed a high phosphorus diet. J Nutr 1971;101:259–64.
16. Swartzman JA, Hintz HF, Schryver HF. Inhibition of calcium absorption in ponies fed diets containing oxalic acid. Am J Vet Res 1978;39:1621–3.
17. McKenzie EC, Valberg SJ, Godden SM, et al. Plasma and urine electrolyte and mineral concentrations in Thoroughbred horses with recurrent exertional rhabdomyolysis after consumption of diets varying in cation-anion balance. Am J Vet Res 2002;63:1053–60.
18. Glade MJ, Krook L, Schryver HF, et al. Calcium metabolism in glucocorticoid-treated pony foals. J Nutr 1982;112:77–86.
19. Glade MJ, Krook L. Glucocorticoid-induced inhibition of osteolysis and the development of osteopetrosis, osteonecrosis and osteoporosis. Cornell Vet 1982;72:76–91.
20. Toribio RE, Kohn CW, Hardy J, et al. Alterations in serum parathyroid hormone and electrolyte concentrations and urinary excretion of electrolytes in horses with induced endotoxemia. J Vet Intern Med 2005;19:223–31.
21. Toribio RE, Kohn CW, Rourke KM, et al. Effects of hypercalcemia on serum concentrations of magnesium, potassium, and phosphate and urinary excretion of electrolytes in horses. Am J Vet Res 2007;68:543–54.
22. Schryver HF, Hintz HF, Craig PH, et al. Site of phosphorus absorption from the intestine of the horse. J Nutr 1972;102:143–7.
23. Schryver HF. Intestinal absorption of calcium and phosphorus by horses. J S Afr Vet Assoc 1975;46:39–45.
24. Caple IW, Doake PA, Ellis PG. Assessment of the calcium and phosphorus nutrition in horses by analysis of urine. Aust Vet J 1982;58:125–31.
25. Coffman J. Percent creatinine clearance ratios. Vet Med Small Anim Clin 1980;75: 671–6.
26. Mundy GR, Guise TA. Hormonal control of calcium homeostasis. Clin Chem 1999; 45:1347–52.
27. Suva LJ, Winslow GA, Wettenhall RE, et al. A parathyroid hormone-related protein implicated in malignant hypercalcemia: cloning and expression. Science 1987; 237:893–6.
28. Wysolmerski JJ, Stewart AF. The physiology of parathyroid hormone-related protein: an emerging role as a developmental factor. Annu Rev Physiol 1998; 60:431–60.
29. Berndt T, Kumar R. Novel mechanisms in the regulation of phosphorus homeostasis. Physiology (Bethesda) 2009;24:17–25.

30. Aguilera-Tejero E, Estepa JC, Lopez I, et al. Polycystic kidneys as a cause of chronic renal failure and secondary hypoparathyroidism in a horse. Equine Vet J 2000;32:167–9.
31. Couetil LL, Sojka JE, Nachreiner RF. Primary hypoparathyroidism in a horse. J Vet Intern Med 1998;12:45–9.
32. Frank N, Hawkins JF, Couetil LL, et al. Primary hyperparathyroidism with osteodystrophia fibrosa of the facial bones in a pony. J Am Vet Med Assoc 1998;212: 84–6.
33. Ronen N, Van Heerden J, van Amstel SR. Clinical and biochemistry findings, and parathyroid hormone concentrations in three horses with secondary hyperparathyroidism. J S Afr Vet Assoc 1992;63:134–6.
34. Elfers RS, Bayly WM, Brobst DF, et al. Alterations in calcium, phosphorus and C-terminal parathyroid hormone levels in equine acute renal disease. Cornell Vet 1986;76:317–29.
35. Marr CM, Love S, Pirie HM. Clinical, ultrasonographic and pathological findings in a horse with splenic lymphosarcoma and pseudohyperparathyroidism. Equine Vet J 1989;21:221–6.
36. Meuten DJ, Price SM, Seiler RM, et al. Gastric carcinoma with pseudohyperparathyroidism in a horse. Cornell Vet 1978;68:179–95.
37. Rosol TJ, Nagode LA, Robertson JT, et al. Humoral hypercalcemia of malignancy associated with ameloblastoma in a horse. J Am Vet Med Assoc 1994;204: 1930–3.
38. Harrington DD, Page EH. Acute vitamin D3 toxicosis in horses: case reports and experimental studies of the comparative toxicity of vitamins D2 and D3. J Am Vet Med Assoc 1983;182:1358–69.
39. Aguilera-Tejero E, Estepa JC, Lopez I, et al. Plasma ionized calcium and parathyroid hormone concentrations in horses after endurance rides. J Am Vet Med Assoc 2001;219:488–90.
40. Beyer MJ, Freestone JF, Reimer JM, et al. Idiopathic hypocalcemia in foals. J Vet Intern Med 1997;11:356–60.
41. Helman RG, Edwards WC. Clinical features of blister beetle poisoning in equids: 70 cases (1983–1996). J Am Vet Med Assoc 1997;211:1018–21.
42. Dart AJ, Snyder JR, Spier SJ, et al. Ionized calcium concentration in horses with surgically managed gastrointestinal disease: 147 cases (1988–1990). J Am Vet Med Assoc 1992;201:1244–8.
43. Garcia-Lopez JM, Provost PJ, Rush JE, et al. Prevalence and prognostic importance of hypomagnesemia and hypocalcemia in horses that have colic surgery. Am J Vet Res 2001;62:7–12.
44. Toribio RE. Disorders of the endocrine system. In: Reed SM, Bayly WM, Sellon DC, editors. Equine internal medicine. St Louis (MO): W.B. Saunders; 2004. p. 1295–379.
45. Kaneps AJ, Knight AP, Bennett DG. Synchronous diaphragmatic flutter associated with electrolyte imbalances in a mare with colic. Equine Pract 1980;2:18.
46. Hudson NP, Church DB, Trevena J, et al. Primary hypoparathyroidism in two horses. Aust Vet J 1999;77:504–8.
47. Carlson GP, Mansmann RA. Serum electrolyte and plasma protein alterations in horses used in endurance rides. J Am Vet Med Assoc 1974;165:262–4.
48. Schoeb TR, Panciera RJ. Blister beetle poisoning in horses. J Am Vet Med Assoc 1978;173:75–7.
49. Baird JD. Lactation tetany (eclampsia) in a Shetland pony mare. Aust Vet J 1971; 47:402–4.

50. Kerr MG, Snow DH. Composition of sweat of the horse during prolonged epinephrine (adrenaline) infusion, heat exposure, and exercise. Am J Vet Res 1983;44:1571–7.
51. Schryver HF, Hintz HF, Lowe JE. Calcium metabolism, body composition, and sweat losses of exercised horses. Am J Vet Res 1978;39:245–8.
52. Mansmann RA, Carlson GP, White NA, et al. Synchronous diaphragmatic flutter in horses. J Am Vet Med Assoc 1974;165:265–70.
53. Durie I, van LG, Hesta M, et al. Hypocalcemia caused by primary hypoparathyroidism in a 3-month-old filly. J Vet Intern Med 2010;24:439–42.
54. Hurcombe SD, Toribio RE, Slovis NM, et al. Calcium regulating hormones and serum calcium and magnesium concentrations in septic and critically ill foals and their association with survival. J Vet Intern Med 2009;23:335–43.
55. Bienfet V, Dewaele A, Van Essch R. A primary parathyroid disorder. Osteofibrosis caused by a parathyroid adenoma in a Shetland pony. Ann Med Vet 1964;108:252–6.
56. Krook L, Lowe JE. Nutritional secondary hyperparathyroidism in the horse. Pathol Vet 1964;65:26–56.
57. Peauroi JR, Fisher DJ, Mohr FC, et al. Primary hyperparathyroidism caused by a functional parathyroid adenoma in a horse. J Am Vet Med Assoc 1998;212:1915–8.
58. Roussel AJ, Thatcher CD. Primary hyperparathyroidism in a pony mare. Compendium on Continuing Education for the Practicing Veterinarian 1987;9:781–3.
59. Wong D, Sponseller B, Miles K, et al. Failure of Technetium Tc 99m sestamibi scanning to detect abnormal parathyroid tissue in a horse and a mule with primary hyperparathyroidism. J Vet Intern Med 2004;18:589–93.
60. Brobst DF, Bayly WM, Reed SM. Parathyroid hormone evaluation in normal horses and horses with renal failure. J Equine Vet Sci 1982;2:150–7.
61. Argenzio RA, Lowe JE, Hintz HF, et al. Calcium and phosphorus homeostasis in horses. J Nutr 1974;104:18–27.
62. Clarke CJ, Roeder PL, Dixon PM. Nasal obstruction caused by nutritional osteodystrophia fibrosa in a group of Ethiopian horses. Vet Rec 1996;138:568–70.
63. Freestone JF, Seahorn TL. Miscellaneous conditions of the equine head. Vet Clin North Am Equine Pract 1993;9:235–42.
64. Bertone JJ. Nutritional secondary hyperparathyroidism. In: Robinson NE, editor. Current therapy in equine medicine. Philadelphia: W.B. Saunders; 1992. p. 119–22.
65. Estepa JC, guilera-Tejero E, Zafra R, et al. An unusual case of generalized soft-tissue mineralization in a suckling foal. Vet Pathol 2006;43:64–7.
66. Boland RL. Solanum malacoxylon: a toxic plant which affects animal calcium metabolism. Biomed Environ Sci 1988;1:414–23.
67. Krook L, Wasserman RH, Shively JN, et al. Hypercalcemia and calcinosis in Florida horses: implication of the shrub, Cestrum diurnum, as the causative agent. Cornell Vet 1975;65:26–56.
68. Muylle E, Oyaert W, de Roose P, et al. Hypercalcaemia and mineralisation of non-osseous tissues in horses due to vitamin-D toxicity. Zentralbl Veterinarmed A 1974;21:638–43.
69. Worker NA, Carrillo BJ. 'Enteque seco', calcification and wasting in grazing animals in the Argentine. Nature 1967;215:72–4.
70. Harrington DD. Acute vitamin D2 (ergocalciferol) toxicosis in horses: case report and experimental studies. J Am Vet Med Assoc 1982;180:867–73.
71. Kasali OB, Krook L, Pond WG, et al. Cestrum diurnum intoxication in normal and hyperparathyroid pigs. Cornell Vet 1977;67:190–221.

72. Sellers RS, Toribio RE, Blomme EA. Idiopathic systemic granulomatous disease and macrophage expression of PTHrP in a miniature pony. J Comp Pathol 2001;125:214–8.
73. Peters M, Graf G, Pohlenz J. Idiopathic systemic granulomatous disease with encephalitis in a horse. J Vet Med A Physiol Pathol Clin Med 2003;50:108–12.
74. Heath SE, Bell RJ, Clark EG, et al. Idiopathic granulomatous disease involving the skin in a horse. J Am Vet Med Assoc 1990;197:1033–6.
75. Nunes H, Bouvry D, Soler P, et al. Sarcoidosis. Orphanet J Rare Dis 2007;2:46.
76. Tan JY, Valberg SJ, Sebastian MM, et al. Suspected systemic calcinosis and calciphylaxis in 5 horses. Can Vet J 2010;51:993–9.
77. Gossett KA, French DD, Cleghorn B, et al. Blood biochemical response to sodium bicarbonate infusion during sublethal endotoxemia in ponies. Am J Vet Res 1990; 51:1370–4.

Magnesium Disorders in Horses

Allison J. Stewart, BVSc (Hons), MS

KEYWORDS

- Hypomagnesemia • Hypermagnesemia • Calcium • Alkalosis
- Parathyroid hormone

Magnesium (Mg) is an essential macroelement that is required for cellular energy-dependent reactions involving ATP, including ion pump function, glycolysis and oxidative phosphorylation, and nucleic acid and protein synthesis. Mg has an important role in the regulation of calcium (Ca) channel function and therefore neurotransmitter release, neuronal excitation, skeletal muscle contraction, vasomotor tone, and cardiac excitability. Because of the importance of Mg in several physiologic processes, homeostatic mechanisms normally maintain intracellular and extracellular concentrations within narrow limits. Severe Mg deficiency results in neuromuscular disturbances, but such overt clinical signs are rarely documented in horses. In contrast, subclinical hypomagnesemia is common in critically ill humans and animals. Subclinical hypomagnesemia increases the severity of the systemic inflammatory response syndrome (SIRS); worsens the systemic response to endotoxins; and can lead to ileus, cardiac arrhythmias, refractory hypokalemia, and hypocalcemia.

CHEMISTRY

Mg concentrations in body fluids are reported as mEq/L, mg/dL, or mmol/L. Because the atomic weight of Mg is 24.3 and its valence is 2^+, 1 mEq (0.5 mmol) = 12.156 mg. The conversion factors are as follows:

mg/dL = mmol/L $\times$ 2.43
mmol/L = mg/dL $\times$ 0.411
mmol/L = mEq/L $\times$ 0.5
mg/dl = mEq/L

Dietary Mg levels are reported in g/kg of feed, in parts per million (ppm), which is expressed as mg/kg = g/kg $\times$ 1000 or as a percentage, by dividing by 10. Oral Mg is commonly available as magnesium oxide (MgO), MgO_x, which contains 60.25% elemental Mg. Magnesium carbonate ($MgCO_3$) and magnesium sulfate ($MgSO_4$) can also be fed. $MgSO_4$ for intravenous (IV) injection is commercially available as

Department of Clinical Science, John Thomas Vaughan Large Animal Teaching Hospital, College of Veterinary Medicine, Auburn University, 1500 Wire Road, Auburn, AL 36849, USA
E-mail address: stewaaj@auburn.edu

Vet Clin Equine 27 (2011) 149–163
doi:10.1016/j.cveq.2010.12.009 vetequine.theclinics.com

$MgSO_4 \cdot 7H_2O$ in a 50% solution. Although the $MgSO_4$ compound contains 20.2% elemental Mg, its solution contains only 9.9% elemental Mg. Each mL of 50% $MgSO_4 \cdot 7H_2O$ solution contains 99 mg (8 mEq = 4 mmol) of elemental Mg. The 50% solution (500 mg/mL = 4 mEq/mL) is hypertonic, with an osmolarity of 4000 mOsm/L and should be diluted to at least a 10% solution before IV administration.

MG DISTRIBUTION WITHIN THE BODY

Mg is the fourth most abundant cation in the mammalian body and the second most abundant intracellular cation after potassium. The body of domestic animals contains 0.05% Mg by weight, of which 60% is in bones, 38% is in soft tissues, and 1% to 2% is in extracellular fluids. Only 30% of the bone Mg is readily exchangeable and therefore available as a reservoir to maintain extracellular Mg concentrations. The remaining 70% of bone Mg has structural functions and is held within the hydroxyapatite lattice and released only during active bone resorption. Although most soft tissue Mg is in the intracellular compartment, intracellular and extracellular ionized Mg (Mg^{2+}) concentrations are similar, with only a very small transmembrane gradient compared with calcium ions (Ca^{2+}). Intracellular Mg^{2+} concentrations are variable, being proportional to the metabolic activity of the cell.

Less than 1% of the total body Mg is contained in the extracellular fluid, therefore serum Mg concentration may not adequately reflect the total body Mg stores. In equine serum, 30% of Mg is protein bound and 10% is complexed to weak acids, with the remaining 60% in the ionized form (Mg^{2+}).[1,2] Only the ionized form is biologically active, therefore it is preferable to measure the concentration of the ionized form in the serum rather than the total Mg (tMg) concentrations. Red blood cells contain approximately 3 times the concentration of Mg in serum; therefore hemolysis can elevate measured serum Mg concentrations.

The serum tMg concentration depends on the protein concentration, whereas the Mg^{2+} concentration depends on the acid-base status. Acidosis increases the Mg^{2+} concentration, whereas alkalosis reduces it. This property is clinically important when treating alkalotic conditions, such as exercise-associated metabolic alkalosis in endurance horses resulting from chloride loss, nasogastric reflux associated with small intestinal obstruction, or duodenitis/jejunitis and respiratory alkalosis associated with hyperventilation. Clinical signs of hypomagnesemia can develop because of low concentrations of Mg^{2+} despite normal tMg concentrations. Feeding an acidic diet with a low dietary cation-anion balance will increase the percentage of Mg^{2+}.[1]

PHYSIOLOGIC ROLE OF MG

Mg serves as an essential cofactor for more than 300 enzymatic reactions involving ATP, such as replication, transcription and translation of genetic information, and cellular energy metabolism reactions of glycolysis and oxidative phosphorylation.[3,4] Mg is necessary for membrane stabilization, nerve conduction, ion transportation, regulation of Ca channel activity, and normal functioning of the sodium-potassium–activated ATP (Na^+/K^+ ATPase) pump, which maintains the Na^+/K^+ gradient across all membranes as well as regulates the intracellular K^+ balance.[5] Ca ATPase and proton pumps also require Mg as a cofactor. Consequently, Mg plays an important role in excitable tissues. Defective function of ATPase pumps and ion channels may result in interference with the electrochemical gradient, alteration in resting membrane potential, and disturbances in repolarization, resulting in neuromuscular and cardiovascular abnormalities.[4,6–8] Mg's role in the regulation of movement of Ca into the myocyte, gives it a pivotal role in cardiac contractile strength, peripheral vascular tone, and visceral peristalsis.[8]

MG ABSORPTION

Mg^{2+} is absorbed by passive, nonsaturable, and concentration-dependent paracellular diffusion and by saturable transcellular active transport. In horses, 25% of the ingested Mg is absorbed in the proximal half of the small intestine; 35% in the distal half of the small intestine; and only 5% in the cecum, large colon, and small colon.[9] Increased dietary Mg leads to increases in bone, tissue, erythrocyte, and serum Mg concentrations. Intestinal Mg absorption increases in proportion to the amount supplied in the diet, but the absorptive efficiency decreases as the dietary Mg content increases until a plateau is reached.[10] The average absorption of Mg from feed by horses is 49.5% (30%–60%),[9] which is higher than that in ruminants.[11] Alfalfa has the highest Mg digestibility of 50%; clover and meadow hay, 31%; and hay and grain, 38%.[12] The diet type does not affect the site of Mg absorption.[9] Oral MgO, $MgSO_4$, and $MgCO_3$ have equivalent digestibilities (50%–70%), with their absorption rates higher than those from organic sources. Mg digestibility is higher in foals.[13] Excessive amounts of fiber, oxalates, phosphates, and fatty acids decrease Mg absorption in horses, whereas phytates, Ca, and aluminum contents have little effect.[9]

MECHANISMS OF RENAL MG EXCRETION AND REABSORPTION

Mg is primarily excreted via the gastrointestinal tract, kidneys, and mammary gland during lactation, with smaller amounts lost in sweat and to the developing fetus.

In an effort to regulate Mg balance and maintain stable serum Mg concentrations, renal excretion of Mg varies directly with dietary changes. With low Mg intake, the kidney avidly conserves Mg and virtually no Mg is excreted into the urine. Conversely, when excess Mg is ingested, it is rapidly excreted into the urine because of diminished renal tubular reabsorption. Ionized and anion-bound fractions of Mg are filtered by the glomerulus (ultrafilterable), whereas protein-bound Mg passes directly through the renal efferent arteriole without passing into the glomerular filtrate. Approximately 70% of blood Mg is filtered by the glomeruli, with 70% to 90% reabsorbed in different segments of the nephron. The proximal tubule reabsorbs 5% to 15% and the thick ascending limb of the loop of Henle 70% to 80% of the Mg filtered by the glomerulus.[14] The distal convoluted tubule only absorbs approximately 10% of the filtered Mg, but this amount is 70% to 80% of that delivered from the loop of Henle. Because there is minimal absorption beyond the distal tubule, this segment is responsible for determining the final urinary Mg excretion.

MG REQUIREMENTS OF HORSES

Obligatory urinary and fecal Mg loss in horses was estimated at 2.8 and 1.8 mg/kg birth weight (BW)/d, respectively.[9] Maintenance Mg requirement for horses has been estimated at 13 mg/kg BW/d and can be provided by a diet containing 0.16% Mg (1600 ppm of feed).[9,10] Growing, lactating, and exercising animals have a higher requirement of dietary Mg. The mammary gland actively secretes 3 to 6 mg/kg/BW/d of Mg into the milk. During the first week of lactation the Mg concentration in milk is 120 to 300 mg/L, then it decreases to 50 to 70 mg/L for the next 2 to 3 months.[15] During lactation, mares require 15- to 30-mg/kg dietary intake of Mg.[16] Hypomagnesemia is more likely to occur in high-producing mares, especially if transported long distances without feed. Substantial amounts of Mg can also be lost in sweat. The

Mg intake should be increased 1.5 to 2 times for maintenance horses undergoing moderate to intense exercise.

Dietary Mg deficiency in horses is very rare unless extreme conditions combine to result in decreased consumption and increased demand, such as long distance transportation of unfed lactating mares or prolonged administration of enteral or parenteral fluid or nutrition solutions deficient in Mg.

MG HOMEOSTASIS

Although the extracellular concentration of Mg depends on gastrointestinal absorption, renal excretion, and bone exchange, there is no precise homeostatic regulating system for Mg.[17] However, parathyroid hormone (PTH), PTH-related protein, arginine vasopressin (AVP, antidiuretic hormone), aldosterone, insulin, and β-adrenergic agonists increase renal reabsorption of Mg.[18] In vitro and in vivo studies have demonstrated that insulin may modulate the shift of Mg^{2+} concentration from the extracellular to intracellular space. Activation of the Ca-sensing receptor in the thick ascending loop of Henle by hypercalcemia increases urinary Ca^{2+} and Mg^{2+} excretion.[16] Reabsorption of Mg^{2+} is impaired with osmotic diuresis (volume expansion), hyperglycemia, hypercalciuria, hypercalcemia, hypermagnesemia, hypophosphatemia, hypokalemia, tubular acidosis, metabolic acidosis, and toxicities caused by amphotericin B or aminoglycosides.[18] Administration of furosemide and induction of hypercalcemia causes reduction in serum tMg and Mg^{2+} concentrations in healthy horses by inhibition of the $Na^+/K^+/2Cl^-$ transporter, which reduces the transepithelial voltage gradient[19] and directly decreases the reabsorption of Ca and Mg. PTH indirectly increases Mg^{2+} release from bone during bone resorption. PTH, vitamin D, calcitonin, AVP, glucagon, and Ca concentrations influence Mg absorption and excretion to some degree.

PTH acts on the renal tubules to increase Mg reabsorption.[20] Micropuncture studies have shown that PTH changes the cortical thick ascending limb of the loop of Henle potential difference, which increases the transepithelial voltage gradient to enhance paracellular Mg reabsorption.[14,21]

PATHOPHYSIOLOGICAL CONSEQUENCES OF HYPOMAGNESEMIA AND INFLAMMATION

Mg has a role in protection against neurotoxicity, cardiotoxicity, inflammation, and free radical damage.[22–25] Hypomagnesemia is associated with increased cytokine production and systemic inflammation.[26,27] Subclinical hypomagnesemia is common in the intensive care unit and is associated with increased risk of death. Experimental endotoxin administration in horses results in an acute decrease in tMg and Mg^{2+} concentrations.[28] It seems that endotoxemia induces acute hypomagnesemia and that Mg administration may have a protective effect in hypomagnesemic endotoxemic patients. Endotoxemic humans with concurrent hypomagnesemia have a worse outcome compared with normomagnesemic endotoxemic patients.[22] Considering that approximately 40% of horses with colic have endotoxemia, and that free radical injury is an important mechanism in intestinal ischemia-reperfusion injury, the role of Mg and its therapeutic importance in equine disease warrants investigation.

INCIDENCE AND OUTCOME OF HYPOMAGNESEMIA IN EQUINE PATIENTS

Hypomagnesemia is commonly observed in the critically ill patient, but whether it contributes to mortality or is merely associated with severe disease is unknown.

A retrospective study found that 48.7% (401/823) of hospitalized horses had tMg values below the reference range.[29] Hypomagnesemia was associated with gastrointestinal disease, infectious respiratory disease, and multiorgan disease.[29] Although there was no association with mortality, the length of hospitalization was longer for horses with hypomagnesemia.[29] In equine surgical colic patients, 54% had low serum Mg^{2+} levels and 17% had low tMg concentrations. Horses with ionized hypomagnesemia had a significantly greater prevalence of postoperative ileus than normomagnesemic equine surgical colic patients.[30] Surgical colic patients that were euthanized at the time of surgery (7/35) had significantly lower preoperative serum concentrations of Mg^{2+} compared with horses that survived, but the serum Mg concentration did not predict hospitalization time or survival.[30] A low Mg^{2+} concentration was documented in 78% (50/64) of horses with enterocolitis.[19] In other species, a clear association has been made between hypomagnesemia, severity of disease, and mortality, but larger studies in severely ill horses may be required to determine if similar associations exist in horses. Although 15% of critically ill foals were found to have low serum Mg^{2+} concentrations, no association between hypomagnesemia and mortality was detected.[31] Hypomagnesemia is also commonly seen in blister beetle toxicosis[32] and horses with synchronous diaphragmatic flutter (SDF).

Sepsis-induced hypocalcemia and hypomagnesemia may be associated with intracellular ionic shift, hemodilution, or sequestration. Mg may function as a Ca antagonist, and low Mg concentrations may enhance intracellular entry of Ca in sepsis and endotoxemia.[22] It is undetermined if Mg administration to acutely hypomagnesemic patients is beneficial in the reduction of mortality or length of hospitalization, but it seems reasonable to therapeutically maintain serum concentrations within reference range during times of severe illness when homeostatic mechanisms are overwhelmed.

ASSOCIATION OF HYPOMAGNESEMIA WITH HYPOKALEMIA

Hypomagnesemia is frequently associated with hypokalemia and kaliuresis in other species.[33–37] Mg deficiency has been associated with the loss of cellular potassium stores, and as is the case in hypocalcemic patients, it may be difficult to restore normokalemia until the concurrent Mg deficiency is corrected.[38] Hypomagnesemia affects the ability of Mg to act as a coenzyme for the Na^+/K^+ ATPase pump, resulting in decreased intracellular K^+ and increased intracellular Na^+ concentrations that lower the resting membrane potential, predisposing cells to spontaneous depolarization and impairment of transmission of electric impulses. Hypomagnesemia can result in the blockade of voltage-gated K^+ channels,[39] which interferes with electric repolarization and the propagation of the action potential. Hypomagnesemia can also lead to increased Purkinje fiber excitability, which predisposes to arrhythmia generation.[40] Clinically, concurrent hypomagnesemia and hypokalemia leads to hyperexcitability, cardiac arrhythmias, seizures, muscle fasciculations, and weakness.

ASSOCIATION OF HYPOMAGNESEMIA WITH HYPOCALCEMIA

Hypocalcemia and hypomagnesemia are concurrently observed in horses with blister beetle poisoning, endotoxemia, enterocolitis, intestinal strangulation, ileus, and SDF; in transported horses; and in lactating mares.[19,28,30,32] Hypocalcemic patients with concurrent hypomagnesemia are often refractory to Ca therapy unless the low serum Mg concentrations are identified and corrected.[41–44] Although the mechanisms by which hypomagnesemia results in hypocalcemia are not completely understood, low serum Mg concentrations can impair PTH synthesis and secretion and induce target tissue resistance to PTH. This mode of action affects renal resorption of Ca^{2+}

and Mg^{2+}, decreases bone resorption, and reduces renal synthesis of 1,25-dihydroxyvitamin D_3.[45] Consequently, parallel determination of Ca and PTH concentrations is important in the investigation of Mg and Ca homeostasis.

Mg is considered nature's physiologic Ca blocker because it reduces the release of Ca from and into the sarcoplasmic reticulum and protects the cell against Ca overload under conditions of ischemia.[46] Mg's Ca channel blocking effect seems to be decreased in the hypomagnesemic state with a subsequent increase in intracellular Ca concentration, leading to enhanced cellular sensitivity to cardiotoxic drugs or ischemic events.

ASSOCIATION OF MG AND ENDOTOXEMIA

Hypocalcemia and hypomagnesemia are common in horses with sepsis and endotoxemia.[19,29,30] Experimental endotoxin infusion in horses resulted in electrolyte abnormalities that included hypomagnesemia, hypocalcemia, hypokalemia, hypophosphatemia, and increased serum PTH and insulin concentrations, but no changes in serum sodium or chloride concentrations.[28] Correction of electrolyte abnormalities is well recognized as part of the care of the critically ill equine patient, and it seems that correction of serum Mg^{2+} concentrations is warranted. Experimental murine studies have implicated Mg in cell messaging and cytokine production. Hypomagnesemic rats exhibit elevated circulating cytokine concentrations (interleukin [IL] 1, IL-6, tumor necrosis factor [TNF]) indicating a generalized inflammatory state.[26,27] Hypomagnesemic rats are acutely sensitive to the effects of experimentally administered endotoxin, and this vulnerability is correlated with higher plasma TNF concentrations.[27] In a murine model, progressive Mg deficiency led to increasing mortality rates from the effects of endotoxin administration, whereas Mg supplementation reduced the endotoxin-induced mortality.[22] Hypomagnesemia also predisposed animals to free radical–associated injury,[23,24] leading to the formation of cardiomyopathic lesions and altered vascular tone.[25,47] These murine studies were performed after chronic dietary-induced hypomagnesemia, and care must be taken when extrapolating this information to the critically ill patients, which have redistribution of serum and cellular Mg rather than a state of whole body Mg depletion.

ASSOCIATION OF MG AND INSULIN RESISTANCE

Although a great deal of controversy exists about the role of Mg in human diabetes, there have been epidemiologic studies linking low Mg status with insulin-dependent and non–insulin-dependent diabetes mellitus.[48] Intracellular Mg^{2+} concentration has been shown to modulate insulin action, and there is an increased incidence of low intracellular Mg^{2+} concentrations in human patients with non–insulin-dependent diabetes mellitus.[49] There have been suggestions that this incidence may result in defective tyrosine kinase activity at the insulin receptor level, resulting in increased intracellular Ca^{2+} concentrations, which can contribute to worsening insulin resistance.[48,49] Daily oral Mg supplementation to human patients with non–insulin-dependent diabetes mellitus has resulted in the restoration of intracellular Mg^{2+} concentrations and improvement of insulin-mediated glucose uptake.[48]

Care should be taken when making inferences from humans to horses because human epidemiologic data are often confounded with poor dietary intake and alcoholism. There has been some discussion as to the usefulness of Mg supplementation to horses with insulin resistance with either equine metabolic syndrome or pituitary pars intermedia dysfunction. It seems unlikely that horses would develop chronic whole body Mg deficiency because efforts to induce Mg depletion have required long-term feeding of severely Mg-deplete artificial diets in young growing animals.[1,9,10] It is the author's opinion that dietary Mg supplementation to horses is infrequently required when a normal diet is fed. However, oral Mg supplementation is unlikely to be harmful because of rapid renal elimination of excessive Mg if renal function is normal. There are anecdotal reports from veterinarians that Mg supplementation in addition to previously attempted dietary modifications to horses with equine metabolic syndrome has been beneficial in reducing neck crestyness and the frequency of laminitis episodes. However, there are no published reports or experimental substantiation of such claims.

EXPERIMENTAL DIETARY MANIPULATION OF MG IN HORSES

Hypomagnesemia was induced in mature ponies by feeding 5 to 6 mg/kg BW/d of Mg (using a 370 ppm diet) while 20 mg/kg BW/d met Mg requirements.[50] A deficiency state can be more readily induced in growing animals because of their higher dietary requirement of Mg. Foals fed an extremely Mg-deficient diet (7–8 ppm or 0.0007%) developed severe mineralization of the aorta, with severe clinical signs of hypomagnesemia becoming apparent after 90 days in 2 of 11 foals.[51]

Urinary excretion of electrolytes is useful for assessing the dietary supply of minerals. The urinary Mg concentration decreased from a baseline of 30 mg/dL to 4 mg/dL after 6 days on a Mg-deficient diet (370 ppm) and increased to more than 300 mg/dL on a high Mg diet supplemented with 36 g of MgO/d.[50] Increasing the Mg content of a diet from 3100 ppm to 8600 ppm increased Mg digestibility, retention, and excretion in urine and feces and increased serum concentrations from 2.21 mg/dL to 3.39 mg/dL.[10] In foals fed a severely Mg-deficient diet (7–8 ppm), serum Mg concentration decreased rapidly from a baseline of 0.78 mmol/L to 0.53 mmol/L after 7 days and then decreased steadily to 0.26 mmol/L after 150 days. The slower rate of reduction in serum Mg concentrations was presumed to be caused by the mobilization of Mg from bone. Bone Mg content decreased in response to Mg depletion, however, there was no effect on tissue (brain, liver, kidney, spleen, lung, cardiac, or skeletal muscle) concentrations of Mg, Ca, or P after 71 to 180 days.[52]

CLINICAL SIGNS AND CONSEQUENCES OF MG DEFICIENCY

In comparison to cattle, clinical signs of hypomagnesemia are rarely reported in horses, but include weakness, muscle fasciculations, ventricular arrhythmias, seizures, ataxia, and coma. Hypocalcemic tetany complicated by hypomagnesemia was reported in Welsh mountain ponies.[53,54] Similar signs were experimentally induced after 90 days in 2/11 foals fed an extremely Mg-deficient diet (7–8 ppm). Signs of hypomagnesemic tetany were precipitated by loud noises, with foals initially exhibiting nervousness, muscular tremors, and ataxia followed by collapse, with profuse sweating, hyperpnea, and convulsions. One foal died during its third seizure on day 150 of the deficiency trial.[51]

Concurrent hypocalcemic and hypomagnesemic tetany was reported in 2 thoroughbred broodmares that had been transported for breeding. The mares were nursing foals that were aged 4 and 7 weeks. Their serum total Ca (tCa) concentration was 4.0 mg/dL and 5.4 mg/dL, whereas their tMg was 1.0 mg/dL and 1.9 mg/dL, respectively. The mares responded to IV calcium borogluconate and magnesium chloride.[55]

Severe hypomagnesemia can lead to ventricular arrhythmias, supraventricular tachycardia, or atrial fibrillation. Characteristic findings on electrocardiogram (ECG) include prolongation of the PR interval, widening of the QRS complex, ST segment depression, and peaked T waves.[56]

Hypomagnesemia and hypocalcemia are common perioperatively in horses requiring exploratory celiotomy for colic, particularly in horses with strangulating intestinal lesions and ileus. Significantly lower serum concentrations of Mg^{2+} occurred in horses that developed postoperative ileus.[30] Horses with strangulating lesions were more likely to be hypomagnesemic and hypocalcemic and have more ECG changes than horses with nonstrangulating lesions.[30] There are probably multiple factors that contribute to the observed ECG disturbances, but the routine detection and correction of electrolyte abnormalities (including Mg^{2+} and Ca^{2+}) is recommended.

Hypomagnesemia and hypocalcemia can contribute to SDF, also known as "thumps." Horses with dehydration; electrolyte derangements; and especially hypochloremic metabolic alkalosis associated with prolonged endurance exercise, gastric outflow obstruction, and sometimes after inappropriate bicarbonate administration are predisposed. Irritation of the phrenic nerve causes unilateral or bilateral contraction of the diaphra\ synchronous with the heartbeat. A state of alkalosis because of massive chloride and hydrogen ion loss caused by prolonged sweating or reflux of gastric origin or inappropriate bicarbonate administration can result in hydrogen ion shifts and exposure of negative charges on serum protein molecules, which subsequently bind Ca^{2+} and Mg^{2+} resulting in a relative ionized hypocalcemia and hypomagnesemia. The tCa and tMg levels are normal, but Mg^{2+} and Ca^{2+} concentrations are low. The condition may resolve spontaneously after resolution of the primary cause or after the correction of electrolyte and acid-base imbalance and rehydration. IV administration of calcium gluconate and $MgSO_4$ often speeds recovery.

MG AND BRAIN INJURY

Mg is important in the regulation of neuroexcitation by blocking signal transmission via inhibition of Ca^{2+} -dependent presynaptic excitation-secretion coupling.[57–60] Depletion of Mg contributes to tetany by increasing acetylcholine release from neuromuscular junction and delaying degradation by acetylcholinesterase. Mg infusions have been advocated in the treatment of human and equine brain and spinal trauma patients, but the efficacy of such treatments is still uncertain.[58–60] Based on evidence from human medicine, Mg infusions are also used in the empiric treatment of hypoxic ischemic encephalopathy (HIE) in neonatal foals.[61]

Cerebral hypoxia impairs maintenance of ionic gradients across cell membranes, resulting in an influx of Ca and glutamate. Intracellular Ca and glutamate overload results in neuronal cell death. Traumatic brain injury induces the activation of the *N*-methyl-D-aspartate (NMDA) subtype of the glutamate receptor[62] and has been implicated in the pathophysiology of HIE.[63] Mg is important in the voltage-dependent blockade of NMDA Ca channels, preventing Ca entry into the cell and decreasing neurotransmitter release. Mg also blocks the entry of Ca through the voltage-gated Ca channels in the presynaptic membrane.[64] Normal blood-brain vessel vasodilation is also dependent on Mg.[65] Lower Mg concentrations increase vascular smooth muscle tone, potentiating vasospasm with reduction of oxygen and substrate delivery to tissues. Focal traumatic brain and spinal cord injury in rats can reduce free Mg concentrations in the brain by as much as 60%, with the reduction proportional to the extent of the injury.[64] Therefore, brain injury reduces brain Mg concentration, which will result in the loss of Mg's protective role and potentiate further brain injury.

The reduction in the voltage-dependant Mg^{2+} blockage of NMDA current in mechanically injured neurons can be restored by increasing extracellular Mg concentration. $MgSO_4$ has been shown to dramatically improve the immediate recovery of rats from hypoxia[66] and improve the motor outcome in rats treated after severe traumatic axonal brain injury.[67] $MgSO_4$ has also been shown to protect the fetal brain during severe maternal hypoxia.[68] The available experimental literature and reasoning suggests that in most cases, Mg therapy may be advantageous in protecting against, and in the treatment of, HIE in foals and horses with traumatic brain injury, but further evidence is still required before the benefits, if any, can be proven.[59,61]

DIAGNOSTIC TESTING

The clinical laboratory evaluation of Mg status is primarily limited to the measurement of serum Mg concentration, 24-hour urinary excretion, and percentage retention after parenteral Mg loading. However, results for these tests do not necessarily correlate with intracellular ionized concentrations. There is no universally accepted, validated, and readily available test to determine the intracellular/total body Mg status.

The easiest way to assess Mg status is using serum tMg or Mg^{2+} concentrations. Serum Mg^{2+} is more useful because it is the active form and is minimally affected by serum protein concentrations. Hypoalbuminemia results in a low measured serum tMg concentration (pseudohypomagnesemia) and does not require Mg supplementation if the serum Mg^{2+} concentration is normal. Formulas to correct tMg concentration based on adjustment for protein concentrations are not accurate, and Mg^{2+} concentration should be measured. pH can affect the availability of serum Mg and the percentage in the active ionized form. Similar to Ca, Mg binds to anionic (negatively charged) protein binding sites, with the binding affinity depending on the pH. During acidosis, the increased hydrogen ion concentration displaces Ca^{2+} and Mg^{2+} from their protein binding sites, increasing the percentage of these cations in their ionized form, resulting in increased serum Ca^{2+} and Mg^{2+} concentrations. In animals with respiratory or metabolic alkalosis, (often observed after prolonged strenuous endurance exercise), Ca^{2+} and Mg^{2+} concentrations may be low because of increased protein binding. Because Mg^{2+} is the physiologically active component, with ionized hypomagnesemia, supplementation is recommended, especially if clinical signs of SDF (thumps); ileus; or rarely muscle fasciculations, ataxia, or tetany are observed. Although not likely to be of consequence in an animal with adequate renal function, resolution of the alkalosis may result in elevations of the serum Mg^{2+} concentration. In contrast, animals with metabolic acidosis secondary to sepsis, SIRS, and severe gastrointestinal disease rarely have serum ionized hypermagnesemia, rather their serum Mg^{2+} concentration tends to be low from altered Mg homeostasis, cellular or third space redistribution, gastrointestinal loss of Mg, or diuresis secondary to aggressive fluid therapy with IV fluids unsupplemented with Mg.

Renal excretion of Mg may be used to evaluate Mg balance. With low dietary Mg intake, urinary Mg excretion decreases to negligible levels.[1] Renal Mg excretion is measured in urine collected over 24 hours (mg/kg/d). The fractional clearance of Mg (FMg) is determined by expressing the renal Mg clearance relative to creatinine clearance. FMg in healthy horses fed grass hay ranges from 15% to 35%,[1,28] and values less than 6% indicate inadequate dietary Mg intake.[1] The Mg retention test to assess they total body status has been evaluated in horses receiving Mg-deficient diets using 10 mg/kg of elemental Mg (100 mg/kg of a 50% $MgSO_4$solution diluted to 10%) administered intravenously over 60 minutes. Percentage retention (%Ret) is calculated as $\% \text{ Ret} = (1 - [\text{Mg excretion in 24 h}]/[\text{Mg infused}]) \times 100$.

However, in the study validating the Mg retention test in horses, the 24-hour excretion of Mg was found to be a more sensitive indicator of reduced Mg intake than the Mg retention test, and the spot FMg reflected the 24-hour excretion of Mg, providing a simple method to assess the Mg status in horses.[1]

Muscle Mg content has been used as an estimate of total body Mg stores in horses.[1,15] In horses fed a moderately Mg-deficient diet, no differences were found in muscle Mg content compared with controls, but intracellular Mg^{2+} concentrations were lower in Mg-deficient horses.[1]

TREATMENT OF HYPOMAGNESEMIA

When supplementing Mg, it is important to carefully determine whether the dose reported is for elemental Mg or for the salt. For $MgSO_4$ solution (9.7% Mg), a dose of 100 mg/kg provides 9.7 mg/kg of elemental Mg, whereas for $MgCl_2$ (25.5%), a dose of 100 mg/kg provides 25.5 mg/kg of elemental Mg. Confusion and subsequent overdose may be fatal.

Recommended dose rates for $MgSO_4$ in adult horses are 25 to 150 mg/kg/d (0.05–0.3 mL/kg of a 50% solution) diluted to a 5% solution in normal saline, dextrose, or a polyionic isotonic solution and given by slow IV infusion. An IV constant rate infusion (CRI) of 150 mg/kg/d of $MgSO_4$ solution (0.3 mL/kg/d of the 50% solution) would provide the horse's daily requirements.[69] For a 500-kg horse receiving 30 L/d of IV fluids, 25 mL of a 50% $MgSO_4$ solution should be added to each 5 L bag, whereas for a horse receiving 60 L/d, 12 mL of $MgSO_4$ solution should be added per 5 L bag. Such therapy should also be considered in horses with postoperative ileus and SDF.

Plasmalyte-A and Normosol-R contain 3 mEq/L (3.6 mg/dL) of elemental Mg. If a horse received 60 mL/kg/d of the replacement fluid, it would receive 2.16 mg/kg/d of elemental Mg (equivalent to 20 mg/kg of $MgSO_4$). Additional Mg is required for long-term fluid support of an animal with inappetence.

$MgSO_4$ is also used to treat refractory ventricular arrhythmias, including those caused by idiosyncratic quinidine reactions (especially torsades de pointes). For ventricular arrhythmias, the intravenous administration of 2 to 6 mg/kg/min of $MgSO_4$ (1.8–5.4 mL of 50% $MgSO_4$/450 kg horse/min) to effect is recommended. Some investigators recommend a maximum dose of 25 g (56 mg/kg) of $MgSO_4$, but the author's studies in normal horses indicate that 100 mg/kg of $MgSO_4$ can be safely administered over 60 minutes, with mild sedation being occasionally noted.[1]

For the treatment of HIE in neonatal foals, Wilkins[61] suggests a CRI of $MgSO_4$ at an initial intravenous dose of 50 mg/kg/hour for 1 hour followed by a 25-mg/kg/h CRI for 24 hours. For a 50-kg foal, 62 mL of 50% $MgSO_4$ solution should be added to a 1 L bag of isotonic fluids and run at 85 mL/h for 1 hour, which is then decreased to 42 mL/h. This dose provides 600 mg/kg/d of $MgSO_4$ and is higher than that required for maintenance. Therapy has been continued for up to 3 days without visible detrimental effects other than possible trembling.[61] $MgSO_4$ has also been recommended as a muscle relaxant as an adjunctive treatment of tetanus. $MgSO_4$ can be infused with a high therapeutic safety index, with the safety depending on the dose and infusion rate, but is contraindicated with undiagnosed disturbances in cardiac conduction, renal failure, or elevated serum Mg concentrations.

The typical equine diet contains sufficient Mg for maintenance, with supplementation rarely required. If necessary, oral Mg can be provided with MgO, $MgCO_3$, or $MgSO_4$, which have equivalent digestibilities of approximately 70%. The maintenance requirement of 13 mg/kg/d of elemental Mg could be provided by 31 mg/kg/d of MgO,

64 mg/kg/d of $MgCO_3$, or 93 mg/kg/d of $MgSO_4$. This information may be important when formulating oral replacement fluids for horses that are inappetent.

$MgSO_4 \times H_2O$ (Epsom salt) is commonly used as an osmotic cathartic in the treatment of large colon impactions. A dose of 0.5 to 1.0 g/kg of $MgSO_4$ in 6 to 8 L of water can be administered by a stomach tube when the horse is metabolically stable. A second dose can be administered 24 to 36 hours later in severe cases only if serum Mg concentrations have returned to normal. Hypermagnesemic neuromuscular paralysis has been reported after the administration of 1.5 to 2 g/kg of $MgSO_4$.[31]

HYPERMAGNESEMIA

Hypermagnesemia is rare in all species and is commonly the result of iatrogenic Mg overdose or excessive supplementation to a patient with renal failure. Serum hypermagnesemia (with hyperkalemia and hyperphosphatemia) occurs after severe cellular damage (rhabdomyolysis, tumor lysis syndrome, hemolysis, severe sepsis).

Hypermagnesemia was reported in 2 horses given excessive Epsom salt in addition to dioctyl sodium sulfosuccinate (DSS) for the treatment of large colon impaction.[31] The 450-kg and 500-kg horses were reportedly given 750 g and 1000 g of Epsom salt, respectively. Four to six hours after the Epsom salt overdose, the horses showed signs of agitation, sweating, muscle tremors followed by recumbency, and flaccid paralysis. Tachycardia and tachypnea developed, peripheral pulses were undetectable, and capillary refill time was prolonged at 4 seconds. Serum tMg concentrations increased to 5 times the reported reference range. The horses were treated with 250 mL of a 23% solution of calcium gluconate (diluted in 1 L of 0.9% NaCl) administered slowly intravenously. One horse was able to stand 10 minutes after the completion of infusion. IV fluids were given to induce diuresis. A second Ca infusion was required when muscle tremors reoccurred 1 hour later in this horse. The second horse remained weak for several hours, being only able to stand for short periods. These 2 horses were given Epsom salt at 1.5 to 2 times the recommended maximum dose, but it is unlikely that this dose of Epsom salt alone would normally be able to induce such severe clinical signs. The investigators suggested that the concurrently administered DSS may have increased the intestinal permeability and the Mg absorption, with exacerbation of the signs of hypermagnesemia because of the concurrent low serum Ca concentration. Epsom salt should only be given to treat large colon impactions after correction of dehydration and metabolic imbalances. Simultaneous administration of excessive doses of Epsom salt with DSS should be avoided.[31]

REFERENCES

1. Stewart AJ, Hardy J, Kohn CW, et al. Validation of diagnostic tests for determination of magnesium status in horses with reduced magnesium intake. Am J Vet Res 2004;65(4):422–30.
2. Lopez I, Estepa JC, Mendoza FJ, et al. Fractionation of calcium and magnesium in equine serum. Am J Vet Res 2006;67(3):463–6.
3. Wacker WE, Parisi AF. Magnesium metabolism. N Engl J Med 1968;278:658–63, 712–7, 772–6.
4. Elin RJ. Magnesium metabolism in health and disease. Dis Mon 1988;34(4): 161–218.

5. Rude RK, Oldham S. Disorders of magnesium metabolism. In: Bohen RD, editor. The metabolic and molecular basis of acquired disease. London: Balliere, Tindall; 1990. p. 1124–48.
6. McLean R. Magnesium and its therapeutic uses: a review. Am J Med 1994;96: 63–76.
7. Marino P. Calcium and magnesium in critical illness: a practical approach. In: Sivak E, Higgins T, Seiver A, editors. The high risk patient: management of the critically ill. Baltimore (MD): Williams & Wilkins; 1995. p. 1183–95.
8. White R, Hartzell H. Magnesium ions in cardiac function. Biochem Pharmacol 1989;38:859–67.
9. Hintz H, Schryver H. Magnesium metabolism in the horse. J Anim Sci 1972;35: 755.
10. Hintz F, Schryver H. Magnesium, calcium and phosphorus metabolism in ponies fed varying levels of magnesium. J Anim Sci 1973;37:927–30.
11. Rook JA. Spontaneous and induced magnesium deficiency in ruminants. Ann N Y Acad Sci 1969;162:727–31.
12. Martens H, Schweigel M. Pathophysiology of grass tetany and other hypomagnesemias. Implications for clinical management. Vet Clin North Am Food Anim Pract 2000;16(2):339–68.
13. Harrington D, Walsh J. Equine magnesium supplements: Evaluation of magnesium oxide, magnesium sulphate and magnesium carbonate in foals fed purified diets. Equine Vet J 1980;1980(12):32–3.
14. Quamme GA, Dirks JH. Renal magnesium transport. Rev Physiol Biochem Pharmacol 1983;265:H281–8.
15. Grace N, Pearce S, Firth E, et al. Content and distribution of macro- and microelements in the body of pasture fed horses. Aust Vet J 1999;77:172–6.
16. Toribio RE, Kohn CW, Rourke KM, et al. Effects of hypercalcemia on serum concentrations of magnesium, potassium, and phosphate and urinary excretion of electrolytes in horses. Am J Vet Res 2007;27(68):543–54.
17. Kayne L, Lee D. Intestinal magnesium absorption. Miner Electrolyte Metab 1993; 19:21–217.
18. Toribio RE. Magnesium and disease. In: Reed SM, Bayley WM, Sellon DC, editors. Equine internal medicine. 3rd edition. St Louis (MO): Saunders; 2010. p. 1291–5.
19. Toribio RE, Kohn CW, Chew DJ, et al. Comparison of serum parathyroid hormone and ionized calcium and magnesium concentrations and fractional urinary clearance of calcium and phosphorus in healthy horses and horses with enterocolitis. Am J Vet Res 2001;62(6):938–47.
20. Rasmussen H, Bordier P. The physiological and cellular basis of metabolic bone disease. Baltimore (MD): Williams & Wilkins; 1974.
21. de Rouffignac C, Mandon B, Wittner M, et al. Hormonal control of renal magnesium handling. Miner Electrolyte Metab 1993;19:226–31.
22. Salem M, Kasinski N, Munoz R, et al. Progressive magnesium deficiency increases mortality from endotoxin challenge: protective effects of acute magnesium therapy. Crit Care Med 1995;23:108–18.
23. Kramer J, Misik V, Weglicki W. Magnesium-deficiency potentiates free radical production associated with postischemic injury to rat hearts: vitamin E affords protection. Free Radic Biol Med 1994;16(6):713–23.
24. Mak I, Stafford R, Weglicki W. Loss of red cell glutathione during Mg deficiency: prevention by vitamin E, D-propranolol, and chloroquine. Am J Physiol 1994; 267(5 Pt 1):C1366–70.

25. Freedman A, Atrakchi A, Cassidy M, et al. Magnesium deficiency-induced cardiomyopathy: protection by vitamin E. Biochem Biophys Res Commun 1990;170:1102–6.
26. Weglicki W, Phillips T, Freedman A, et al. Magnesium-deficiency elevates circulating levels of inflammatory cytokines and endothelin. Mol Cell Biochem 1992; 110:169–73.
27. Malpuech-Brugere C, Nowacki W, Rock E, et al. Enhanced tumour necrosis factor-alpha production following endotoxin challenge in rats is an early event during magnesium deficiency. Acta Biochem Biophys 1999;1453(1):35–40.
28. Toribio RE, Kohn CW, Hardy J, et al. Alterations in serum parathyroid hormone and electrolyte concentrations and urinary excretion of electrolytes in horses with induced endotoxemia. J Vet Intern Med 2005;19(2):223–31.
29. Johansson AM, Gardner SY, Jones SL, et al. Hypomagnesemia in hospitalized horses. J Vet Intern Med 2003;17(6):860–7.
30. Garcia-Lopez JM, Provost PJ, Rush JE, et al. Prevalence and prognostic importance of hypomagnesemia and hypocalcemia in horses that have colic surgery. Am J Vet Res 2001;62(1):7–12.
31. Henninger RW, Horst J. Magnesium toxicosis in two horses. J Am Vet Med Assoc 1997;211(1):82–5.
32. Helman R, Edwards W. Clinical features of blister beetle poisoning in equids: 70 cases (1983–1996). J Am Vet Med Assoc 1997;211(8):1018–21.
33. Whang R, Oei TO, Aikawa JK, et al. Predictors of clinical hypomagnesemia. Hypokalemia, hypophosphatemia, hyponatremia, and hypocalcemia. Arch Intern Med 1984;144(9):1794–6.
34. Reinhart RA, Desbiens NA. Hypomagnesemia in patients entering the ICU. Crit Care Med 1985;13(6):506–7.
35. Ryzen E. Magnesium homeostasis in critically ill patients. Magnesium 1989; 8(3–4):201–12.
36. Whang R, Whand D, Ryan M. Refractory potassium repletion: a consequence of magnesium deficiency. Arch Intern Med 1992;152:40–5.
37. Martin L, Matteson V, Wingfield W. Abnormalities of serum magnesium in critically ill dogs: incidence and implications. J Vet Emerg Crit Care 1994;1:15–20.
38. al-Ghamdi SM, Cameron EC, Sutton RA. Magnesium deficiency: pathophysiologic and clinical overview. Am J Kidney Dis 1994;24(5):737–52.
39. Roden DM, Iansmith DH. Effects of low potassium or magnesium concentrations on isolated cardiac tissue. Am J Med 1987;82:18–23.
40. Tobey RC, Birnbaum GA, Allegra JR, et al. Successful resuscitation and neurologic recovery from refractory ventricular fibrillation after magnesium sulfate administration. Ann Emerg Med 1992;21:92–6.
41. Ryzen E, Wagners P, Singer F, et al. Magnesium deficiency in a medical ICU population. Crit Care Med 1985;13(1):19–21.
42. Fatemi S, Ryzen E, Flores J, et al. Effect of experimental human magnesium depletion on parathyroid hormone secretion. Endocrinol Metab 1991;73:1067–72.
43. Leicht E, Schmidt-Gayk H, Langer HJ. Hypomagnesemia induced hypocalcemia: Concentrations of parathyroid hormone, prolactin and 1,25-dihydroxyvitamin D during magnesium replenishment. Magnes Res 1992;5:33–6.
44. Shah BR, Santucci MD, Finberg L. Magnesium deficiency as a cause of hypocalcemia in the CHARGE association. Arch Pediatr Adolesc Med 1994;148; 486–9.
45. Abbot L, Rude R. Clinical manifestations of magnesium deficiency. Miner Electrolyte Metab 1993;19:314–22.

46. Shechter M, Sharir M, Labrador MJP. Oral magnesium therapy improves endothelial function in patients with coronary artery disease. Circulation 2000; 102(19):2353–8.
47. Freedman A, Cassidy M, Weglacki W. Captopril protects against myocardial injury induced by magnesium deficiency. Hypertension 1991;18:142–7.
48. Nielsen FH. Magnesium, inflammation, and obesity in chronic disease. Nutr Rev 2010;68(6):333–40.
49. Barbagallo M, Dominguez LJ, Galiato A, et al. Role of magnesium in insulin action, diabetes and cardio-metabolic syndrome X. Mol Aspects Med 2003;24:39–52.
50. Meyer H, Ahlswede L. Untersuchungen zum Mg-Stofwechsel des pferdes. [Magnesium metabolism in the horse]. Zentrabl Veterinarinacrmed 1977;24: 128–39 [in German].
51. Harrington DD. Pathological features of magnesium deficiency in young horses fed purified rations. Am J Vet Res 1974;35:503.
52. Harrington D. Influence on magnesium deficiency on horse foal tissue concentrations of magnesium, calcium and phosphorus. Br J Nutr 1975;34:45.
53. Montgomerie RF, Savage WH, Dodd EC. Tetany in Welsh mountain ponies. Vet Rec 1929;9:319.
54. Green HH, Allcroft WM, Montgomerie RF. Hypomagnesemia in equine transit tetany. J Comp Path Ther 1935;48:74.
55. Meijer P. [Two cases of tetany in the horse (author's transl)]. Tijdschr Diergeneeskd 1982;107(9):329–32 [in Dutch].
56. Marr CM. Cardiac emergencies and problems of the critical care patient. Vet Clin North Am Equine Pract 2004;20(1):217–30.
57. Hoenderop JG, Bindels RJ. Epithelial Ca2+ and Mg 2+ channels in health and disease. J Am Soc Nephrol 2005;16:15–26.
58. Arango MF, Bainbridge D. Magnesium for acute traumatic brain injury. Cochrane Database Syst Rev 2008;4:CD005400.
59. MacKay RJ. Brain injury after head trauma: pathophysiology, diagnosis, and treatment. Vet Clin North Am Equine Pract 2004;20(1):199–216.
60. Sen AP, Gulati A. Use of magnesium in traumatic brain injury. Neurotherapeutics 2010;7(1):91–9.
61. Wilkins PA. Magnesium infusion in hypoxic ischemic encephalopathy. Paper presented at American College of Veterinary Internal Medicine. Denver (CO), June, 2001.
62. Zhang L, Rzigalinski BA, Ellis EF, et al. Reduction of voltage-dependant Mg2+ blockade of NMDA current in mechanically injured neurons. Science 1996;274: 1291–923.
63. Thordstein M, Bagenholm R, Thiringer K, et al. Scavengers of free oxygen radicals in combination with magnesium ameliorate perinatal hypoxic-ischemic brain damage in the rat. Pediatr Res 1993;34:23–6.
64. Leonard SE, Kirby R. The role of glutamate, calcium and magnesium in secondary brain injury. J Vet Emerg Crit Care 2002;12:17–32.
65. Seelig JM, Wei EP, Kontos HA, et al. Effect of changes in magnesium ion concentration on cat cerebral arterioles. Am J Physiol 1983;245:H22–6.
66. Seimkowicz E. Pretreatment with magnesium sulfate protects against hypoxic-ischemic brain injury but post-asphyxial treatment worsens brain injury in 7-day old rats. Resuscitation 1997;35:53–9.
67. Heath DL, Voink R. Pretreatment with magnesium sulfate protects against hypoxic-ischemic brain injury but post-asphyxial treatment worsens brain injury in 7-day old rats. Am J Obstet Gynecol 1999;180:725–30.

68. Hallak M, Hotra JW, Kupsky WJ. Magnesium sulfate protection of fetal rat brain from severe maternal hypoxia. Obstet Gynecol 2000;96:124–8.
69. Mogg TD. Magnesium disorders - their role in equine medicine. Paper presented at American College of Veterinary Internal Medicine 19th Annual Veterinary Medical Forum. Denver (CO), 2001.

The Endocrine Disruptive Effects of Ergopeptine Alkaloids on Pregnant Mares

Tim J. Evans, DVM, MS, PhD

KEYWORDS

- Agalactia • Ergopeptine alkaloids
- Ergotism • Fescue toxicosis

During equine gestation, ergopeptine alkaloid exposure is not uncommon, and pregnant mares are particularly sensitive to the endocrine disruptive effects of these compounds on lactogenesis and steroidogenesis. Many pregnant mares reside in geographic areas where toxigenic *Neotyphodium coenophialum* (endophyte)-infected tall fescue is the dominant grass in pastures and hays. A large variety of grasses and cereal grains can be infected by *Claviceps purpurea* (ergot), and fungal sclerotia can contaminate forage and, especially, ground and pelleted feeds. Ergopeptine alkaloids produced by the fescue endophyte and/or contained within ergot bodies interact with D_2-dopamine receptors on lactotropes within the anterior pituitary and induce hypoprolactinemia. Decreased prolactin secretion by pituitary lactotropes or, possibly, ergopeptine alkaloid interactions with receptors in other cells within the fetus and/or placenta can induce alterations in steroidogenic pathways. Agalactia, prolonged gestation, abortion, dystocia, and placental and fetal abnormalities are all clinical manifestations of changes in the endocrine milieu induced by the ingestion of ergopeptine alkaloid-contaminated feedstuffs by mares during late gestation. An understanding of the endocrine disruptive effects of gestational exposure to ergopeptine alkaloids is necessary for the diagnosis of potential exposures to these compounds and for effective prophylaxis and therapy.

ENDOCRINE DISRUPTION

Endocrine disruption refers to the effects of any synthetic or naturally occurring xenobiotic that can affect the endocrine system of exposed individuals (ie, the balance of normal hormonal functions) and cause exposure-related physiologic alterations.[1] This definition encompasses any exogenous agent or xenobiotic that interferes with the

Department of Veterinary Pathobiology, Veterinary Medical Diagnostic Laboratory, College of Veterinary Medicine, 1600 East Rollins Street, Columbia, MO 65211, USA
E-mail address: evanst@missouri.edu

Vet Clin Equine 27 (2011) 165–173
doi:10.1016/j.cveq.2010.12.003
vetequine.theclinics.com
0749-0739/11/$ – see front matter

synthesis, release, transport, distribution, binding, actions, metabolism, and/or elimination of endogenous hormones involved in homeostasis or the regulation of developmental processes. Within the broad scope of this definition, gestation and lactation are 2 physiologic states that are profoundly susceptible to the adverse effects of chemicals that can interfere with normal endocrine function.

ERGOPEPTINE ALKALOIDS

Ergot alkaloids are a complex class of compounds with at least 3 separate systems of nomenclature. Most of the naturally occurring ergot alkaloids have been isolated from fungal species belonging to the *Claviceps* and *Neotyphodium* genera.[2,3] These compounds are generally either ergoline alkaloids, such as lysergic acid, lysergol, lysergic acid amide, and ergonovine, or are classified as ergopeptine alkaloids, which include ergotamine, ergocristine, ergosine, ergocryptine, ergocornine, and ergovaline.[4,5] Lysergic acid amide, lysergic acid diethylamide, and ergonovine (ergometrine) are also classified as carboxamides because of the nonpeptidic amidation of the C-8 carboxy group of lysergic acid. Peptidic amidation of this same carboxy group results in the biosynthesis of the ergopeptine alkaloids. Ergopeptine alkaloids, which are also referred to as peptide ergot alkaloids, are essentially tetrapeptides consisting of lysergic acid and 3 other, "classical" amino acids.[3]

SOURCES OF ERGOPEPTINE ALKALOIDS

Ergovaline is thought to be the most physiologically active ergot alkaloid produced by the fungal endophyte, *N coenophialum* (previously known as *Acremonium coenophialum* or *Epichlöe typhina*).[2,6,7] This endophyte grows within the intercellular spaces of tall fescue (*Festuca arundinacea* or *Lolium arundinaceum*) and is part of a symbiotic, grass/endophyte relationship. More than 35 million acres in the upper southeastern and lower regions of the United States contain endophyte-infected tall fescue, and it has been estimated that this grass is the primary forage for over 700,000 horses.[2,6,8,9] While ergovaline concentrations are highest in the seed heads, this ergopeptine alkaloid is also found in other parts of tall fescue grass infected by toxigenic *N coenophialum*.[2,5,6,8,9] Concentrations of ergovaline generally range between 0.2 and 0.6 mg/kg (ppm) in tall fescue, with seed head concentrations of ergovaline often exceeding 1 mg/kg (ppm).[5,10]

The ergopeptine alkaloids ergotamine, ergocristine, ergosine, ergocornine, and ergocryptine are the predominant toxins contained within the black, dark brown, or purple ergot bodies (sclerotia) of *C purpurea*.[2,4,8,9] Unlike endophytic mycelia, fungal sclerotia are externally visible and replace the individual seeds in the seed head of common pasture grasses, including fescues, bluegrasses, and bromegrasses or cereal grains, such as oats, barley, wheat, and especially rye and triticale. The germination and growth of *C purpurea* is facilitated by the cool, wet springs in the northwestern United States and the northern Great Plains.[2,9] Horses are most likely to be exposed to ergot bodies found in contaminated pastures or hays or fragments of fungal sclerotia hidden in processed feeds or concentrated within the screenings from ergotized grains.[4,9] The total concentration of ergopeptine alkaloids in *C purpurea* sclerotia generally range from 2000 to 10,000 mg/kg (ppm).[4,11]

MECHANISM OF ACTION OF ERGOPEPTINE ALKALOIDS

Ergopeptine alkaloids cause vasoconstriction through interactions with dopaminergic, adrenergic, and serotonergic receptors.[2,8,9] However, the pathogeneses of the decreased lactation or agalactia and the impaired reproductive function associated with equine "fescue toxicosis" are generally thought to primarily involve the endocrine disruptive stimulation of D_2-dopamine receptors by ergopeptine alkaloids and the subsequent, dramatic decrease in prolactin secretion by lactotropes located in the anterior pituitary gland or adenohypophysis.[2,4–6,8,9,12] In addition to the endocrine regulation of lactogenesis, prolactin also facilitates certain aspects of steroidogenesis and, possibly, other endocrine pathways.[8,9,13] The initiation of parturition in the mare depends on the maturation and proper function of the fetal hypothalamic-pituitary-adrenal axis.[14] Prolonged gestation in mares exposed to ergopeptine alkaloids might be related to hypoprolactinemia-induced alterations in uterofetoplacental steroid metabolism or might, potentially, be mediated by direct or indirect inhibition of D_2-dopamine receptors on corticotropes in the fetal anterior pituitary.[8,9,14]

CLINICAL SIGNS OF EQUINE FESCUE TOXICOSIS AND ERGOTISM

Equine fescue toxicosis is most commonly recognized as a disease syndrome of late-gestational and early post-parturient mares.[6] However, embryonic death has been associated with ergopeptine alkaloid exposure very early in pregnancy, and short-term, experimental exposures to relatively low concentrations of ergot alkaloids between days 65 and 100 of gestation have resulted in alterations in catecholamine metabolism, even when prolactin concentrations did not appear to differ between treatment groups.[15]

The clinical signs of fescue toxicosis and ergotism in late-gestational mares include, almost without exception, agalactia and, less frequently, prolonged gestation, abortion, dystocia, fetal asphyxia, weakness, dysmaturity and mortality; placental abnormalities, such as premature placental separation; and thickening and edema, as well as retention of fetal membranes.[2,5,6,8,9,12] Agalactia can apparently be observed in mares fed total dietary concentrations of ergovaline as low as 0.05 mg/kg (ppm), and other investigators have reported clinical cases of fescue toxicosis in mares consuming fescue hay with ergovaline concentrations greater than 0.1 mg/kg (ppm).[5] Mares ingesting processed feeds containing screenings of ergotized grain with total ergopeptine alkaloid concentrations ranging from 0.5 to 1.5 mg/kg (ppm) also exhibited signs of agalactia.[9] Reflecting hypoprolactinemia, the signs of impending parturition in pregnant mares, such as the rapid increase in udder development and the commonly observed "waxing" or accumulation of colostrum at the teat orifices, as well as increases in the calcium concentrations in mammary secretions, are often absent or minimal in those late-gestational mares that have consumed ergopeptine alkaloids. Without these prolactin-dependent indicators of approaching parturition, foal deliveries are frequently unexpected, and therefore unattended.[4–6,9]

While ergopeptine alkaloid-induced abortions can certainly occur, they appear to be less common than prolonged gestation in mares ingesting toxigenic endophyte-infected tall fescue.[8,12] Abortions are generally more common with ingestion of high doses of ergot alkaloids produced by *C purpurea*, which can include the ergoline alkaloid ergonovine (also referred to as ergometrine because of its oxytocic effects), in addition to ergopeptine alkaloids.[4] Ergot alkaloid–induced abortions are most likely associated with stimulation of the myometrium as well as probably impaired placental circulation.

Fetal growth frequently continues during the prolonged gestation observed in pregnant mares consuming ergopeptine alkaloids, and the increased size of the foal, despite often less than optimal placental function, appears to contribute to the fetal dysmaturity or, rather, overmaturity often observed in these situations.[9] As parturition is initiated by the foal and requires appropriate fetal presentation, position, and posture, increased fetal size with dysmaturity/overmaturity, associated with maternal consumption of ergopeptine alkaloids, contribute to the development of dystocias and their sequelae in both mares and foals.[6,9] In addition, failure of passive transfer, neonatal septicemia, and decreased viability commonly occur in foals from agalactic mares exposed to ergopeptine alkaloids.

ENDOCRINE DISRUPTIVE EFFECTS OF ERGOPEPTINE ALKALOIDS IN PREGNANT MARES

Hypoprolactinemia During Late Gestation

Prolactin is secreted by lactotropic cells in the adenohypophysis and is most often thought of in conjunction with its role in lactogenesis.[9,14] Prolactin secretion is tonically inhibited by endogenous dopamine interacting with D_2-dopamine receptors on lactotropes. Large increases in prolactin secretion normally occur a few days before parturition in the mare and can stay elevated for several weeks postpartum. Because a placental lactogen is not produced during equine pregnancy, lactogenesis and lactation in mares, unlike that in cattle and many other species, are completely dependent on the production and secretion of prolactin by the adenohypophseal lactotropes.[14] Ergopeptine alkaloids produced by *N coenophialum* or *C purpurea* mimic the actions of dopamine on lactotropic D_2 receptors, and induce hypoprolactinemia (**Fig. 1**A) and, therefore, agalactia in pregnant mares. Hypoprolactinemia is considered by many to be the hallmark endocrine biomarker for ergopeptine alkaloid exposure in pregnant mares, and agalactia or dysgalactia are almost always present in late-gestational, ergopeptine alkaloid–exposed pregnant mares.[2,4–6,8,9,12]

Suppression of Maternal Progestagen Concentrations During Late Gestation

Beginning on or about day 40 of gestation, the utero-feto-placental unit begins to secrete progestagens known as 5-α pregnanes, which differ structurally from

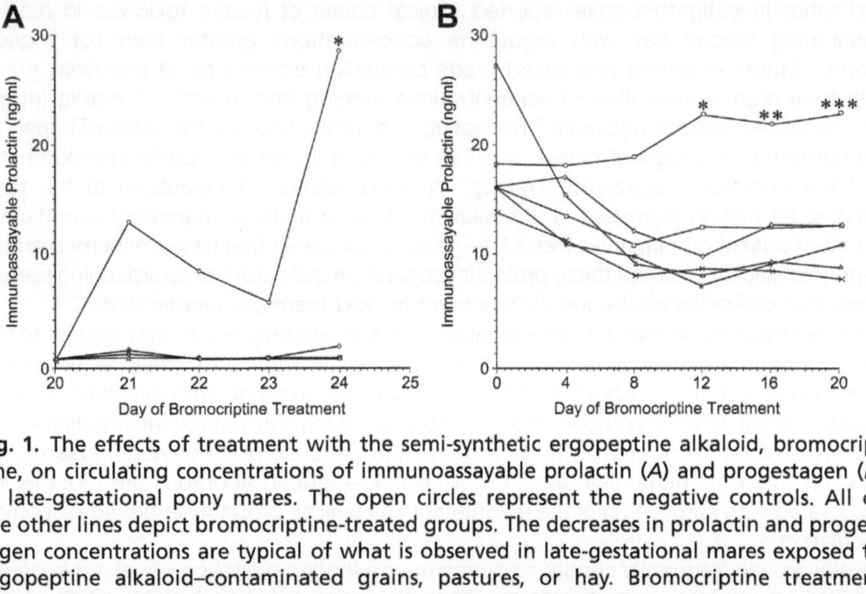

Fig. 1. The effects of treatment with the semi-synthetic ergopeptine alkaloid, bromocriptine, on circulating concentrations of immunoassayable prolactin (*A*) and progestagen (*B*) in late-gestational pony mares. The open circles represent the negative controls. All of the other lines depict bromocriptine-treated groups. The decreases in prolactin and progestagen concentrations are typical of what is observed in late-gestational mares exposed to ergopeptine alkaloid–contaminated grains, pastures, or hay. Bromocriptine treatment began on day 300 of gestation and continued until after foaling. Asterisks denote the concentrations of statistical significance (*$P<.05$, **$P<.01$, and ***$P<.001$, respectively) between bromocriptine treatment groups and negative controls.

progesterone (4-pregnene-3,20-dione).[9,14] The predominant 5-α pregnane found in the peripheral blood of mares during late gestation, 3,20-dione (5α-DHP), may be found in extremely large concentrations (mg/ml vs ng/ml for progesterone).[9] The 5-α pregnanes cross-react with the radioimmunoassay for progesterone, but these compounds are undetectable with enzyme-linked immunosorbent assays (ELISA), which measure progesterone.[9,14] The existence of a unique steroidogenic pathway in pregnant mares is suggested by the predominance of 5-α pregnanes in mid- to late-term pregnant mares and the manner in which these mares metabolize exogenous progestagens.[9,14,16] Production of 5-α pregnanes by the utero-fetal-placental unit reaches a plateau by approximately mid-gestation, and there is normally a dramatic increase in maternal concentrations of immunoassayable progestagens 30 days before parturition. This surge in maternal progestagen concentrations peaks 2 to 3 days prepartum and declines precipitously within 24 hours of parturition.[14] In cases of ergopeptine alkaloid exposure, the metabolism of progestagens is altered and the dramatic increase in maternal, circulating progestagens observed during the last 30 days of pregnancy is suppressed or absent (**Fig.** 1B).[4–6,8,9,12,14] This suppression of the late-gestational surge in immunoassayable progestagens is frequently concurrent with prolonged gestation, and may be related to maternal hypoprolactinemia and/or alterations in fetal cortisol concentrations.[4,6,8,9,12] Administration of D_2-dopamine receptor antagonists to ergopeptine alkaloid-exposed pregnant mares results in resolution of the hypoprolactinemia and resurgence of maternal concentrations of circulating progestagens.[6,8,13]

Decreased Maternal Relaxin Concentrations During Gestation

The placenta is thought to be the sole source of relaxin in the pregnant mare.[14,17] Relaxin decreases the collagen content in the extracellular matrices of the pubic symphysis and uterine cervix, inhibits uterine contractility, and may also play a role in mammary gland development.[9,14] Placental secretion of relaxin begins on about day 80 of pregnancy and peaks initially at approximately day 175. Following a subsequent, slight decline in blood relaxin concentrations, maternal concentrations of relaxin begin to increase gradually from about day 225 of gestation until parturition.[14,17] Relaxin has been demonstrated to be an indicator of placental health in the mare. In late-gestational mares exposed to endophyte-infected fescue, maternal, circulating concentrations of relaxin are decreased and may indicate placental dysfunction.[9,17]

Alterations in Maternal Estrogen Concentrations

As luteal estrogen production begins to decline around days 60 to 90 of pregnancy, fetoplacental estrogen secretion begins to increase. Estrogens of fetoplacental origin increase gradually until day 200 of pregnancy and then decrease very gradually until parturition.[14] It has been suggested that circulating concentrations of immunoassayable estrogens are increased in mares exposed to ergopeptine alkaloids during late gestation.[8] However, this endocrine alteration appears to be less consistent during the last 30 days of gestation than alterations in prolactin, progestagens, and relaxin.[9,13]

Alterations in Maternal Thyroid Hormones

There has been much debate regarding the diagnosis of equine thyroid dysfunction. A wide variety of external factors appear to influence the hypothalamic pituitary thyroid axis. Dopamine also inhibits thyroid-stimulating hormone release by the pituitary thyrotropes, and it has been suggested that mares exposed to endophyte-infected fescue during late gestation, as well as their foals, have decreased circulating concentrations of thyroxine (T_4). This effect of ergopeptine alkaloids may be worthy of further investigation.[7]

ERGOPEPTINE ALKALOID–INDUCED ENDOCRINE DISTURBANCES IN NEONATAL FOALS

Neonatal foals from mares exposed to ergopeptine alkaloids during late gestation frequently exhibit signs of dysmaturity.[4–6,13] Plasma concentrations of immunoassayable progestagens, cortisol, thyroxine (T_4), and tri-iodothyronine (T_3) are generally decreased in the foals of mares grazing endophyte-infected tall fescue pastures.[4–7,18] These endocrine alterations in the neonate may reflect the effects of ergopeptine alkaloids on blood supply to the fetus, placental structure and metabolism, and/or fetal hypothalamic and pituitary function.

DIAGNOSIS OF ERGOPEPTINE ALKALOID EXPOSURE IN HORSES

Endocrine alterations in pregnant mares during the last 30 days of gestation might be helpful in diagnosing ergopeptine alkaloid exposure, but assays for immunoassayable progestagens, prolactin, and relaxin might not be available at all diagnostic laboratories.[4,5,9] In many cases, prolonged gestation and, especially, decreased mammary development and agalactia might be the best diagnostic criteria available for ergopeptine alkaloid exposure.[4–6] Calcium concentrations in mammary secretions rarely exceed 50 ppm in mares exposed to ergopeptine alkaloids.[9] ELISA testing for urinary excretion of fescue ergot alkaloids, if performed within 24 to 48 hours of animal removal from suspect pasture, hay, or grain-containing products, has provided a method of definitively confirming exposure to ergot alkaloids in cattle and horses.[4,5,15] The determination of ergopeptine alkaloid concentrations by ELISA or high-performance liquid chromatography does not confirm ingestion of ergopeptine alkaloids by horses, but it might be very useful in establishing exposure to these compounds, especially in geographic areas where fescue pastures and *Claviceps purpurea* infection are uncommon.[4–6,9,10]

PROPHYLACTIC AND THERAPEUTIC CONSIDERATIONS IN ERGOPEPTINE ALKALOID TOXICOSIS

Knowledge of breeding dates, confirmation of pregnancy, and careful monitoring of mammary gland development are critical steps in the identification of mares most susceptible to the effects of exposure to ergopeptine alkaloids.[4,5,9] Exposure of pregnant mares to heavily ergotized feedstuffs should be avoided. Pastures, hays, and grains should be monitored for the presence of *C purpurea* sclerotia, and grain screenings should not be incorporated in feedstuffs intended for consumption by horses.[2,4,5,9] Analysis for ergopeptine alkaloid concentrations in suspect forages or rations may be advisable.[4,5]

Avoidance of the use of toxigenic *N coenophialum*–infected tall fescue in pastures or hays may be the best prophylactic approach to fescue toxicosis, but might be extremely challenging. Complete pasture renovation and reseeding with endophyte-free fescue or other grass species is limited by the symbiotic nature of tall fescue grass/*Neotyphodium* interactions. Endophyte-free tall fescue might not grow as well under some environmental conditions as fescue infected with *N coenophialum*.[2,4,5,9] The Continental genotype of tall fescue (the most common in the United States), infected with a genetically altered, nontoxigenic, "friendly" endophyte, has shown promise in the prevention of the clinical signs of fescue toxicosis in pregnant mares.[9] However, this approach to prevention and control of fescue toxicosis may be limited by economic and time constraints, as well as the possible reintroduction of "unfriendly," toxigenic endophyte-infected fescue grass.[5] In addition, recent reports of a potentially fatal, fescue-associated edema syndrome in Australian horses grazing genetically-altered, "nontoxigenic" endophyte-infected Mediterranean tall fescue might be cause for some additional caution when considering the use of genetically modified varieties of fescue in valuable broodmares.[19]

Strategic timing of withdrawal of horses from endophyte-infected pasture or hay for periods as long as 60 to 90 days before anticipated foaling dates has been recommended for pregnant mares. However, because the most significant endocrine alterations associated with ergopeptine alkaloid exposure occur after day 300 of gestation, the removal of pregnant mares from potential sources of ergopeptine alkaloids at least 30 days before the expected foaling date is absolutely critical and has generally been successful in controlling the incidence of equine fescue toxicosis.[4–6,8] Frequent mowing, heavy grazing pressure, and chemical treatment to prevent or retard seed head development have been recommended as ways to decrease ergopeptine alkaloid concentrations in fescue pastures. Seeding fescue pastures with at least 20% palatable legumes such as clovers may also be a means of decreasing concentrations of ergopeptine alkaloids.[4,5]

Successful treatment of fescue toxicosis and ergotism in horses is dependent on the early recognition of the clinical signs, as well as preparturient monitoring and assistance during foaling. D_2-dopamine receptor antagonists, such as domperidone (1.1 mg/kg by mouth, once a day), sulpiride (3.3 mg/kg by mouth, once a day), perphenazine (0.3 to 0.5 mg/kg by mouth, twice a day), and acepromazine (20 mg/horse intramuscularly, 4 times a day) have been used with some success in the treatment of agalactia in mares exposed to ergopeptine alkaloids (**Fig. 2**A).[4–6,8,9,12,20] The Rauwolfian alkaloid, reserpine (2.5–5.0 mg/450 kg horse, once a day), which depletes brain depots of dopamine, serotonin, and/or norepinephrine, can be used for the treatment

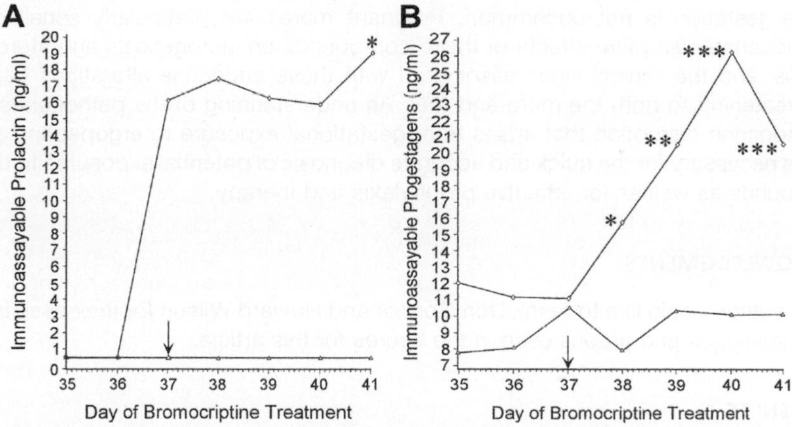

Fig. 2. Decreased circulating concentrations of immunoassayable prolactin (*A*) and progestagens (*B*) rapidly increased after the initiation of domperidone therapy (*open diamonds*) in bromocriptine-treated pony mares with prolonged gestation and agalactia. No significant alterations in these endocrine parameters were observed in bromocriptine-treated pregnant pony mares, exhibiting similar clinical signs, which were treated with reserpine (*open triangles*). Domperidone or reserpine administration began on day 337 of gestation. Asterisks denote statistically significant differences (*$P<.05$, **$P<.01$, and ***$P<.001$, respectively) between treatments.

of postpartum but not prepartum agalactia in mares with a history of exposure to ergopeptine alkaloids, but its use may be associated with sedation and diarrhea (see **Fig. 2**A).[4–6,13] Domperidone does not cross the blood-brain barrier like other D_2 antagonists, thereby diminishing the incidence of unpredictable, extrapyramidal signs, and has been demonstrated to be effective for the treatment of ergopeptine alkaloid-related prolonged gestation and the associated decrease in maternal immunoassayable progestagen concentrations in mares (**Fig. 2**B).[4–6,8,13] Similar to what was discussed with regard to the treatment of preparturient ergopeptine alkaloid-induced agalactia, prepartum administration of reserpine does not appear to resolve prolonged gestation and alterations in maternal immunoassayable progestagen concentrations caused by maternal ingestion of ergopeptine alkaloids (see **Fig. 2**B).[4–6,13]

Pharmacologic intervention can also be used in late-gestational mares to prevent the clinical signs of ergopeptine alkaloid toxicosis. This prophylactic approach may be advisable in environments favoring the growth endophyte-infected fescue and the germination and development of *C purpurea*. Domperidone, sulpiride, and perphenazine have all been used experimentally at their therapeutic doses, beginning on day 300 of gestation, to prevent the endocrine alterations and clinical signs associated with ergopeptine alkaloid toxicosis in pregnant mares.[4–6,8,20] In clinical settings, administration of domperidone 10 to 14 days before the expected foaling date has proven to be a useful prophylactic approach to ergopeptine alkaloid toxicosis in the pregnant mare, as long as udder development is monitored carefully and the dosage regimen modified if the mare begins dripping colostrum.[4–6,9] The D_2-dopamine receptor antagonist, fluphenazine (25 mg intramuscularly in pony mares on day 320 of gestation), has also been used to prevent decreases in relaxin related to ergopeptine alkaloid–induced placental dysfunction.[4,5,9,17]

SUMMARY

It should be clear from this discussion that ergopeptine alkaloid exposure during equine gestation is not uncommon. Pregnant mares are particularly sensitive to the endocrine disruptive effects of these compounds on lactogenesis and steroidogenesis, and the clinical signs associated with these endocrine alterations can be life-threatening to both the mare and foal. An understanding of the pathogenesis of the endocrine disruption that arises from gestational exposure to ergopeptine alkaloids is necessary for the quick and accurate diagnosis of potential exposures to these compounds as well as for effective prophylaxis and therapy.

ACKNOWLEDGMENTS

The author would like to thank Don Connor and Howard Wilson for their assistance with the images and graphs used in the figures for this article.

REFERENCES

1. Evans TJ. Reproductive toxicity and endocrine disruption. In: Gupta RC, editor. Veterinary toxicology: basic and applied principles. New York: Academic Press/Elsevier, Inc; 2007. p. 206–44.
2. Burrows GE, Tyrl RJ. Toxic plants of North America. Ames (IA): Iowa State University Press; 2001.
3. Roberts CA, Kallenbach RL, Hill NS, et al. Ergot alkaloid concentrations in tall fescue hay during production and storage. Crop Sci 2009;49:1496–502.

4. Evans TJ, Rottinghaus GE, Casteel SW. Ergotism. In: Plumlee KH, editor. Clinical veterinary toxicology. St Louis (MO): Mosby; 2004. p. 239–43.
5. Evans TJ, Rottinghaus GE, Casteel SW. Fescue toxicosis. In: Plumlee KH, editor. Clinical veterinary toxicology. St Louis (MO): Mosby; 2004. p. 243–50.
6. Brendemuehl JP. Reproductive aspects of fescue toxicosis. In: Robinson NE, editor. Current therapy in equine medicine. 4th edition. Philadelphia: Saunders; 1997. p. 571–3.
7. Messer NT, Riddle T, Traub-Dargatz JL, et al. Thyroid hormone levels in Thoroughbred mares and their foals at parturition. Proc Am Assoc Equine Pract 1998;44:248–51.
8. Cross DL, Redmond LM, Strickland JR. Equine fescue toxicosis; signs and solutions. J Anim Sci 1995;73:899–908.
9. Evans TJ. Endocrine alterations associated with ergopeptine alkaloid exposure during equine pregnancy. Vet Clin North Am Equine Pract 2002;18:371–8.
10. Rottinghaus GE, Garner GB, Cornell CN, et al. An HPLC method for quantitating ergovaline in endophyte-infested tall fescue: seasonal variation of ergovaline levels in stems with leaf sheaths, leaf blades, and seed heads. J Agric Food Chem 1991;39:112–5.
11. Rottinghaus GE, Schultz LM, Ross PF, et al. An HPLC method for the detection of ergot in ground and pelleted feeds. J Vet Diagn Invest 1993;5:242–7.
12. Ireland FA, Loch WE, Worthy K, et al. Effects of bromocriptine and perphenazine on prolactin and progesterone concentrations in pregnant mares during late gestation. J Reprod Fertil 1991;92:179–86.
13. Evans TJ, Youngquist RS, Loch WE, et al. A comparison of the relative efficacies of domperidone and reserpine in treating equine "fescue toxicosis". Proc Am Assoc Equine Pract 1999;45:207–9.
14. Evans TJ, Constantinescu GM, Ganjam VK. Clinical reproductive anatomy and physiology of the mare. In: Youngquist RS, editor. Current therapy in large animal theriogenology. Philadelphia: Saunders; 1997. p. 43–70.
15. Youngblood RC, Filipov NM, Rude BJ, et al. Effects of short-term early gestational exposure to endophyte-infected tall fescue diets on plasma 3,4-dihydroxylphenyl acetic acid and fetal development in mares. J Anim Sci 2004;82:2919–29.
16. Holtan DW, Houghton E, Silver M, et al. Plasma progestagens in the mare, fetus, and newborn foal. J Reprod Fertil Suppl 1991;44:517–28.
17. Ryan PL, Bennet-Wimbush K, Vaala WE, et al. Systemic relaxin in pregnant pony mares grazed on endophyte-infected fescue: effects of fluphenazine treatment. Theriogenology 2001;56:471–83.
18. Boosinger TR, Brendemuehl JP, Bransby DL, et al. Prolonged gestation, decreased tri-iodothyronine concentration, and thyroid gland histomorphologic features in newborn foals of mares grazing *Acremonium coenophialum* infected fescue. Am J Vet Res 1995;56:66–9.
19. Bourke CA, Hunt E, Watson R. Fescue-associated oedema of horses grazing on endophyte-inoculated tall fescue grass (*Festuca arundinacea*) pastures. Aust Vet J 2009;87:492–8.
20. Redmond LM, Cross DL, Strickland JR, et al. Efficacy of domperidone and sulpiride as treatments for fescue toxicosis in horses. Am J Vet Res 1995;55:722–9.

Water Homeostasis and Diabetes Insipidus in Horses

Harold C. Schott II, DVM, PhD

KEYWORDS

- Polyuria • Polydipsia • Primary polydipsia
- Water deprivation test • Desmopressin
- Pituitary pars intermedia dysfunction

Diabetes insipidus (DI) is a rare disorder of horses characterized by moderate to severe polyuria and polydipsia (PU/PD). Before the problems that may result in DI are discussed, a review of body water balance and factors affecting water intake and renal water loss is warranted.

BODY WATER BALANCE

Water accounts for 60 to 65% of total adult body mass, equivalent to 300 to 325 L in a 500-kg horse.[1–3] About 200 to 220 L of total body water is intracellular fluid, and the remaining 100 to 110 L is extracellular fluid (ECF). ECF is divided between plasma (5–6% of body weight, ~25 L), interstitial fluid and lymph (8–10% of body weight, ~45 L), and transcellular fluid (6–8% of body weight, ~35 L, the majority in the lumen of the gastrointestinal tract). Despite marked differences in ionic composition, ECF and intracellular fluid compartments exchange water freely to maintain osmotic equilibrium.[1–4]

Appropriate water balance maintains plasma osmolality (P_{osm}) in a narrow range (270–300 mOsm/kg) and is achieved by matching daily water intake with water loss.[1,4–6] Water is provided from 3 sources: (1) free water intake (drinking); (2) water in feed; and (3) metabolic water. For horses on a dry forage (hay) diet, most water is consumed by drinking (about 85%), but feed and metabolic water provide about 5% and 10% of daily water, respectively. Water can be lost by 3 routes: (1) in urine; (2) in feces; and (3) as insensible losses (evaporation) across the skin and respiratory tract. Studies of water balance in horses have revealed a daily maintenance water requirement of 55 to 65 mL/kg/d, of which 45 to 55 mL/kg is provided by drinking, equal to 22.5 to 27.5 L/d for a 500-kg horse.[5,6] These values are consistent with the recommendation that stalled horses under temperate environmental conditions should be provided with 5 to 10 gallons of fresh water daily.[7] Urinary and fecal water

Department of Large Animal Clinical Sciences, College of Veterinary Medicine, D-202 Veterinary Medical Center, Michigan State University, East Lansing, MI 48824-1314, USA
E-mail address: schott@cvm.msu.edu

Vet Clin Equine 27 (2011) 175–195
doi:10.1016/j.cveq.2011.01.002 vetequine.theclinics.com
0749-0739/11/$ – see front matter

losses range from 20 to 55% and 30 to 55%, respectively, of the total daily water loss.[5,6] The remaining (insensible) loss accounted for up to 15 to 40% of daily water loss, despite mild ambient conditions and the lack of sweating in these studies of water balance. In contrast to horses consuming hay diets, horses grazing pasture acquire most water from feed and may drink only once a day (or less frequently). Further, the maintenance water requirement of horses that are off feed because of a variety of medical problems is considerably lower; horses receiving intravenous fluid support at a rate of 0.75 to 1.0 mL/kg per hour (9–12 L/d for a 500-kg horse) consistently produce moderately dilute urine (specific gravity 1.010–1.020).

Although balance of daily water intake and output is critical for maintenance of homeostasis, it warrants mention that equidae tolerate water deprivation.[8–11] For example, after horses were deprived of water for 72 hours (which resulted in body mass loss in excess of 10%), most of the weight lost (90% of which was assumed to be water) was recovered within the first hour of being provided with access to water.[11] Similarly, even greater body mass losses (approaching 20%) induced by water deprivation and desert walking in donkeys and burros were largely replaced within the first few minutes after water was provided.[9,10] Thus, in terms of water balance, equidae (especially donkeys and burros) can truly be considered desert-adapted animals.[9,10,12,13] An important reason for their ability to tolerate water deprivation seems to be a substantial intestinal reserve of water and electrolytes (transcellular fluid) that can be called on during periods of dehydration for the maintenance of plasma and effective circulating volumes.

CONTROL OF BODY WATER BALANCE

Drinking and production of concentrated or dilute urine are the mechanisms by which water balance is finely tuned. Both thirst and renal water conservation are triggered primarily by increases in plasma osmolality (P_{osm}) (directly related to plasma sodium concentration) and secondarily by decreases in effective circulating volume and blood pressure. The initial response to a mild increase in P_{osm} is secretion of arginine vasopressin (AVP or antidiuretic hormone) from the neurohypophysis, resulting in enhanced renal water conservation, whereas thirst, resulting in drinking, is a secondary response to even greater increases in plasma tonicity (**Fig. 1**). Despite being a less sensitive defense to a decrease in total body water, thirst and drinking responses are reviewed first.

Thirst and Drinking Behavior

There are 2 main stimuli for thirst in mammals: increased P_{osm} and hypovolemia/hypotension.[4,14] The former is mediated through osmoreceptors in the anterior hypothalamus that have a high threshold for activation (about 295 mOsm/kg in humans). Hemodynamic stimuli are mediated by afferent input to hypothalamic osmoreceptors from both low- and high-pressure baroreceptors. Both osmotic and hemodynamic stimuli can produce their dipsogenic effect, in part, by activating a local renin-angiotensin-aldosterone system in the central nervous system.[4,14,15] Studies in horses, ponies, and donkeys have shown that both increased P_{osm} (induced by water deprivation or infusion of hypertonic saline) and hypovolemia (induced by furosemide administration) are stimuli for thirst.[16–20] As mentioned earlier, after a period of water deprivation, dehydrated equids seem to be able to replace water deficits within 15 to 30 minutes of gaining access to water. The increase in P_{osm} associated with water deprivation is also corrected in this same period, indicating that imbibed water is rapidly absorbed from the gastrointestinal tract.[16] Drinking also seems to directly

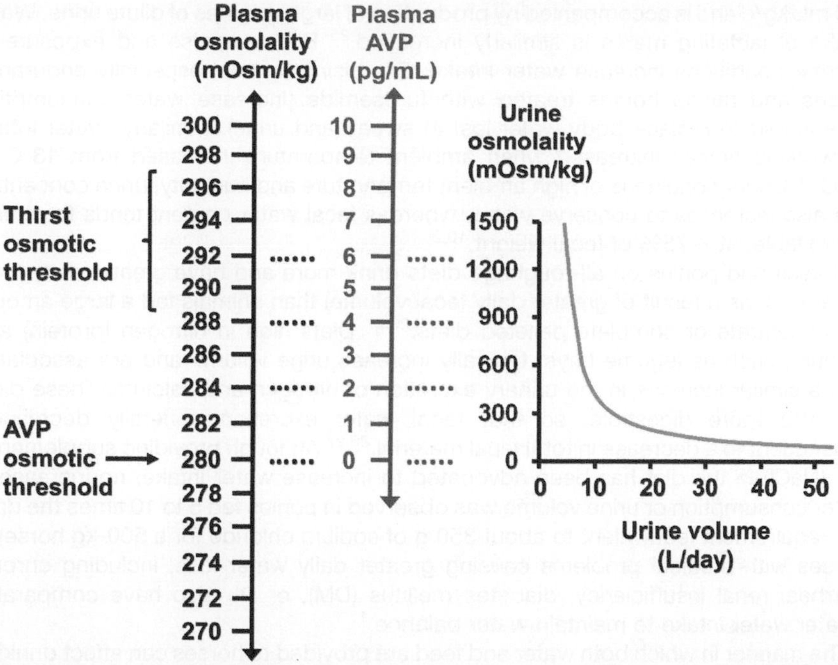

Fig. 1. Relationship of P_{osm}, plasma AVP concentration, U_{osm}, and urine volume in horses. Note that the osmotic threshold for AVP secretion defines the point at which U_{osm} begins to increase, but the osmotic threshold for thirst is significantly higher and approximates the point at which maximal U_{osm} has already been achieved. Note also that because of the inverse relation between U_{osm} and urine volume, changes in plasma AVP concentrations have greater effects on urine volume at low plasma AVP concentrations than at high plasma AVP concentrations. (*Adapted from* Berl T, Verbalis J. Pathophysiology of water metabolism. In: Brenner BM, editor. The Kidney, vol. 1. 7th edition. Philadelphia: WB Saunders; 2004. p. 857–919; with permission.)

stimulate pharyngeal receptors that signal the hypothalamus to decrease AVP secretion before a decrease in P_{osm} has been achieved.[4]

Despite rapid fluid replacement by equidae that have been dehydrated by water deprivation, horses that become dehydrated as a consequence of prolonged exercise or diarrheal disease (colitis) often do not drink. This situation can be attributed to the fact that these conditions produce loss of both body water and electrolytes in sweat or diarrhea. With loss of electrolyte-containing body fluids, the increase in P_{osm} is smaller and osmotic thirst stimulus is blunted compared with water deprivation. In human endurance athletes this state of mild to moderate dehydration that does not induce adequate thirst has been called both voluntary and involuntary dehydration,[21,22] and, although less well documented, a similar response seems to occur in horses performing endurance exercise.[23] Another form of involuntary dehydration, which may be accompanied by increases in P_{osm} and protein concentration, has also been anecdotally described in postfoaling mares.

Drinking responses can vary widely between individual horses and are affected by age, pregnancy and lactation, environmental conditions, level of exercise, diet, and disease state. For example, neonatal foals may consume milk in excess of 20% of their body weight daily.[24] This amount equates to a fluid intake approaching

250 mL/kg/d and is accompanied by production of large volumes of dilute urine. Water intake of lactating mares is similarly increased.[25] Both exercise and exposure to warmer conditions increase water intake. Exercising horses, especially endurance horses and racing horses treated with furosemide, increase water consumption several-fold to replace body water lost in sweat (and urine). Similarly, water intake by working horses increased when ambient temperature increased from 13°C to 25°C.[25] Under conditions of high ambient temperature and humidity, urine concentration also increases to conserve water, whereas fecal water content tends to remain fairly stable, at ~75% of fecal weight.[10,26]

Horses and ponies on all-roughage diets drink more and have greater daily fecal water loss (as a result of greater daily fecal volume) than animals fed a large amount of concentrate or complete pelleted diets.[26,27] Diets high in nitrogen (protein) and calcium, such as legume hays, typically increase urine volume and are associated with a similar increase in the urinary excretion of nitrogen and calcium. These diets are also more digestible, so that fecal water excretion generally decreases, consequent to a decrease in total fecal material.[26,27] Although providing supplemental salt (NaCl) in the diet has been advocated to increase water intake, no increase in water consumption or urine volume was observed in ponies fed 5 to 10 times the daily salt requirement (equivalent to about 350 g of sodium chloride for a 500-kg horse).[28] Horses with medical problems causing greater daily water loss, including chronic diarrhea, renal insufficiency, diabetes mellitus (DM), or DI, also have comparably greater water intake to maintain water balance.[1]

The manner in which both water and feed are provided to horses can affect drinking behavior and water balance. It is commonly believed that horses should always have access to fresh water, yet feral horses and ponies usually drink only once or twice daily.[29] When stalled horses are provided with hay meals twice a day, most water is drunk within the hour after feeding.[30] Thus, it is unlikely that horses require continuous access to water, and 1 study found no difference in total water consumption or water balance between groups of pregnant mares that were either provided with water for 5 minutes 3 times daily, or had continuous access to water.[31] Both the type of water container and fill rate can affect water intake. In a study comparing preference for drinking from 23.7-L (5-gallon) buckets versus 2 types of automatic watering devices (one with a pressure valve and the other with a float valve), horses preferred drinking from buckets, and daily water intake was lower when an automatic waterer with a float valve was used.[32] Temperature of water offered also affects intake. For example, ponies stabled in a cold environment (near freezing) consumed a greater volume when warm (31–48°C) water was offered, compared with when cold (0–4°C) water was offered.[33] Similarly, after dehydration induced by endurance exercise, horses preferred and drank a greater volume of rehydration fluid at 20°C, compared with rehydration fluids at either 10°C or 30°C.[34]

Vasopressin Secretion and Renal Water Reabsorption

AVP is a 9–amino acid peptide produced in the neurohypophysis (pars nervosa or posterior pituitary) in the distal axons of magnocellular neurons that comprise the neurohypophysis. The cell bodies of these neurosecretory neurons are located in the paired supraoptic and paraventricular nuclei within the hypothalamus.[4] Once synthesized, AVP is stored in granules within these axons until specific stimuli result in release of the hormone into the venous circulation. Secretion of AVP is triggered by propagation of an action potential along the axon, influx of calcium, and a calcium-dependent exocytotic process. Stores of AVP in the posterior pituitary are substantial and can provide a week's supply of hormone under conditions required to produce maximal antidiuresis.[4]

As for thirst, increases in P_{osm} and hypovolemia/hypotension are the stimuli for AVP release. Osmoreceptors located in the anterior hypothalamus, likely in or near the circumventricular organ called the organum vasculosum of the lamina terminalis, yet outside the blood-brain barrier, are responsive to changes in plasma solutes.[4] However, osmoreceptors are not equally sensitive to all plasma solutes. For example, increases in plasma sodium concentration and infusion of mannitol are potent stimuli, whereas increases in plasma glucose and urea concentrations are weak stimuli.[4] This differential response to various solutes is observed because osmoreceptor activation is caused by an osmotic water shift that produces cell shrinkage (which is greater for sodium and mannitol than for glucose or urea). Cell shrinkage activates a stretch-inactivated noncationic membrane channel that initiates depolarization of the osmoreceptor. Subsequent release of various neurotransmitters leads to secretion of AVP from the neurohypophysis but this process remains incompletely understood.[4]

P_{osm} must exceed a set point or threshold value for activation of hypothalamic osmoreceptors.[4] The threshold for AVP release in humans is lower than that for thirst; however, it is variable between individuals (275–290 mOsm/kg) because of genetic differences and other factors that may influence osmoreceptor sensitivity, most notably changes in blood pressure and effective circulating volume. Other factors that can affect osmoreceptor sensitivity include phase of the estrus cycle and pregnancy. Once the threshold is exceeded, osmoreceptors are highly sensitive to changes in P_{osm}, with each 1 mOsm/kg increase leading to an increase in plasma AVP concentration of 0.5 to 1.0 pg/mL. The renal response to increasing AVP concentration is an increase in urine osmolality (U_{osm}) that is directly proportional to AVP concentrations from 0.5 to 5.0 pg/mL, with the latter value producing a maximal increase in U_{osm}. Thus, a small increase in P_{osm} (as little as 1%) can increase AVP concentration and U_{osm}. Further, because urine volume and U_{osm} are inversely related, the antidiuretic response (ie, decrease in urine volume) to an initial increase in AVP concentration from 1 to 2 pg/mL is greater than that produced by a further increase in AVP concentration from 4 to 5 pg/mL.[4] As a consequence, small increases in P_{osm} and AVP concentration can have a substantial effect on renal water conservation (see **Fig. 1**).

In contrast to increases in P_{osm}, hemodynamic changes including decreases in effective circulating volume and blood pressure are weaker stimuli for AVP release. There is little AVP release in response to modest hemodynamic changes; however, progressively larger hemodynamic changes lead to exponential increases in plasma AVP concentration. These hemodynamic influences on AVP secretion are mediated, in part, by afferent baroreceptor neural pathways. With normal blood volume and pressure, baroreceptor afferent signals seem to be inhibitory to AVP release and this neural regulation may modulate the sensitivity of hypothalamic osmoreceptors to changes in P_{osm}. Loss of this inhibitory influence with more severe hemodynamic changes is believed to be the reason for substantially greater increases in plasma AVP concentration that are found with more severe hypovolemia and hypotension.

Although most information about AVP release comes from studies of laboratory animals, increases in plasma AVP concentration have been measured in horses and ponies during water deprivation.[16,17] However, in equidae AVP also seems to be a stress hormone because substantially greater concentrations (10-fold > those induced by water deprivation) have been measured after application of a nose twitch, nasogastric intubation, or exercise.[35,36] Thus, the magnitude of the increase in plasma AVP concentration consequent to water deprivation may be variable in horses, and it may sometimes be difficult to separate osmotic effects from stress effects.

Once released, AVP acts on vasopressin (V_2) receptors on the basolateral membrane of principal cells of the collecting duct, leading to translocation and insertion of intracellular vesicles containing water channels (transmembrane proteins termed aquaporin 2 [AQP2]) into the apical membrane.[37] Aquaporins are a family of water channel proteins that increase membrane water permeability and have actions in several other tissues as well as the kidney.[38] AQP1 is found in proximal tubular and thin descending limb of Henle epithelia cells, whereas AQP3 and 4 are expressed constitutively in basolateral membranes of collecting duct epithelia. Again, AVP action leads to insertion of AQP2 into the apical membrane of principal cells and results in increased renal water reabsorption across collecting duct epithelia in the presence of medullary hypertonicity, and recent work has reported similar localization of AQP1 to AQP4 in renal tissue of the horse.[39] V_2 receptors are also present on the basolateral membrane of tubular epithelial cells in the thick medullary ascending limb, and stimulation of these receptors leads to enhanced reabsorption of NaCl, an essential step in generation of a hypertonic medullary interstitium. Further, AVP stimulates transepithelial movement of urea in the inner collecting ducts, another important factor in generating and maintaining a hypertonic medullary interstitium.[37]

The V_2 receptor is coupled to a transmembrane G protein that stimulates adenyl cyclase, with resultant increase in cytosolic cyclic adenosine monophosphate (cAMP) concentration. Increased cAMP activates protein kinase A, leading to phosphorylation and translocation of AQP2-containing vesicles.[37] V_2 receptor activation can be antagonized by activation of adjacent α_2-adrenoceptors and by a prostaglandin E_2 (PGE_2)-mediated effect on an inhibitory G protein.[40,41] Although effects of these antagonists vary with species and have not been studied in horses, it is likely that the diuresis associated with administration of α_2-agonists to horses is caused by antagonism of V_2 receptor activation.[42–44]

URINARY EXCRETION OF SOLUTE AND WATER

Renal function is traditionally thought of in terms of glomerular filtration, tubular modification of the filtered fluid, and excretion of the final urine. This concept accommodates excretion of nitrogenous and organic wastes and the major aspects of regulation of total body water and ECF ionic composition. In normal horses, glomerular filtration rate (GFR) exceeds 1000 L/d, a volume that is 10 times greater than the total ECF volume; however, more than 99% of this water is reabsorbed in the renal tubules and collecting ducts, resulting in production of between 5 and 10 L of urine daily. The result is urine that is 3 to 4 times more concentrated than plasma (U_{osm} 900–1200 mOsm/kg and specific gravity 1.025–1.050). Further, urea (in urine) has replaced sodium (in plasma) as the most important solute. However, if only 98% of water were to be reabsorbed, urine volume would double and the additional water would result in more dilute urine (U_{osm} 450–600 mOsm/kg urine and specific gravity 1.015–1.025). If water reabsorption decreased to 96% of filtered water, approximately 40 L of urine would be produced, with a U_{osm} of 200 to 300 mOsm/kg and a specific gravity of 1.005 to 1.010. In the latter scenario, urine is more dilute than plasma (hyposthenuria) and the kidneys are actively excreting water. Under certain conditions, active water excretion by the kidneys is important for maintenance of P_{osm} in the normal range. The best example is a neonatal foal that may ingest a volume of milk in excess of 20% of its body weight daily. As stated earlier, this finding equates to intake of a hypotonic fluid approaching 250 mL/kg/d, and failure to produce a large volume of hyposthenuric urine could result in water retention, decreased P_{osm}, and clinical hyponatremia (usually manifested by neurologic signs).

Urine concentration and volume are also affected by solute intake and excretion. Thus, another way to think about renal function is in terms of total daily solute and water excretion. For example, a typical horse may produce 6 L of urine daily with an osmolality of 1000 mOsm/kg to excrete 6000 mOsm of solute. However, if the solute intake were doubled to 12,000 mOsm (perhaps by greater feed intake and salt supplementation [eg, 100 g of NaCl would constitute nearly 3500 mOsm]), 12 L of urine with an osmolality of 1000 mOsm/kg or 9 L of urine with an osmolality of 1500 mOsm/kg would need be produced to eliminate the additional solute. Thus, U_{osm} reflects the ability of the kidney to dilute or concentrate the final urine but does not actually provide an accurate estimate of the quantitative ability to excrete solute or retain water. These functions are more accurately assessed by calculating osmolal (C_{osm}) and free water clearances (C_{H2O}).[45] Like other clearances, these calculations require determination of urine flow rate (via timed urine collection) and measurement of both P_{osm} and U_{osm}.

These measures of renal solute and water handling can be conceptualized by considering urine to have 2 components: (1) that which contains all the urinary solute in a solution that is isosmotic to plasma (C_{osm}, usually expressed in mL/min or L/d); and (2) that which contains free water without any solute (C_{H2O}, also expressed in mL/min or L/d). The sum of these 2 components is the urine flow rate in mL/min or L/d. Because urine is typically more concentrated than plasma, C_{H2O} typically has a negative value, which indicates water conservation. The inverse of free water clearance is termed renal water reabsorption. Returning to the earlier example, excretion of 6000 osmol would require production of 20 L of urine that is isosmotic with plasma (using a value of 300 mOsm/kg for P_{osm}). However, because 6 L of concentrated urine was produced during the period measured, the kidneys have quantitatively reabsorbed 14 L of free water per day. In contrast, despite production of urine with an identical U_{osm} (1000 mOsm/kg), excretion of 12,000 mOsm would require production of 40 L of urine isosmotic with plasma. Free water clearance would be ~28 L/d (ie, 28 L/d of free water would be reabsorbed by the kidneys). Under the influence of higher plasma AVP concentrations, U_{osm} may increase to 1500 mOsm/kg, again requiring production of 9 L of urine. With the more concentrated urine, C_{H2O} would be ~31 L/d, and less water intake (by 3 L) would have been needed to eliminate the higher solute load. Although concentrated urine always has a negative C_{H2O} value, which indicates renal water reabsorption, and dilute urine always has a positive value for C_{H2O}, which indicates renal water excretion, quantitative assessment of renal solute and water handling requires measurement of both osmolal and free water clearances.

One of the features of the kidney is that it can conserve water as well as eliminate excess water from the body. Excretion of free water by the kidney occurs by generation of hypotonic tubular fluid in the ascending limb of Henle and distal tubule. Further, the amount or volume of free water that can be excreted depends on the amount of fluid presented to this nephron segment, which is dependent on GFR. Free water is consequently excreted by keeping the collecting ducts relatively impermeable to water (lack of AVP). Assessment of C_{H2O} is most helpful in patients with hyponatremia and hypoosmolality that cannot be attributed to another primary disease process (diarrhea or bladder rupture). For hyponatremia to develop, water excretion must be defective. For example, hyponatremia can develop with renal failure secondary to a reduction in GFR and the amount of filtrate presented to the loop of Henle. Hyponatremia and hypoosmolality may also develop with use of loop diuretics because less free water is generated in the ascending limb of Henle loop as a result of blockade of the apical $Na^{+}/K^{+}/2Cl^{-}$ cotransporter (less solute is removed). Other causes of hyponatremia may include the syndromes of inappropriate AVP secretion (syndrome of inappropriate antidiuretic hormone secretion [SIADH]) and pseudohypoaldosteronism. With SIADH excessive AVP activity and water reabsorption may be driven by hemodynamic stimuli, and this syndrome may contribute to development of hyponatremia in horses and foals with diarrhea and hypovolemia.[46] With the latter condition it has been speculated that the distal tubule is unresponsive to aldosterone, leading to increased clearances of sodium and chloride.[47]

DI

The term diabetes was derived from the Greek verb diabainein, formed by combining the prefix *dia*, meaning across or apart, and the verb *bainein*, meaning to stride or stand. Taken together, the verb had the meaning to stand with legs asunder or apart as if in the position for urination. The term was originally used to describe DM (mellitus meaning honey in Latin) to characterize the sweet character of urine passed by people afflicted with DM. In ancient times, DM was recognized as an incurable disease that considerably shortened life span. DI (insipidus coming from a Latin word meaning tasteless urine) seems to have been recognized and described considerably later. According to Scottish folklore, familial DI, now recognized to be caused by several genetic mutations, was caused by a gypsy curse when a housewife refused to provide water for the gypsy's thirsty son. The curse by the gypsy woman caused the housewife's sons to crave water and condemned her daughters to pass the curse on to future generations (now recognized as a V_2 receptor gene defect associated with an X-linked recessive inheritance pattern).

Previous medical literature has varied in the use of the term DI: some investigators have used DI in a broad sense to include PU/PD associated with renal disease, metabolic disorders (DM, hypercalcemia, and hypokalemia), medullary washout, and primary PD, whereas others have limited use of DI to more specific disorders in which AVP production and/or action is disturbed.[4,48,49] Regardless, the hallmarks of DI are excretion of dilute urine in combination with excessive thirst, or PU/PD. Polyuria is defined in human medicine and small-animal practice as urine output in excess of 40 to 50 mL/kg/d and PD as water intake of more than of 100 mL/kg/d.[50,51] These values equate to more than 20 to 25 L of urine production and more than 50 L of water consumption for a 500-kg horse, compared with normal values for daily urine production and water consumption of 5 to 10 L and 20 to 30 L, respectively. When urine production and drinking are this dramatic, the problem is usually recognized by owners of stalled horses. However, when horses are group housed in a pen or turned out at pasture with a common water source, PU/PD may not be so easily recognized. The major causes of PU/PD in horses include renal insufficiency, pituitary pars intermedia dysfunction (PPID or equine Cushing disease), and primary or psychogenic PD. Less common causes include excessive salt consumption, central and nephrogenic DI, DM, sepsis and/or endotoxemia, and iatrogenic causes (sedation with α_2-agonists, corticosteroid therapy, or diuretic use). Discussion of all the causes of PU/PD is beyond the scope of this article and readers are referred to previous reviews for further information.[52,53] The remainder of this article focuses on conditions resulting in PU/PD in which abnormalities of AVP production and/or action have been implicated or suggested (**Box 1**).

Renal Insufficiency

In horses with acute kidney injury (AKI), there may be a transient period of anuria or oliguria. If horses survive the primary disease and acute phase of renal injury, glomerular and tubular damage results in a period during which impaired concentrating ability results in PU.[51–53] Urine is frequently hyposthenuric (specific gravity <1.008) during

Box 1
Potential causes of DI in horses

Neurogenic (central) DI

- Congenital
  - Cerebral malformations, hydrocephalus
  - Hypoxic-ischemic encephalopathy
- Acquired
  - Head trauma
  - Brain or pituitary gland mass
  - Infection (viral encephalopathy, protozoal encephalopathy, pituitary abscess)
  - Postoperative
  - Drug-induced
  - Idiopathic

Nephrogenic DI

- Congenital
  - X-linked recessive (suspected)
- Acquired
  - Renal disease
    - After acute kidney injury (AKI)
    - With chronic kidney failure
    - Postobstructive uropathy
    - Medullary washout
  - Drug-induced
  - Idiopathic

Primary PD

- Behavior problem
- Altered thirst
- Excessive salt consumption

this period of nephron recovery, and return of concentrating ability may take several weeks in horses recovering from AKI. However, an occasional horse may manifest PU/PD for several months after AKI and fail to produce concentrated urine in response to water deprivation (author's unpublished observations). Although there are no well-documented published reports, it is possible that affected horses may have transient nephrogenic DI, in part consequent to a compromised response to AVP in multiple nephron segments.

With chronic kidney disease (CKD) horses typically have a variable degree of azotemia, and urinalysis reveals isosthenuria (urine is isosmotic with plasma [270–300 mOsm/kg] with a specific gravity of 1.008–1.014).[51–53] When recognized, PU/PD is usually mild compared with more dramatic increases in urine production observed with primary PD or true DI. The mechanism(s) of PU consequent to CKD are not clear but likely include increased solute load and tubular flow rate in surviving nephrons, loss of medullary hypertonicity, and impaired response to AVP (again, a form of acquired nephrogenic DI).[54]

PPID

PPID or equine Cushing's disease may develop in as many as 15% to 20% of equids more than 15 years of age.[55]

Although the most consistent clinical sign is hirsutism, PU/PD (sometimes referred to as DI) may be recognized in one-third or more of affected animals.[56] The earliest diagnoses of DI in horses seem to have been made in horses with PPID,[57] and these investigators described DI to be a consequence of infiltration and compression of the neurohypophysis by neoplastic pars intermedia melanotropes. Their diagnosis of DI was supported by showing an increase in urine specific gravity and a decrease in water intake after administration of exogenous AVP. However, these investigators did not assess the response to water deprivation, and measurement of endogenous AVP concentration was not possible to further document a diagnosis of central DI. Further, hyperglycemia and glycosuria were also detected, leading to possible contribution of an osmotic diuresis to the observed PU/PD. Subsequently, larger case series of horses with PPID examined both prevalence and potential causes of PU/PD. For example, in 1 report of 17 horses with PPID, PU/PD was found in 13 (76%)[58]; however, in another series of 21 cases, PU/PD was not a historical complaint in any of the affected horses.[59]

Although the cause(s) of DI with PPID is not well understood, PU has been attributed to hyperglycemia and an associated osmotic diuresis. However, glycosuria was found in only 1 of 5 and 2 of 19 affected horses in 2 reports.[59,60] Further, horses with hyperglycemia and glycosuria may still be able to concentrate their urine in response to water deprivation or exogenous AVP administration, supporting functional AVP activity on collecting ducts[57,61] (author's unpublished observations). A second mechanism implicated in the development of PU is antagonism of the action of AVP on the collecting ducts by cortisol. Although frequently cited as the mechanism of PU in canine hyperadrenocorticism, experimental evidence to support this mechanism is lacking in both dogs and horses. Further, there is considerable species heterogeneity in the effects of corticoids on AVP activity, and in some species a primary dipsogenic effect may be more important. As mentioned earlier, it has also been suggested that growth of a pituitary macroadenoma may lead to impingement (crushing) of the neurohypophysis, the site of AVP storage. Decreased AVP storage and release could result in a form of neurogenic DI.[57,62] However, central DI is not the cause of PU in all cases because some affected horses can concentrate their urine when deprived of water[61] (author's unpublished observations). Consequently, PU/PD seen in many, but not all, horses with PPID is likely the combined result of several mechanisms.

Primary PD or Dipsogenic DI

Primary or psychogenic PD is probably the most common cause of PU/PD in adult horses, for which clients have a primary complaint of excessive water consumption and urination.[51,52] This observation can be attributed to the fact that horses that have this problem are generally in good body condition and are not azotemic. Further, the magnitude of PU typically is greater than that observed with either renal insufficiency or PPID. Owners may report that horses with primary PD drink 3 to 5 times more water than their stablemates and their stalls can be flooded with urine. In some instances, primary PD seems to be a stable vice that reflects boredom in affected horses, whereas in other cases it may develop after a change in environmental conditions, stabling, diet, or medication administration. It is reported to be more common in southern states during periods of high temperature and humidity. In humans, primary PD can be a compulsive behavior associated with mental illness or it may be caused by a primary abnormality in regulation of thirst, in which case it is referred to as dipsogenic DI.[4,48,49] The latter may be caused by a lower osmotic threshold for thirst (idiopathic), or it may be secondary to neurologic disease affecting hypothalamic osmoreceptors regulating thirst. Excessive water consumption causes expansion and dilution of body fluids, leading to a decrease in P_{osm} and suppression of AVP release. In humans, the magnitude of PU/PD varies considerably between affected individuals, and similar variation, although undocumented, likely occurs in affected horses as well.

A diagnosis of primary PD is made by exclusion of other disorders, including renal insufficiency and PPID. In addition, other potential causes such as excessive salt eating[63] and medication administration must be excluded. Neurogenic and nephrogenic DI are excluded by showing urine concentrating ability after water deprivation.[64–66] Specific gravity should exceed 1.025 after water deprivation of sufficient duration (12–24 hours) to produce a 5% loss in body weight. In cases of long-standing PU, the osmotic gradient between the lumen of the collecting tubule and the medullary interstitium may be diminished (medullary washout). In these cases AVP activity may not lead to an increase in urine specific gravity to values greater than 1.020. Consequently, in horses with primary PD of several weeks' duration that fail to concentrate their urine after 24 hours of water deprivation, a modified water-deprivation test may be tried. This test is performed by restricting water intake to approximately 40 mL/kg/d for 3 to 4 days. By the end of this time, urine specific gravity should exceed 1.025 in a horse that has had medullary washout. If the urine specific gravity remains in the isosthenuric range (1.008–1.014), the polyuric horse should be further evaluated for early CKD, in which urine concentrating ability may be compromised before the onset of azotemia. Horses with primary PD typically produce hyposthenuric urine, which is an unlikely finding with CKD.

Management of horses with primary PD is empirical. Because it is a diagnosis of exclusion, once it has been established that the horse is not suffering from a significant renal disease, it is safe to consider restricting water intake to meet maintenance, work, and environmental requirements of the horse. Typically, water is initially restricted to twice the estimated maintenance needs and can be further reduced to maintenance needs over the ensuing weeks. In addition, steps should be taken to improve the attitude of the horse by reducing boredom. Increasing the amount of exercise or turning the horse out to pasture are possible options, as is providing a companion or toys in the stall. Also, increasing the frequency of feedings or the amount of roughage in the diet may increase the time spent eating and thus reduce the habitual drinking.

Central or Neurogenic DI

In humans, lack of AVP, or neurogenic DI, is the more common form of DI; both hereditary and acquired forms have been described.[4,48,49] The hereditary form seems to result from decreased numbers of magnocellular neurons in the supraoptic nuclei of the hypothalamus and is inherited in an autosomal-dominant fashion. However, PU/PD often does not develop until after the first few years of life in affected children, suggesting progressive loss of AVP production. Several diverse mutations in the gene that codes for the neurophysin-AVP precursor peptide have been reported in human patients with autosomal-dominant central DI.[4] It has been speculated that all identified mutations result in production of an abnormal precursor protein that accumulates and eventually kills magnocellular neurons because it cannot be correctly processed, folded, and transported out of the endoplasmic reticulum. However, only 1 allele is affected, allowing some AVP production in the first few years of life. Progressive loss of magnocellular neurons would explain the delayed onset of PU/PD because experimental studies have shown that 80% to 90% of magnocellular neurons must be destroyed before significant PU develops.[4]

To better understand the nearly total loss of AVP production or activity that is necessary for significant PU to develop, it is important to remember that there is an inverse relationship between U_{osm} and urine volume. A decrease in the maximal AVP response to an increase in P_{osm} does not typically cause an observable increase in urine volume because an AVP response that is only 25% to 50% of normal still results in production of concentrated urine and only a modest increase in urine volume. For U_{osm} to decrease to less than 300 mOsm/kg, the AVP response to an increase in P_{osm} must decrease by 80% to 90%.[4] An increase in urine volume is generally clinically recognized because urine becomes more hypotonic than plasma (**Fig. 2**). Production of dilute urine results in an increase in P_{osm} and stimulation of thirst, with the result that a new set point for P_{osm} is established near the threshold for stimulation of thirst.[4]

Acquired forms of neurogenic DI result from degeneration of magnocellular neurons in the supraoptic nuclei secondary to trauma, vascular abnormalities, infection, or a variety of tumors.[4,48,49] As with the hereditary form, PU/PD is not usually manifested

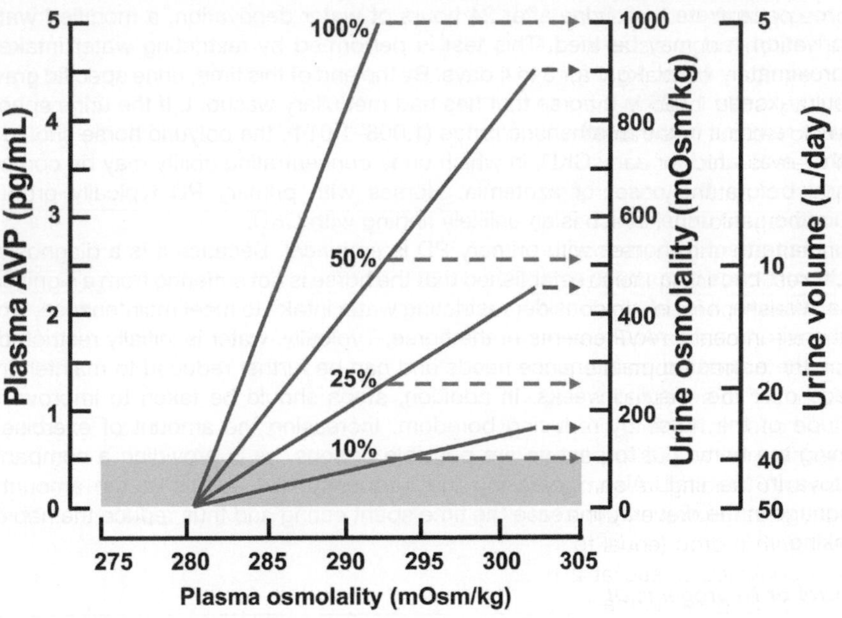

Fig. 2. Relation between plasma AVP concentration, U_{osm}, and P_{osm} in subjects with normal neurohypophyseal function (100%) compared with patients with graded reductions in hypothalamic magnocellular neurons (to 50%, 25%, and 10% of normal). Note that a patient with a 50% reduction in AVP secretory capacity can achieve only half the plasma AVP concentration and half the U_{osm} of normal subjects at a P_{osm} of 290 to 295 mOsm/kg, but with increasing P_{osm} the same patient can eventually stimulate sufficient AVP secretion to reach a near maximal U_{osm}. In contrast, patients with more severe degrees of magnocellular neuron loss are unable to produce urine with maximal osmolality at any level of P_{osm}. (*Adapted from* Berl T, Verbalis J. Pathophysiology of water metabolism. In: Brenner BM, editor. The Kidney, vol. 1. 7th edition. Philadelphia: WB Saunders; 2004. p. 857–919; with permission.)

until 80% to 90% of the neurosecretory neurons are destroyed. Similar to PPID, compression and destruction of the neurohypophysis has been suggested to cause central DI in humans. However, it has been subsequently shown through surgical ablation and magnetic resonance imaging (MRI) studies that destruction of distal magnocellular neuronal axons or compression of the neurohypophysis is unlikely to cause central DI. With surgical ablation of the pituitary stalk at the level of the diaphragm sella (considered a low-stalk section), only transient DI was produced because AVP production and secretion ware maintained by the surviving proximal aspect of magnocellular neurons. However, when a high-stalk section was performed (cutting the axons in the infundibulum closer to the cell bodies), retrograde neuronal cell death occurred and permanent central DI was produced.[67] A pituitary bright spot representing AVP storage is recognized in the neurohypophysis on T1-weighted noncontrast MRI studies in normal individuals.[68] However, with a pituitary adenoma that is large enough to destroy the neurohypophysis, the bright spot moves dorsally to the infundibulum, and AVP secreted at that level is believed to diffuse into blood vessels of the median eminence at the base of the brain. Thus, for neoplasms to produce central DI, they typically have to be more invasive than a pituitary macroadenoma (eg, craniopharygioma, lymphoma, or metastatic cancers). A recent case series of neurogenic DI in children revealed that more than half of the cases were classified as idiopathic.[69] However, further investigation revealed lymphocytic infundibuloneurohypophysitis in some patients with idiopathic DI, leading to suspicion of autoimmune destruction of the neurohypophysis as a cause of central DI in some of these patients.[4,69]

In equidae, central DI has also been experimentally produced by transaction of the pituitary stalk in pony mares.[70] Similar to findings in other species, marked PU/PD developed but was transient, lasting about 48 hours, likely because of AVP production and release higher up by the magnocellular neurons. There have also been several reports of naturally occurring central DI in equids.[71–76] Three well-documented cases of neurogenic DI have been described.[71–73] None of the affected animals could concentrate urine in response to water deprivation, but administration of exogenous AVP resulted in an increase in urine concentration and a decrease in urine volume. In a Welsh pony in which the condition was considered idiopathic, absence of an increase in plasma AVP concentration after water deprivation (compared with control ponies) further supported a diagnosis of neurogenic DI.[72] Acquired neurogenic DI secondary to encephalitis was supported by detection of hypothalamic inflammation at necropsy in another horse.[71] Next, a 10-day-old Fresian filly with very dilute urine (specific gravity 1.001) failed to increase urine specific gravity in response to limiting access to nursing its dam. AVP concentration was below the detection limit of the assay used. However, urine specific gravity did increase to 1.019 4 hours after treatment with a drop (equal to 10 μg of desmopressin) of desmopressin nasal spray in each conjunctival sac at 2 hours intervals. Long-term treatment was not pursued and the filly grew normally over the subsequent 2 years, but dramatic PU persisted. In a fourth case, a filly was evaluated for dramatic PD and hyposthenuria. U_{osm} increased after administration of exogenous AVP but a water-deprivation test was not performed to exclude primary PD.[74] Two similar reports of suspected central DI in horses also likely described cases of primary PD, because both animals showed an ability to concentrate urine during water deprivation or had urine specific gravity exceeding 1.020 on randomly collected urine samples.[75,76]

Nephrogenic DI

Nephrogenic DI results from failure of AVP activity on cortical- and medullary-collecting ducts.[4,48,49] In the absence of systemic disease, it is most commonly a familial disorder in humans, with a sex-linked pattern of inheritance. The disorder is carried by females and expressed in male offspring. PU is present from birth, plasma AVP concentration can be normal to increased (depending on P_{osm}), and resistance to AVP activity is virtually complete. More than 100 mutations have been found in the gene encoding the V_2 receptor in affected human patients but the phenotypic effect can be categorized into 1 of 4 functional abnormalities: (1) the mutant receptor is not inserted into the cell membrane; (2) the mutant receptor is inserted into the cell membrane but it does not bind AVP; (3) the mutant receptor is inserted into the cell membrane and binds AVP but does not activate adenyl cyclase; or (4) the mutant receptor is inserted into the cell membrane and binds AVP but with subnormal stimulation of adenyl cyclase activity.[4] In the last instance partial urine concentrating ability may be present and the magnitude of PU may be less. Congenital nephrogenic DI can also result from mutations in the gene encoding AQP2. More than 20 mutations have been recognized and most are inherited in an autosomal-recessive pattern.[4] Regardless of the type of mutation, the phenotypic effect of dramatic PU/PD is similar with most forms of hereditary nephrogenic DI.

Nephrogenic DI has been reported in sibling Thoroughbred colts in which PU/PD had been noted since birth, suggesting that an inherited form of nephrogenic DI may occur in horses.[77] These colts were in fair body condition, and only modest increases in U_{osm} (50–100 mOsm/kg increases to a high value of 202 mOsm/kg) were achieved after overnight water deprivation (during which weight loss was 10–15%), although they did show appropriate increases in plasma AVP concentration. Further, minimal response to exogenous AVP administration confirmed resistance of the collecting ducts to the antidiuretic action of AVP. Treatment was not attempted and both colts were killed after diagnostic evaluation, but no significant gross or microscopic renal lesions were detected. Nephrogenic DI was also documented in a Quarter Horse colt that presented at 5 months of age for evaluation of poor growth and PU/PD.[78] It had been acquired only 2 weeks previously by the owner, and further history was unknown. PD was dramatic (58 L/d or >500 mL/kg/d) with marked hyposthenuria (specific gravity 1.004 and U_{osm} 76 mOsm/kg). The colt lost more than 11% of its body weight during a 12-hour water-deprivation test, during which urine specific gravity increased from 1.003 to 1.004, whereas plasma AVP concentration increased from 7.4 to 11.1 pg/mL. Subsequent challenges with hypertonic saline and exogenous AVP failed to produce significant increases in U_{osm}, confirming a diagnosis of nephrogenic DI. Ultrasonographic images of both kidneys were normal but a renal biopsy revealed vacuolization and intracellular eosinophilic granular changes in collecting duct epithelial cells. With proper nutrition the colt's body condition improved over a 3-month period, during which water was limited to 30L/day and access to salt was limited to that present in feed. Long-term follow-up was not reported but repeat renal biopsies showed no significant lesions, leading the investigators to suggest that it was likely a case of congenital nephrogenic DI.

Nephrogenic DI may also be acquired consequent to a variety of metabolic, infectious, or mechanical (postobstruction) disorders as well as an adverse drug reaction (eg, lithium use in people with psychiatric disorders).[4,48,49] Anomalous (eg, renal dysplasia or polycystic kidney disease) or neoplastic disorders resulting in structural deformation of the kidneys are another potential cause of nephrogenic DI. In addition to damage to the normal renal anatomy leading to altered V_2 receptor activation in multiple nephron segments, downregulation of AQP2 expression may accompany many of these disorders.[79] Downregulation of AQP2 has also been found with AKI and CKD and likely contributes to PU observed with renal insufficiency. Further, AQP2 downregulation seems to also occur with conditions resulting in medullary washout and likely contributes to the delay in reestablishment of full urinary-concentrating ability after a period of diuresis, regardless of the cause of PU.

Gestational DI

Another cause of transient DI in humans is gestational DI, observed in a small percentage of women in the third trimester. The condition is caused by increased activity of a placental vasopressinase that degrades AVP. Because placental vasopressinase is metabolized and inactivated by the liver, hepatic dysfunction during late term pregnancy seems to be an important contributing factor for this disorder.[80,81] Gestational DI has not yet been documented in pregnant equids.

DIAGNOSTIC EVALUATION OF HORSES WITH SUSPECTED DI

When physical examination findings are otherwise normal, azotemia has been excluded, and renal size and structure appear normal on ultrasonography, it is important to document the magnitude of PD by isolating the horse and measuring water intake over a 3- to 5-day period, because documenting the volume of urine production is more challenging.[51,52] This step can often be performed at the home stable by the horse owner or manager and allows differentiation from conditions causing more frequent urination (pollakiuria), including cystitis or cystolithiasis. It is also important to instruct clients about the difference between water offered and water imbibed because spillage can lead to substantial overestimation of water intake in an occasional horse. Once PD has been documented, water deprivation is the next test to pursue. This test can also be performed in the home environment. With PU/PD, urination is more frequent and owners are often able to collect a free-catch urine sample to document baseline urine specific gravity. As an alternative, a urine collection device consisting of an inverted plastic gallon bottle with the bottom removed can be suspended 2.5 to 5 cm (1–2 in) below the sheath of male horses[51] or a bladder catheter can generally be passed without sedation in mares. Once the baseline sample has been collected the horse is deprived of water for 12 to 24 hours, typically starting with the overnight period. Feed can still be provided. Collection of the second urine sample typically requires use of the urine collection device in male horses or passing a bladder catheter in the mare. An increase in urine specific gravity to 1.025 or greater is the goal after a body weight loss of about 5%.

In horses with normal renal function, urine specific gravity and U_{osm} continue to increase to values of more than 1.040 and more than 1300 mOsm/kg, respectively, after 48 hours of water deprivation, with maximal values exceeding 1.050 and 1500 mOsm/kg in some horses.[64–66,82] Normal horses are able to tolerate 48 to 72 hours of water deprivation with few clinical problems under moderate as ambient conditions. As mentioned earlier, horses with long-standing PU are unlikely to be able to produce such concentrated urine because of medullary washout and downregulation of AQP2 expression. However, if urine specific gravity increases to 1.025 or greater after overnight water deprivation of a horse with PU/PD, a diagnosis of primary PD is supported rather than a diagnosis of neurogenic or nephrogenic DI. If urine specific gravity does not exceed 1.020, an overnight water-deprivation test can be repeated after 3 to 5 days of limiting water intake to about 75 mL/kg/d (a modified water-deprivation test), with body-weight monitoring to prevent losses exceeding 5%. A word of caution is warranted about subjecting horses with suspected DI to water deprivation. Because urine concentrating ability may show minimal improvement with either form of DI, affected horses may continue to excrete excess water in the face of water deprivation. As a result, they may become substantially dehydrated (10–15%) within the first

12 hours of water deprivation, as illustrated by the cases described earlier. Thus, horses with suspected DI should be carefully monitored during the period of water deprivation to decrease the risk of inducing serious hypertonic dehydration.

In equids that fail to achieve a significant increase in urine concentrating ability after water deprivation, measurement of P_{osm} and plasma AVP concentration in samples collected at the start and end of the water-deprivation test are the next logical diagnostic tests. Measurement of AVP in equine plasma is not commercially available; thus, if samples are submitted to a laboratory using an AVP assay that has not been validated for use on equine plasma, control horse samples should be collected from a normal horse subjected to an identical water-deprivation test. An appropriate increase in plasma AVP concentration is to a value greater than 10 pg/mL when P_{osm} exceeds 300 mOsm/kg and provides support of a diagnosis of nephrogenic DI. In contrast, a lack of a significant AVP response establishes a diagnosis of central or neurogenic DI. Another test that is sometimes pursued to stimulate an increase in plasma AVP concentration in patients with suspected DI is infusion of hypertonic saline to induce a rapid increase in P_{osm} (Hickey-Hare test).[78] This test can be pursued when there are concerns about water deprivation in an individual patient. The appropriate urinary response to hypertonic saline infusion is an increase in urine output to excrete the sodium load but the effect on urine specific gravity and U_{osm} can be variable, in part depending on the initial urine concentration.

The final diagnostic test to confirm a diagnosis of nephrogenic DI in patients that fail to concentrate urine in response to water deprivation, and as a simple alternative to measuring plasma AVP concentrations, is administration of exogenous AVP. In the past, extracts of the neurohypophysis (Pitressin and others) were available but these products are no longer on the market. As an alternative, desmopressin acetate (1-desamino-8-D-AVP, available as DDAVP and others) can be used. Desmopressin is a modified form of AVP in which the first amino acid has been deaminated and the arginine at the eighth position is in the *dextro* rather than the *levo* form. It is available as intravenous, nasal spray, and tablet formulations although shortages of the intravenous formulation have been a problem. The nasal spray (100 μg DDAVP/mL) can be used intravenously as a diagnostic tool for evaluation of horses with DI. Intravenous administration of 20 μg DDAVP (0.2 mL of the nasal spray, equal in antidiuretic activity to 80 IU of AVP) produced an increase in urine specific gravity to values greater than 1.020 and a 5-fold decrease in urine volume in normal horses in which PU and hyposthenuria (specific gravity <1.005) had been induced by repeated nasogastric intubation with water.[83] Similar increases in urine specific gravity and decreases in urine volume have been produced after DDAVP administration to clinical cases as a diagnostic test in the evaluation of PU/PD associated with primary PD, PPID, and possible transient central DI (Harold C. Schott II, DVM, PhD, unpublished observations, 2006–2010).

TREATMENT OF DI

Treatment of DI is directed at managing PU/PD and minimizing the risk of significant alterations in P_{osm} or electrolyte concentrations.[4,48,49] With neurogenic DI, recovery of AVP secretion is rare once the magnocellular neurons have degenerated to the degree that PU/PD becomes apparent; however, spontaneous recovery has been observed in some cases of idiopathic (possibly autoimmune) disease.[69] Generally, treatment of neurogenic DI consists of hormone replacement. Oral desmopressin acetate tablets are administered to older children and adults, whereas the nasal spray is used in younger children.[48,49,69] There is variation in the effective dose between patients to control PU, and treatment is initiated with a low dose, which may be increased over several weeks until the lowest effective dose is determined. Dilutional hyponatremia is the only significant adverse effect if excessive doses are administered over a prolonged course. Successful use of desmopressin acetate for treatment of neurogenic DI in dogs and cats has been reported.[84,85]

With nephrogenic DI, replacement hormone therapy is largely ineffective except in a subset of patients that may have receptor mutations that allow a partial response to AVP. In these patients, higher doses of desmopressin acetate may limit PU/PD. For the remaining majority of patients, treatment of nephrogenic DI includes dietary sodium restriction and administration of thiazide diuretics.[4,48,49] This treatment may reduce PU by 50% in many cases. Although it may seem paradoxic to treat PU with a diuretic agent, thiazides inhibit sodium reabsorption in the distal tubule (diluting segment of the nephron) and, when combined with dietary sodium restriction, may cause mild hypovolemia. Limiting the ability to produce hyposthenuric urine in the diluting segment decreases free water clearance (or enhances water reabsorption), whereas hypovolemia reduces renal blood flow and GFR and enhances proximal tubular solute and water reabsorption. In addition, thiazide diuretics also seem to directly enhance water reabsorption in the inner medullary collecting ducts via a mechanism independent of AVP.[86] Thiazide diuretics may be combined with prostaglandin inhibitors (indomethacin) to further decrease renal blood flow and GFR. Amiloride (a potassium-sparing diuretic) can be used in combination with a thiazide diuretic to further diminish PU, with the added benefit of being able to limit use and associated adverse effects of prolonged indomethacin treatment.[4,48,49] In a dog with congenital nephrogenic DI, treatment with hydrochlorothiazide, coupled with a low-sodium diet, was successful in decreasing PD by more than 75%, and PU was well controlled over the next 2 years.[87]

REFERENCES

1. Carlson GP. Fluid therapy in horses with acute diarrhea. Vet Clin North Am Equine Pract 1979;1(2):313–29.
2. Rose RJ. A physiologic approach to fluid and electrolyte therapy in the horse. Equine Vet J 1981;13(1):7–14.
3. Schott HC, Hinchcliff KW. Fluids, electrolytes, and bicarbonate. Vet Clin North Am Equine Pract 1993;9(3):577–604.
4. Berl T, Verbalis J. Pathophysiology of water metabolism. In: Brenner BM, editor. The Kidney, vol. 1. 7th edition. Philadelphia: WB Saunders; 2004. p. 857–919.
5. Tasker JB. Fluid and electrolyte studies in the horse. III. Intake and output of water, sodium, and potassium in normal horses. Cornell Vet 1967;57(4):649–57.
6. Groenendyk S, English PB, Abetz I. External balance of water and electrolytes in the horse. Equine Vet J 1988;20(3):189–93.
7. Hinton M. On the watering of horses: a review. Equine Vet J 1978;10(1):27–31.
8. Tasker JB. Fluid and electrolyte studies in the horse. IV. The effects of fasting and thirsting. Cornell Vet 1967;57(4):658–67.
9. Yousef MK, Dill DB, Mayes MG. Shifts in body fluids during dehydration in the burro, *Equus asinus*. J Appl Physiol 1970;29(3):345–9.
10. Maloiy GMO. Water economy of the Somali donkey. Am J Physiol 1970;219(5):1522–7.
11. Carlson GP, Rumbaugh GE, Harrold D. Physiologic alterations in the horse produced by food and water deprivation during periods of high environmental temperatures. Am J Vet Res 1979;40(7):982–5.

12. Sneddon JC, van der Walt JG, Mitchell G. Water homeostasis in desert-dwelling horses. J Appl Physiol 1991;71(1):112–7.
13. Sneddon JC. Physiological effects of hypertonic dehydration on body fluid pools in arid-adapted mammals. How do Arab-based mammals compare? Comp Biochem Physiol Comp Physiol 1993;104(1):201–13.
14. Fitzsimons JT. Angiotensin, thirst, and sodium appetite. Physiol Rev 1998;78(3): 583–686.
15. Andersson B, Augustinsson O, Bademo E, et al. Systemic and centrally mediated angiotensin II effects in the horse. Acta Physiol Scand 1987;129(2):143–9.
16. Houpt KA, Thorton SN, Allen WR. Vasopressin in dehydrated and rehydrated ponies. Physiol Behav 1989;45(3):659–61.
17. Jones NL, Houpt KA, Houpt TR. Stimuli of thirst in donkeys *(Equus asinus)*. Physiol Behav 1989;46(4):661–5.
18. Houpt KA, Northrup A, Wheatley T, et al. Thirst and salt appetite in horses treated with furosemide. J Appl Physiol 1991;71(6):2380–6.
19. Houpt KA. Drinking: the behavioral sequelae of diuretic treatment. Equine Pract 1987;9(9):15–7.
20. Irvine CHG, Alexander SL, Donald RA. Effect of an osmotic stimulus on the secretion of arginine vasopressin and adrenocorticotropin in the horse. Endocrinology 1989;124(6):3102–8.
21. Hubbard RW, Sandick BL, Matthew WT, et al. Voluntary dehydration and alliesthesia for water. J Appl Physiol 1984;57(3):868–73.
22. Greenleaf JE. Problem: thirst, drinking behavior, and involuntary dehydration. Med Sci Sports Exerc 1992;24(6):645–56.
23. Butudom P, Schott HC, Davis MW, et al. Drinking salt water enhances rehydration in horses dehydrated by furosemide administration and endurance exercise. Equine Vet J 2002;(Suppl 34):513–8.
24. Martin RG, McMeniman NP, Dowsett KF. Milk and water intakes of foals sucking grazing mares. Equine Vet J 1992;24(4):295–9.
25. Caljuk EA. Water metabolism and water requirements of horses. Nutr Abstr Rev 1962;32:574.
26. Fonnesbeck PV. Consumption and excretion of water by horses receiving all hay and hay-grain diets. J Anim Sci 1968;27(5):1350–6.
27. Cymbaluk NF. Water balance of horses fed various diets. Equine Pract 1989; 11(1):19–24.
28. Schryver HF, Parker MT, Daniluk PD, et al. Salt consumption and the effect of salt on mineral metabolism in horses. Cornell Vet 1987;77(2):122–31.
29. Keiper RR, Keenan MA. Nocturnal activity patterns of feral ponies. J Mammal 1980;61(1):116–8.
30. Sufit E, Houpt KA, Sweeting M. Physiological stimuli of thirst and drinking patterns in ponies. Equine Vet J 1985;17(1):12–6.
31. Freeman DA, Cymbaluk NF, Schott HC, et al. Clinical, biochemical, and hygiene assessment of stabled horses provided continuous or intermittent access to drinking water. Am J Vet Res 1999;60:1445–50.
32. Nyman S, Dahlborn K. Effect of water supply method and flow rate on drinking behavior and fluid balance in horses. Physiol Behav 2001;73(1):1–8.
33. Kristula M, McDonnell S. Effect of drinking water temperature on consumption and preference of water during cold weather in ponies. In: Proceedings of the 40th Annual Convention of the American Association of Equine Practitioners. Seattle (WA); 1994. p. 95–6.

34. Butudom P, Barnes DJ, Davis MW, et al. Rehydration fluid temperature affects voluntary drinking in horses dehydrated by furosemide administration and endurance exercise. Vet J 2004;167(1):72–80.
35. McKeever KH, Hinchcliff KW, Schmall LM, et al. Plasma renin activity and aldosterone and vasopressin concentrations during incremental treadmill exercise in horses. Am J Vet Res 1992;53(8):1290–3.
36. Nyman S, Hydbring E, Dahlborn K. Is vasopressin a "stress hormone" in the horse? Pferdeheilkunde 1996;12(4):419–22.
37. Brown D, Nielsen S. The cell biology of vasopressin action. In: Brenner BM, editor. The Kidney, vol. 1. 7th edition. Philadelphia: WB Saunders; 2004. p. 573–97.
38. Verkman AS. Aquaporins: translating bench research to human disease. J Exp Biol 2009;212(11):1707–15.
39. Floyd RV, Mason SL, Proudman CJ, et al. Expression and nephron segment-specific distribution of major renal aquaporins (AQP1-4) in *Equus caballus*, the domestic horse. Am J Physiol Regul Integr Comp Physiol 2007;293(1):R492–503.
40. Kinter LB, Huffman WF, Stassen FL. Antagonists of the antidiuretic activity of vasopressin. Am J Physiol 1988;254(2 Pt 2):F165–77.
41. Gellai M. Modulation of vasopressin antidiuretic action by renal α_2-adrenoceptors. Am J Physiol 1990;259(1 Pt 2):F1–8.
42. Thurmon JC, Steffey EP, Zinkl JG, et al. Xylazine causes transient dose-related hyperglycemia and increased urine volume in mares. Am J Vet Res 1984;45(2):224–7.
43. Trim CM, Hanson RR. Effects of xylazine on renal function and plasma glucose in ponies. Vet Rec 1986;118(3):65–7.
44. Nuñez E, Steffey EP, Ocampo L, et al. Effects of alpha2-adrenergic receptor agonists on urine production in horses deprived of food and water. Am J Vet Res 2004;65(10):1342–6.
45. Rose BD. Regulation of plasma osmolality. In: Clinical physiology of acid-base and electrolyte disorders. 5th edition. New York: McGraw-Hill; 2001. p. 285–98.
46. Lakritz J, Madigan J, Carlson GP. Hypovolemic hyponatremia and signs of neurologic disease associated with diarrhea in a foal. J Am Vet Med Assoc 1992;200(8):1114–6.
47. Arroyo LG, Vengust M, Dobson H, et al. Suspected transient pseudohypoaldosteronism in a 10-day-old quarter horse foal. Can Vet J 2008;49(5):494–8.
48. Baylis PH, Cheetham T. Diabetes insipidus. Arch Dis Child 1998;79(1):84–9.
49. Majzoub JA, Srivatsa A. Diabetes insipidus: clinical and basic aspects. Pediatr Endocrinol Rev 2006;4(Suppl 1):60–5.
50. Nichols R. Polyuria and polydipsia. Diagnostic approach and problems associated with patient evaluation. Vet Clin North Am Small Anim Pract 2001;31(5):833–44.
51. Roussel AJ, Carter GK. Polydipsia and polyuria. In: Brown CM, editor. Problems in equine medicine. Philadelphia: Lea & Febiger; 1989. p. 150–60.
52. MacKenzie EM. Polyuria and polydipsia. Diagnostic approach and problems associated with patient evaluation. Vet Clin North Am Equine Pract 2007;23(3):641–53.
53. Koterba AM, Coffman JR. Acute and chronic renal disease in the horse. Compend Contin Educ Pract Vet 1981;3(12):S461–9.
54. Taal MW, Luyckx VA, Brenner BM. Adaptation to nephron loss. In: Brenner BM, editor. The Kidney, vol. 2. 7th edition. Philadelphia: WB Saunders; 2004. p. 1955–97.

55. McGowan TW, Hodgson DR, McGowan CM. The prevalence of equine Cushing's syndrome in aged horses [abstract 113]. J Vet Intern Med 2007;21(3):603.
56. Schott HC. Pituitary pars intermedia dysfunction: equine Cushing's disease. Vet Clin North Am Equine Pract 2002;18(3):237–70.
57. Loeb WF, Capen CC, Johnson LE. Adenomas of the pars intermedia associated with hyperglycemia and glycosuria in two horses. Cornell Vet 1966;56(4):623–39.
58. Hillyer MH, Taylor FGR, Mair TS. Diagnosis of hyperadrenocorticism in the horse. Equine Vet Educ 1992;4(3):131–4.
59. van der Kolk JH, Kalsbeek HC, van Garderen E, et al. Equine pituitary neoplasia: a clinical report of 21 cases (1990–1992). Vet Rec 1993;133(24):594–7.
60. Schott HC. Urinalysis and urine culture results in aged mares with and without pituitary pars intermedia dysfunction [abstract 365]. J Vet Intern Med 2010; 24(3):782.
61. Green EM, Hunt EL. Hypophyseal neoplasia in a pony. Compend Contin Educ Pract Vet 1985;7(4):S249–57.
62. Love S. Equine Cushing's disease. Br Vet J 1993;149(2):139–53.
63. Buntain BJ, Coffman JR. Polyuria and polydipsia in a horse induced by psychogenic salt consumption. Equine Vet J 1981;13(4):266–8.
64. Rumbaugh GE, Carlson GP, Harrold D. Urinary production in the healthy horse and in horses deprived of feed and water. Am J Vet Res 1982;43(4):735–7.
65. Brobst DF, Bayly WM. Responses of horses to a water deprivation test. Equine Vet Sci 1982;2(2):51–6.
66. Genetzky RM, Lopanco FV, Ledet AE. Clinical pathologic alterations in horses during a water deprivation test. Am J Vet Res 1987;48(6):1007–11.
67. Maccubbin DA, Van Buren JM. A quantitative evaluation of hypothalamic degeneration and its relation to diabetes insipidus following interruption of the human hypophyseal stalk. Brain 1963;86(3):443–64.
68. Fujisawa I. Magnetic resonance imaging of the hypothalamic-neurohypophyseal system. J Neuroendocrinol 2004;16(4):297–302.
69. Maghnie M, Cosi G, Genovese E, et al. Central diabetes insipidus in children and young adults. N Engl J Med 2000;343(14):998–1007.
70. Sharp DC, Grubaugh W, Berglund LA, et al. Effect of pituitary stalk transaction on endocrine function in pony mares. J Reprod Fertil Suppl 1982;32:297–302.
71. Filar J, Ziolo T, Szalecki J. Diabetes insipidus in the course of encephalitis in the horse. Med Weter 1971;27(4):205–7.
72. Breukink HJ, Van Wegen P, Schotman AJ. Idiopathic diabetes insipidus in a Welsh pony. Equine Vet J 1983;15(3):284–7.
73. Kranenburg LC, Thelen MHM, Westermann CM, et al. Use of desmopressin eye drops in the treatment of equine congenital central diabetes insipidus. Vet Rec 167(20):790–1.
74. Vente JP, Wijsmuller JM. Diabetes insipidus in a filly. Tijdschr Diergeneeskd 1983; 108(5):210.
75. Chenault L. Diabetes insipidus in the equine. Southwest Vet 1969;22(4):321–3.
76. Satish C, Sastry KNV. Equine diabetes insipidus–a case report. Indian Vet J 1978; 55(7):584–5.
77. Schott HC, Bayly WM, Reed SM, et al. Nephrogenic diabetes insipidus in sibling colts. J Vet Intern Med 1993;7(2):68–72.
78. Brashier M. Polydipsia and polyuria in a weaning colt caused by nephrogenic diabetes insipidus. Vet Clin North Am Equine Pract 2006;22(1):219–27.
79. Nielsen S, Kwon TH, Christensen BM, et al. Physiology and pathophysiology of renal aquaporins. J Am Soc Nephrol 1999;10(3):647–63.

80. Kalelioglu I, Uzum AK, Yildirim A, et al. Transient gestational diabetes insipidus diagnosed in successive pregnancies: review of pathophysiology, diagnosis, treatment, and management of delivery. Pituitary 2007;10(1):87–93.
81. Aleksandrov N, Audibert F, Bedard MJ, et al. Gestational diabetes insipidus: a review of an underdiagnosed condition. J Obstet Gynaecol Can 2010;32(3): 225–31.
82. Kohn CW, Chew DJ. Laboratory diagnosis and characterization of renal disease. Vet Clin North Am Equine Pract 1987;3(3):585–615.
83. Barnes DM, Schott HC, Davis MW, et al. Antidiuretic responses of horses to DDAVP (desmopressin acetate) [abstract 199]. J Vet Intern Med 2002;16(3):376.
84. Harb MF, Nelson RW, Feldman EC, et al. Central diabetes insipidus in dogs: 20 cases (1986–1995). J Am Vet Med Assoc 1996;209(11):1884–8.
85. Aroch I, Mazaki-Tovi M, Shemesh O, et al. Central diabetes insipidus in five cats: clinical presentation, diagnosis and oral desmopressin therapy. J Feline Med Surg 2005;7(6):333–9.
86. Cesar KR, Magaldi AJ. Thiazide induces water reabsorption in the inner medullary collecting duct of normal and Brattleboro rats. Am J Physiol 1999;277(5 pt 2): F756–60.
87. Takemura N. Successful long-term treatment of congenital nephrogenic diabetes insipidus in a dog. J Small Anim Pract 1998;39(12):592–4.

Endocrine Alterations in the Equine Athlete: An Update

Kenneth Harrington McKeever, PhD

KEYWORDS

• Pituitary • Stress • Thyroid • Growth hormone • Insulin
• Leptin • Training

Whatever the activity, the performance of work or exercise is a major physiologic challenge, a disturbance to homeostasis, that invokes an integrative response from multiple organ systems.[1] The adjustments to acute exercise require the coordination of several systems, including the respiratory, cardiovascular, muscular, integumentary, renal, and hepatic systems and the gastrointestinal (GI) tract.[1–5] Each tissue or organ called on to facilitate movement must function in coordination with others in a variety of feedback loops. Multiple layers of control exist to facilitate work. The first muscle contractions associated with work cause local changes that are sensed peripherally. Longer work causes system-wide alterations that are integrated with neural and endocrine mediation. The mechanisms that facilitate a coordinated response to acute exercise comprise integration of signals in the periphery with the nervous system to adjust the respiratory and cardiovascular systems.[3–5] Some have suggested that the rapid adjustments in cardiopulmonary function at the onset of exercise occur primarily by parasympathetic withdrawal together with sympathetic activation.[4,5] As exercise progresses beyond a few seconds, more sophisticated mechanisms that involve endocrine, paracrine, and cytokine pathways fine-tune the initial response.

Fine-tuning to acute exercise relies on the regulation of cardiopulmonary, vascular, and metabolic response to exercise to maintain the internal environment within narrow limits to preserve optimal cell function.[3–5] This type of integrative response is slower than a neural response because it requires communication between systems that rely on the secretion of endocrine and paracrine factors.[3–5]

Equine Science Center, Department of Animal Science, School of Environmental and Biological Sciences, Rutgers, The State University of New Jersey, 84 Lipman Drive, New Brunswick, NJ 08901-8525, USA
E-mail address: mckeever@aesop.rutgers.edu

Vet Clin Equine 27 (2011) 197–218
doi:10.1016/j.cveq.2011.01.001 vetequine.theclinics.com

ENDOCRINE SYSTEM AND HORMONES

By definition, a hormone is a substance produced and released by 1 organ or tissue and transported via the blood to a remote target organ or tissue, where it causes a physiologic response. Most hormones fall into 2 major categories: steroid hormones and nonsteroid hormones. Steroid hormones are lipophylic and include cortisol, aldosterone (ALDO), and the reproductive hormones (testosterone, estrogen, progesterone). Nonsteroid hormones are not lipophylic, cannot pass through the cell membrane, and bind in a lock-and-key fashion to specific cell membrane receptors.

The release of most hormones is under the control of positive and negative feedback mechanisms that keep hormone levels within narrow limits. Inputs from exercise are sensed by a controller that modifies various homeostatic responses via nervous and endocrine signals to control the effectors, which could be other glands, organs, and muscle.

Regulation refers to maintaining the output of a system relatively constant under different conditions. For example, mean arterial pressure, plasma osmolality, blood pH, pco_2 and po_2, plasma electrolyte (Na^+, K^+, and Cl^-) concentrations, blood glucose concentration, and body temperature are variables that are regulated and held within narrow limits during exercise. Regulation of these variables is accomplished through a combination of neural and endocrine mechanisms. Rapid responses to maintain homeostasis are usually mediated by neural control mechanisms, whereas less rapid responses are typically mediated by endocrine mechanisms.

MAJOR ENDOCRINE GLANDS AND HORMONES

The Pituitary Gland

The pituitary is found at the base of the brain and is divided into 3 lobes: the anterior, intermediate, and posterior. Hormones of importance during exercise are produced and released by the anterior and posterior lobes. The pituitary is vitally linked to the hypothalamus, an area of the ventral brain with specific neural tracts that act as feedback sensors. The hypothalamus also acts as the integrator to the systems exerting control over the pituitary through neural and endocrine mechanisms. The latter include various releasing and inhibitory hormones and other substances. The strategic location of this hypothalamic-pituitary axis makes it ideal for centrally mediating the control of a variety of functions.

Anterior pituitary hormones

Hormones produced by the anterior lobe of the pituitary include somatotropin (growth hormone [GH]), thyrotropin (thyroid-stimulating hormone [TSH]), adrenocorticotropin (adrenocorticotropic hormone [ACTH], corticotropin), endorphins, enkephalins, dynorphins, follicle-stimulating hormone (FSH), luteinizing hormone (LH), and prolactin.[2,5] GH, TSH, and ACTH play important roles in growth and development in young animals and metabolism in adult animals. Endorphins, enkephalins, and dynorphins are opiate-like peptide hormones that modulate nociception and influence the hypothalamic-pituitary axis.[6] FSH, LH, and prolactin are essential for reproduction and lactation, and severe or prolonged exertion can alter their release, and thus normal reproductive cycles.[5] Prolactin may play a role in the response to stress by interacting with many metabolic hormones.[5]

Somatotropin

GH affects all cells in the body, stimulating development and growth in younger animals. In mature animals, GH participates in muscle metabolism through its effects on protein synthesis and fat and carbohydrate use.[2,5] The importance of GH in normal physiology can be seen in young adult humans, in whom some signs of GH deficiency (appearance, decreased lean body mass, decreased immune function) can be slowed or even reversed.[7] Treatment of these individuals with recombinant human GH (rhGH) increased lean body mass and muscle mass, and decreased body fat. Chronic rhGH administration seems to increase strength and the ability to better perform on weightlifting exercises in aged men.[7] Although there have been no reported effects of GH on aerobic capacity, the increase in muscle mass and strength has been shown to benefit the quality of life in humans by increasing their ability to perform daily tasks such as walking and climbing stairs. This type of information has been used to justify studies assessing rhGH to prevent or delay the functional decline of aging in geriatric humans and horses.[7–10]

Equine researchers have asked quality of life questions similar to those posed with aged humans. Although equine studies have shown that recombinant equine GH (reGH) increases nitrogen retention and improves appearance in geriatric horses, they have not shown any effect of chronic reGH administration on body weight or muscle mass dimensions.[9] Chronic reGH administration did not alter aerobic capacity, muscle strength, or commonly used indices of exercise performance, at least not in unfit aged mares.[10] Studies on geriatric men have shown that rhGH can increase muscle mass and strength.[7] Studies with younger horses showed that reGH can prevent some of the bone demineralization that occurs with initial training.[11] However, reGH did not alter aerobic capacity or markers of performance. Other studies found no benefits of administering reGH to prevent tendon or cartilage injuries or to promote wound healing.[12,13]

Thyrotropin (TSH)

The release of TSH from the pituitary gland is induced by TSH-releasing hormone from the hypothalamus. Studies of humans and other species have shown variable TSH responses to exercise. TSH secretion seems to be linked to exercise intensity, with mild and moderate exertion having minimal effect on TSH release, whereas intensity exceeding 50% of Vo_{2max} or beyond 40 minutes increased TSH secretion.[14] This increase during steady-state exertion is similar to the response of other metabolic hormones aimed at mobilizing substrates to prevent fatigue. In humans, repeated daily exercise induces TSH release, suggesting a conditioning effect of the metabolic function to training.[5,14]

Adrenocorticotropin (ACTH)

The release of ACTH is stimulated by corticotropin-releasing hormone from the hypothalamus. Several studies have documented that exercise increases ACTH release in the horse[15]; however, most studies report postexercise values.[14,16] High-intensity and endurance exercise causes an increase in ACTH that is followed by an increase in cortisol.[14] A poor cortisol response to ACTH suggests adrenal insufficiency or exhaustion.

In horses, ACTH increases in a curvilinear fashion that is proportional to exercise intensity, catecholamine, and lactate concentrations.[17] When horses were exercised at steady speeds (80 or 110% Vo_{2max}) the ACTH response was rapid, and postexercise concentrations fell rapidly to baseline within 60 to 120 minutes.[17] Liburt and colleagues[18] found that ACTH concentrations increased in a curvilinear fashion in mature and old horses, and during recovery old horses had lower ACTH and cortisol concentrations, suggesting an aging effect on the hypothalamic-pituitary-adrenal axis (HPAA). Pre- and posttraining endocrine stimulation tests suggested that the age-related changes in the HPAA were at the pituitary and adrenal gland levels.[19]

Endorphins, enkephalins, and dynorphins

These peptides are released from the pituitary gland and hypothalamus in response to pain, pleasure, or stress. They are naturally occurring pain suppressors that may allow horses to tolerate high-intensity exercise.[6] In horses there is a threshold to evoke a β-endorphin response to exercise, corresponding to ~60% of the speed eliciting Vo_{2max}.[6] This is the same point at which there is a curvilinear increase for plasma renin activity (PRA), catecholamine, and lactate concentrations, suggesting interactions between these factors in the transition from low-intensity aerobic to higher-intensity anaerobic exercise. Duration of exercise also affects the β-endorphin response, with greater plasma concentrations as horses approach fatigue.[6] Training also alters β-endorphin release to acute exertion with greater concentrations measured between 5 and 10 minutes after exertion.[20]

Posterior pituitary hormones

Hormones released from the posterior lobe of the pituitary include arginine vasopressin (AVP) (antidiuretic hormone) and oxytocin. These hormones are synthesized by neurons of the supraoptic and paraventricular nuclei of the hypothalamus and stored in the neurohypophysis as secretory granules. AVP participates in the regulation of fluid and electrolyte balance. Oxytocin causes contraction of smooth muscle cells in the epididymis of males and uterus of females, and mammary myoepithelial cells of lactating females to induce milk ejection. AVP participates in short- and long-term cardiovascular function during and after exercise, whereas oxytocin does not seem to be involved in the response to exercise. For additional information on AVP function see the article by Hurcombe elsewhere in this issue.

AVP and exercise

AVP is a hormone of the neurohypophysis involved in the regulation of blood pressure, plasma volume, and fluid and electrolyte balance. AVP is released in response to hyperosmolality (osmoreceptors in the supraoptic and paraventricular nuclei of the hypothalamus) and hypotension (baroreceptors in the atria, carotid sinuses, aortic arch). Minimal increases in plasma osmolality (2–4 mOsm/kg) or volume depletion (1%–2%) trigger AVP release. Physical activity causes an increase in plasma AVP that is associated with duration and intensity of exercise.[15,21,22] AVP is secreted during exercise in concentrations more than the threshold required for antidiuresis, suggesting that its extrarenal actions are more important during exertion.[3,22] AVP-mediated vasoconstriction is likely to be important in the control of blood pressure during exercise and preventing splenic blood vessels from resequestering the splenic reserve in the horse.[23] Drinking cold hypotonic water during exercise may suppress thirst and AVP release, leading to hypohydration.[22,23] It is likely that increases in AVP levels after exercise stimulate drinking, decrease renal water excretion, and may enhance the uptake of sodium and water from the colon.[23] In exercising horses, plasma AVP concentration increased from ~4.0 pg/mL at rest to ~95 pg/mL at a speed of 10 m/s, with a curvilinear relationship between AVP concentration and exercise intensity.[24] One study in horses reported that AVP increased during steady-state submaximal exercise without changes in free water clearance; however, the AVP increase did not become significant until 20 to 40 minutes of exertion.[25] Increased AVP concentrations from prolonged exercise are associated with sweat losses, volume depletion, and altered plasma osmolality.[3] In humans, training alters the slope of the AVP response to acute exercise, suggesting changes in sensitivity to the exercise challenge.[22]

The Thyroid

The thyroid gland is a major player in the control of metabolic rate. Thyroid hormones include triiodothyronine (T_3) and thyroxine (T_4), of which T_3 is the most active, whereas T_4 is mainly a precursor for T_3. The function of the thyroid hormones is to increase metabolic rate and promote cellular differentiation. The thyroid gland also produces calcitonin, which is involved in calcium homeostasis.

T_3 and T_4

The secretion of thyroid hormones is stimulated by TSH, which is released in response to the increased metabolic demands of exercise.[5,14] T_3 and T_4 are released in proportion to intensity and duration of exercise in humans and horses.[5,14,26] Information on the thyroid hormone response to endurance exercise is mixed, with no change or transient decreases in plasma-free T_4, free T_3, T_3, and T_4 after rides between 40 and 56 km.[27] Longer rides (160 km) decreased thyroid hormones, with values returning to normal by 24 hours after the ride.[27]

Calcitonin

The thyroid gland is also involved in calcium homeostasis. Thyroid parafollicular cells (C cells) synthesize calcitonin, a blood calcium-lowering hormone. Calcitonin decreases bone resorption by inhibiting osteoclastic activity and increases renal calcium excretion by inhibiting tubular reabsorption of calcium. Calcitonin may be important in fracture healing. Chiba and colleagues[28] found high calcitonin concentrations in racehorses with various types of fractures. In humans, calcitonin has skeletal analgesic properties,[29] and calcitonin has been used empirically to treat bone pain in horses; however, no controlled study has critically evaluated these actions in the horse.

The Parathyroid Glands

The parathyroid glands, located close to the thyroid gland, regulate calcium homeostasis by secreting parathyroid hormone (PTH) in response to low plasma calcium concentration. The main targets for PTH are the kidneys and bone. See the article by Toribio elsewhere in this issue. In the kidney, PTH increases calcium reabsorption and stimulates phosphate elimination, whereas in bone PTH increases osteoclastic activity and bone resorption (bone loss). Compared with calcitonin, some information is available on PTH in exercising horses. Horses under intense exercise often develop hypocalcemia, which can be explained by metabolic alkalosis, sweat losses, or low PTH concentrations. One study found that exercising horses with hypocalcemia had an increase in serum PTH concentrations, an expected response.[30] In several horses with hypocalcemia the increase in PTH did not restore normocalcemia. In another study, some exercising horses with hypocalcemia did not have the expected increase in PTH concentrations, suggesting dysfunction of the parathyroid gland.[31] Relevant exercise physiology is that hypocalcemia can lead to cardiac arrhythmias, synchronous diaphragmatic flutter (thumps), ileus (colic), and death.

The Adrenals

The adrenal glands have 2 different structures: the medulla and the cortex. The medulla secretes catecholamines (epinephrine, norepinephrine), which have metabolic and cardiovascular actions. The adrenal cortex contains 3 specialized zones: the zona glomerulosa, which produces mineralocorticoids (ALDO); the zona fasciculate, which produces glucocorticoids (cortisol); and the zona reticularis, which synthesizes gonadocorticoids (androgens, estrogens).

The adrenal medulla (catecholamines)

The release of catecholamines has its origin in the fight-or-flight response.[32] This stress response involves the local release of norepinephrine from the sympathetic nerve endings and a systemic release of epinephrine and norepinephrine from the adrenal medulla. Epinephrine potentiates the response to exercise, causing profound effects on central cardiovascular and respiratory function, increasing muscle blood flow and mobilizing glycogen and free fatty acids to fuel exertion. Catecholamines receptors are specialized and divided into 2 groups: α- and β-adrenergic receptors. These are further divided into α_1-, α_2-, β_1-, and β_2-adrenergic receptors.

Sympathetic activity increases with intensity and duration of exercise; however, measurable changes in plasma catecholamine concentrations are not apparent at less than 50% to 70% of maximal aerobic capacity.[32] It has been reported that plasma catecholamine concentrations increase in a curvilinear fashion with intensity of exercise and are correlated with plasma lactate concentrations.[17,26,33] This increase coincides with the intensity at which one expects complete parasympathetic withdrawal. Catecholamines enhance heart rate (HR), cardiac contractility and cardiac output.[3,32] Catecholamines also induce splenic contraction and the delivery of 6 to 12 L of blood into the central circulation at the onset of exercise. Even with this mobilization of reserved blood volume the demands of exercise may exceed cardiovascular capacity in the horse. Thus, during high-intensity or long-duration exercise, catecholamine-induced vasoconstriction decreases blood flow to nonobligate tissues.[3,32] Catecholamines are also involved in respiratory response to exercise. At the onset of exercise, β_2-adrenergic receptors relax tracheal and bronchial smooth muscles, increasing airway diameter, decreasing airway resistance, and thus facilitating air movement and gas exchange.[32] Although the sympathetic system is not directly responsible for controlling ventilation, the ventilatory drive associated with the motor cortex can be enhanced during exercise by catecholamines, which can also sensitize chemoreceptors in the carotid bodies.[32]

Catecholamines affect metabolic pathways associated with substrate use during exercise by increasing the activity of the hormone-sensitive lipase, which releases free fatty acids into circulation. Catecholamines also accelerate glycogen breakdown to increase blood glucose levels. It has been proposed that 1 way warm-up exercises benefit athletes is through activation of these metabolic pathways, increasing blood glucose and free fatty acids before a race, thus facilitating substrate delivery without a significant lag time.[5,14,32]

The responses outlined earlier have been documented during acute exercise, and there are data to suggest that training alters adrenergic receptor numbers and sensitivity in selected tissues.[5,14,32,33] For example, β-adrenergic receptor number is unchanged in cardiac muscle with training, whereas α-adrenergic and muscarinic receptor number is reduced.[5,14,32] Both β-adrenergic receptor number and sensitivity increase with exercise in skeletal muscle and vascular and bronchial smooth muscle.[5,14,32] This finding may also be relevant to drug sensitivity in trained versus untrained animals.[5,14,32]

Adrenal cortex hormones

Of the many steroid hormones secreted by the adrenal gland cortex, ALDO (mineralocorticoid) and cortisol (glucocorticoid) are the most important in regard to exercise.[2,5,14]

ALDO

ALDO is essential for electrolyte homeostasis, in particular sodium and potassium balance. ALDO acts on the renal tubules to enhance sodium (and chloride) reabsorption and potassium excretion. In the intestine, ALDO facilitates the uptake of electrolytes and water. ALDO secretion is stimulated by hyponatremia, hyperkalemia, acidemia, ACTH, and angiotensin II.[3,34] Increased plasma K^+ concentration is considered the most potent stimulus for ALDO release.[3,34] There is some evidence that increased angiotensin II from increased PRA rather than low Na^+ concentrations is the initial stimulus for ALDO secretion in exercising horses.[35,36]

ALDO participates in the hypervolemic response to exercise training. ALDO remained increased for 24 hours after submaximal exercise, with the magnitude of increase being greater after each session and associated with decreased urine volume and sodium excretion.[37,38] A relationship between plasma ALDO and exercise intensity was documented in horses running on a treadmill; ALDO increased from 20 to 50 pg/mL at rest to ~200 pg/mL at a speed of 10 m/s.[24,39] The increase in ALDO during submaximal exercise paralleled changes in PRA; however, the relative increase in PRA (66%) was less than that of ALDO (709%).[25] The investigators concluded that factors other than PRA affect ALDO release in these horses.[25] Increased plasma K^+ concentration is a potent stimulus for ALDO release in horses.[3] An increase in plasma K^+ as small as 0.3 mEq/L can trigger ALDO secretion, independent of PRA.[3] ALDO has a minimal role in the acute response to exercise in horses; however, the ALDO increase that follows exercise may affect the long-term renal and intestinal handling of sodium and water.[38–40]

Cortisol

Cortisol is the major glucocorticoid secreted by the adrenal glands; however, cortisone, corticosterone, and deoxycorticosterone are also released to a lesser extent.[5,14] Cortisol, cortisone, and corticosterone can be found in equine plasma at a ratio of 16:8:0.5.[14] In horses, cortisol has diurnal variations, with peaks in the morning (6:00–10:00 AM) and lowest levels in the evening and early morning.[5,14]

Glucocorticoids are stress hormones; however, they are involved in multiple functions, from metabolism to immune modulation. The effects of cortisol fall into 2 categories: substrate mobilization and immune modulation. Exercise is a challenge in which cortisol stimulates substrate mobilization by enhancing gluconeogenesis and free fatty acid release. At the same time, cortisol decreases glucose use, sparing it to be used by the central nervous system.[5,14] One could speculate that these actions could delay the onset of central fatigue that occurs during endurance exertion when glucose concentrations decrease.[38,41] Cortisol increases protein catabolism and amino acid release to be used for energy, tissue repair, and enzyme synthesis. Cortisol is an immune modulator by acting as an antiinflammatory agent and suppressing immune function. These actions may be of benefit in the response to training. Overload from exercise intensity, resistance, or duration is necessary for training to stimulate an adaptive response to exercise. Minor disruptions in the function and structure of muscle fibers result in protein accretion, substrate uptake and deposition, and remodeling to increase functional capacity. The immune modulatory functions of cortisol may provide a permissive environment for tolerating the slight amount of muscle damage needed for training-induced remodeling. Cortisol increases in horses under a variety of exercise activities, including racing, polo, and endurance rides, and its release seems to be affected by intensity and duration of exercise.[8,14,42] However, the excessive cortisol increase after exertion can be a marker of too much exercise. Prolonged cortisol recovery times as well as inappropriately high or low cortisol concentrations could be a marker of overtraining. Several equine studies have followed cortisol concentrations for extended periods after exercise, showing that exercise can increase cortisol secretion 6-fold, plasma cortisol concentrations 2- to 3-fold, and urinary cortisol 3-fold.[43,44] The investigators also noted a substantial increase in hepatic clearance of cortisol.

Data are mixed on the effects of training on the cortisol response. Previous studies indicate that peak postexercise cortisol concentrations occur earlier in trained horses, with peaks at about 30 minutes after exertion, and that trained horses have faster cortisol recovery times.[14,45]

The Pancreas

The pancreas has exocrine and endocrine functions. The acinus is the exocrine component, secreting digestive enzymes and bicarbonate into the small intestine via the pancreatic duct. The endocrine functions are mediated by cells of the islets of Langerhans. These cells are classified into 3 types: α cells (glucagon), β cells (insulin) and δ cells (somatostatin). Of these hormones, insulin is the most important during exercise.

Insulin

Insulin is synthesized by the pancreatic β cells and is primarily a glucose storage hormone because it facilitates cellular glucose uptake, promotes glycogenesis, and inhibits gluconeogenesis. At rest insulin is the key that opens the cellular door for glucose entrance; however, during exercise, muscle fibers uptake glucose without the effect of insulin.[5,14] Thus, it seems that insulin is important during the recovery from exercise when glycogen repletion is most active.[5,14,46,47] The insulin response to acute exercise is well documented in the horse and other species, with exercise suppressing insulin secretion.[14,45,48–52] This suppression seems to have a threshold of 50% of $\dot{V}O_{2max}$, which coincides with the catecholamine increase that occurs during exercise.[1,14] Recent studies have shown a link between exercise-induced sympathetic drive and changes in insulin and glucagon secretion in the horse.[50,51] This link likely allows an increase in gluconeogenesis to maintain normoglycemia during exercise. Glucose mobilized during exercise can be taken up by muscle through insulin effects; however, endurance performance seems to be limited by central fatigue mechanisms more than peripheral fatigue.[5,14,50,51] Suppression of insulin release and maintenance of normoglycemia may prevent the onset of central fatigue.[53] Much of the work on the insulin response to exertion has centered on the composition and timing of preexercise feeding, as well as mechanisms associated with postexercise glycogen repletion.[54,55] High-carbohydrate feeds are beneficial for optimal muscle glycogen synthesis to fuel exercise; however, the increase in blood glucose after a horse eats a high-carbohydrate ration usually evokes insulin secretion.[56–58] Research has been focused on understanding how to prevent this feed-induced spike in insulin that would decrease blood glucose before or during exercise.[56–59]

Training increases insulin sensitivity and seems to alter the insulin response to acute exercise, enhancing the ability to synthesize glycogen during recovery.[14,60–62] The horse seems to differ from humans in some of the mechanisms for glycogen repletion,[50,51,55] and these differences may be related to the herbivore nature of horses for carbohydrate acquisition.

Glucagon

The functions of glucagon are in opposition to insulin because it stimulates gluconeogensis and inhibits glycogenesis.[5,14] Glucagon is one of many hormones needed for substrate mobilization and increases during exercise in the horse.[63] Glucagon is crucial for maintaining glucose concentrations during exercise, a role that is important during endurance activities when a drop in blood glucose may lead to central fatigue.[2,5,14] Glucagon secretion is altered by exercise intensity and sympathetic activity.[51] Training affects the glucagon response to exercise, enhancing the ability to mobilize glucose during exertion.[5,14]

Other pancreatic hormones

Other pancreatic hormones that may participate in substrate disposition during and after exercise include pancreatic polypeptide (PP), somatostatin, amylin, and galanin.[64]

PP does not seem to affect insulin or glucagon concentrations; however, it affects digestion.[64] PP inhibits pancreatic exocrine function and bile secretion, an observation that is considered appropriate for a horse during long-term exercise when food intake tends to be minimal.[65] Information on the effects of exercise on PP in the horse is minimal. In 1 equine study, PP increased from 20 pmol/L at rest to 102 pmol/L after an 80-km endurance ride.[65] These results are similar to those in other species.[64]

Somatostatin is produced in the hypothalamus, GI tract, and pancreas. It is well known that hypothalamic somatostatin inhibits GH and TSH release. Pancreatic somatostatin alters pancreatic function, reduces intestinal blood flow, and restricts nutrient absorption, which fits well with the reduction in splanchnic blood flow that occurs during exercise.[65] A small but significant increase in GH concentration has been documented during endurance exercise in horses, with no difference caused by duration (42 vs 80 km).[65] This finding is consistent with studies of humans and other species.[64] To the author's knowledge, no study has examined the effect of exercise intensity on concentrations of somatostatin in the horse.

Amylin and galanin are produced by the pancreas and influence insulin secretion.[64] Amylin is a 37–amino acid protein produced by the β cells, whereas galanin is a 29–amino acid protein secreted by nerve cells in the GI tract and pancreas. Galanin functions as a neuropeptide and inhibits basal and stimulated insulin release, as well as somatostatin and PP secretion.[66] Galanin increased in acute exercising middle-aged humans, and it appeared to be involved in the regulation of GH secretion.[67]

Circulating GI (Gut) Hormones

Several other substances with endocrine and paracrine function are secreted by the GI tract. These factors alter digestive function and may influence digestion, absorption, and substrate use during exercise.[64] Included in this group are gastric inhibitory peptide (GIP), vasoactive intestinal polypeptide (VIP), gastrin, somatostatin, secretin, enterglucagon, motilin, cholecystokinin (CCK, see also later discussion), enkephalins, endorphins, substance P, gastrin-releasing peptide, neuropeptide Y, peptide YY, neurotensin, and ghrelin.

GIP is a 42–amino acid peptide that inhibits gastric acid production and stimulates insulin secretion.[64] Exercise does not alter GIP concentrations in humans; however, glucose consumption during recovery decreases GIP concentrations. In horses, Hall and colleagues[65] reported no changes in plasma GIP concentrations during endurance exercise (42 and 80 km); however, with longer endurance competition GIP concentrations decreased from 75 pmol/L before exercise to ~50 pmol/L after 80 km.[65] This decline in GIP was consistent with the decrease in insulin concentrations in the same horses.

VIP is a 28 amino acid neurotransmitter secreted by nerve fibers in the central nervous system and GI tract. VIP actions include vasodilation, stimulation of glucagon secretion, and stimulation of substrate release through lipolysis and hepatic glycogenolysis.[64] Endurance exercise affects VIP secretion, with increases that are associated with exercise duration.[64,65] This finding fits with the energy substrate needs associated with prolonged exercise.

Gastrin is a 10–amino acid peptide that stimulates gastric acid secretion that is affected by previous ingestion of food. Exercise, training, and feeding increased gastrin concentrations in horses.[68,69] Plasma gastrin concentrations were not altered by a 42-km endurance ride, but increased after a longer 80-km ride.[65] One would speculate that this gastrin increase could contribute to excessive acid production and gastric ulcer formation when food is withheld from horses for a long period.

Other GI endocrine or paracrine factors

Most of these substances have been classified as neurotransmitters that act in the GI tract to alter membrane transport, modify motility, and modulate acid production. Gastrin-releasing peptide (27 amino acids, known as bombesin) stimulates GI motility and gastrin release, and its concentrations increase with exercise.[70] Secretin and enterglucagon are both 29–amino acid hormones that inhibit gastric acid secretion. They increase in peripheral blood after exercise in humans and dogs.[64] Motilin is a 22–amino acid peptide that stimulates GI motility, and its concentrations increase with exercise in humans.[64] Enkephalins and opioids decrease motility.[64] Substance P, neuropeptide Y, and peptide YY alter GI tract motility but little is known about their changes during exercise. The actions of these hormones may be relevant for the uptake of water, electrolytes, and energy substrates during and after exercise.[64] Neurotensin is a 10–amino acid peptide produced in the central nervous system and GI tract; in the intestine it promotes mucosal healing and its concentrations are increased in exercising humans.[64,70]

Hormones Related to Appetite and Energy Balance

The energy expended during exercise directly affects energy homeostasis because horses have to increase caloric intake to compensate for energy lost during exercise and energy required for recovery and tissue repair. The neuroendocrine control of energy balance is just beginning to be examined in horses. Endocrine mediators of energy balance include leptin, adiponectin, ghrelin, and CCK.

Leptin

Leptin (16-kDa) is an adipocyte-derived hormone product of the *ob* gene that influences food intake and energy use, and can be used as an indicator of energy balance.[71,72] High levels of leptin increase energy expenditure and decrease food intake and vice versa[73] The feeding or orexigenic system consists of neuropeptide Y, agouti-related protein, and other hormones that increase food intake. The satiety system involves hypothalamic neurons and α-melanocyte-stimulating hormone to decrease food intake.[74] Leptin stimulates the sympathetic system in brown adipose tissue and increases the expression of uncoupling protein 1 and uncoupling protein 3 in skeletal muscle.[75] Leptin stimulates triglyceride and fatty acid cycling by increasing lipolysis and fatty acid oxidation and is secreted in proportion to fat mass, although massively obese humans seem to be resistant to leptin.[72,76]

In horses, plasma leptin is positively correlated with percent fat mass and body condition score.[77,78] Leptin has seasonal variations in young and old mares, with plasma leptin levels increasing in the summer and decreasing in the winter, in correlation to body weight and fat mass.[79,80] Furthermore, 24-hour fasting decreases plasma leptin levels in young and mature mares.[81] One study showed that serum concentrations of leptin were higher in geldings and stallions versus mares, which differs from humans, in whom females have higher leptin concentrations.[77,82] Male rats had higher blood leptin concentrations than female rats.[83]

In regards to exercise, in the horse acute incremental exercise does not change plasma leptin concentrations.[52] This finding is similar to humans under short-term exercise (<60 minutes), in whom no changes in leptin concentrations were found.[84] Studies that reported changes in leptin concentration with short-term exercise attributed the differences to hemoconcentration or circadian rhythm.[85] It is possible that short-term exercise does not cause a sufficient caloric deficit to disrupt long-term energy balance. Also, interactions with other hormones (eg, cortisol, insulin, glucose, epinephrine, and norepinephrine) that fluctuate during exercise are likely to affect leptin secretion.

Long-term exercise (≥60 minutes) has been shown to decrease or cause no change in leptin concentrations.[86,87] It is possible that long-term exercise results in an energy deficit sufficient to decrease leptin levels, leading to increased food intake.

Training regimens have had different effects on leptin release. Training for less than 12 weeks caused no changes in leptin levels, although type 2 diabetic individuals had lower leptin concentrations after 6 weeks of low-intensity walking and cycling, independent of body condition.[88,89] Training reduces fat mass and lowers leptin levels, independent of fat mass.[90,91] It seems that females are more sensitive to the training effect of leptin, with lower leptin concentrations in response to training than males.[92] Training affects leptin concentration in horses, with lower concentrations in fit versus unfit animals.[52]

Leptin has potential health benefits in exercising horses. Leptin can be used to determine if a horse is in a positive or negative energy balance, providing data on body condition and percent fat mass. Understanding how exercise and training affect leptin concentrations in horses can be used to adjust energy balance and training regimens.

Adiponectin

Adiponectin is another hormone secreted by adipocytes that regulates glucose and fat metabolism.[93] In contrast to leptin, adiponectin levels are lower in obese and insulin-resistant humans and animals.[94] Adiponectin may play a role in the increased insulin sensitivity result of training and exercise in humans and horses.[95,96] Old mares with impaired glucose tolerance were able to improve their insulin sensitivity with 12 weeks of training.[18,19,95]

In yearling fillies and mature mares, adiponectin was negatively correlated with percent fat mass.[78] Adiponectin may be involved in the development of insulin resistance of horses with pituitary adenomas and metabolic syndrome. It would be of interest to determine if adiponectin has a role in the insulin-sensitizing effect of exercise.

Ghrelin

This peptide hormone is secreted from the hypothalamus and P/D1 cells of the stomach.[97] Ghrelin is a potent GH-releasing factor that is receiving increasing attention because of its role in initiating food intake in humans and animals. Contrary to leptin, ghrelin promotes hunger (orexigenic). Ghrelin increases before feeding in anticipation of a meal and during fasting.[98] In rats, ghrelin stimulates gastric acid secretion.[99] Ghrelin levels did not change during submaximal aerobic exercise in humans.[100] Ghrelin may help horses maintain energy balance, and exercise alters its secretion.[52] High-performing equine athletes often have problems with inappetance and gastric ulcers that may be related to abnormal ghrelin concentrations.[52]

Humans with anorexia have higher ghrelin concentrations than their normal counterparts, with a presumed ghrelin resistance contributing to the cachexia of this eating disorder.[101]

CCK

CCK is secreted from the small intestine and is involved in energy metabolism by signaling satiety and decreasing food intake.[102] There are few data on CCK in horses; however, equine researchers speculate that increased CCK concentrations may be involved in the development of anorexia that occurs in heavily exercised horses.

There are interactions between many of the hormones mentioned. For example, CCK enhances the effect of leptin on weight loss and together may decrease food intake.[103] Leptin and adiponectin, although expressed in opposite fashions, may be similarly regulated in the short-term but differently in the long-term. Ghrelin is upregulated during leptin therapy, but the ghrelin increase cannot overcome leptin-mediated satiety.[104] Hence, it is clear that to better understand these endocrine mediators they should not be studied in isolation, but collectively.

The regulation of energy balance and how it is affected by exercise and endocrine factors is a field in its infancy in the horse when compared with other species. Conditions such as gastric ulcers and inappetance often seen in heavily exercised horses, as well as insulin resistance of older or obese horses, could benefit from better information, because management practices can be modified to improve energy balance, performance, and health.

The Kidneys

The kidney has important endocrine functions that relate to exercise, tissue perfusion, and oxygenation, including initiating the response of the renin-angiotensin-aldosterone system (RAAS) and synthesis of erythropoietin (EPO). The juxtaglomerular apparatus (JGA) consists of a series of specialized cells associated with the glomeruli and distal tubules, and its function is to sense blood flow (and pressure), sodium and chloride concentrations, and arterial po_2. The RAAS is responsible for maintaining blood pressure and tissue perfusion. The kidney also produces EPO, which acts on erythroid precursors in the bone marrow to promote erythropoiesis. Both the RAAS and EPO play important functions on cardiovascular function and tissue oxygenation.

PRA

Poor renal perfusion and/or decreased sodium and chloride in the distal tubules are sensed by the JGA, which releases renin, the enzyme that cleaves hepatic angiotensinogen into angiotensin I. Angiotensin I is further converted in the lungs to active angiotensin II by angiotensin-converting enzymes (ACEs). PRA is measured as the rate of angiotensin I generation in vitro. Angiotensin II is a potent vasoconstrictor that also stimulates the adrenal gland to secrete ALDO and the neurohypophysis to release vasopressin. After exercise, angiotensin II stimulates thirst and drinking, thus altering postexercise fluid and electrolyte balance.[21,22,24] Mechanisms for increased PRA during exercise include sympathetic renal stimulation, decreased renal blood flow, and low sodium and chloride concentrations, leading to JGA activation.

A linear correlation between work intensity and duration, HR, and increased PRA was found in horses at treadmill speeds of ~9 m/s.[24] More than 9 m/s, HR and PRA reached a plateau with no further increases.[24] PRA increased from 1.9 ± 1.0 at rest to a peak of 5.2 ± 1.0 ng/mL/h at 9 m/s.[24] The concurrent plateau in PRA and HR rate suggests that PRA in exercising horses is linked to sympathetic activity.[22,34] In steady-state submaximal exercise, sympathetic drive is the major stimulation for early increases in PRA.[22,34] However, the secondary PRA increase after 40 minutes of exercise is likely caused by decreases in plasma Cl^- concentrations.[34] The result of increased PRA is increase of plasma angiotensin II concentrations. Horses given the ACE inhibitor enalapril had lower plasma angiotensin II and ALDO concentrations and pulmonary artery pressures during exercise compared with horses given a placebo.[35] This finding confirms that the RAAS plays a key role in blood pressure regulation during exercise in the horse.

EPO

EPO is a glycoprotein produced by renal peritubular endothelial cells in response to hypoxemia. Conditions associated with low oxygen (blood loss, anemia, acute exercise, altitude) stimulate EPO production to enhance erythropoiesis and normalize oxygen delivery. Acute exercise does not seem to stimulate EPO release in horses (McKeever KH, Wickler S, Smith T. Altitude not exercise increases plasma EPO in horses. J Appl Physiol, unpublished). A similar observation was made in humans in which neither intensity nor duration of acute exercise, altered plasma EPO concentrations.[105] This makes sense because if acute exercise increases EPO secretion, then repeated physical activity leads to sustained EPO release, erythropoiesis, polycytemia and increased blood viscosity.

Altitude causes a transient increase in EPO production in humans and horses (McKeever KH, Wickler S, Smith T. Altitude not exercise increases plasma erythropoietin in horses. J Appl Physiol, unpublished).[5] In horses, EPO increased only in the first 3 hours of the first day at 3800 m of altitude, similar to humans, in whom there is a temporary increase in EPO in mountain climbing. An explanation for the rapid EPO return to baseline is cardiorespiratory compensation to limit changes in Pa_{O_2}. Horses exercising at high altitudes did not have a secondary increase in plasma EPO concentration, suggesting that hypobaric hypoxia affects EPO production only in the first day.[37,38] Administration of recombinant human EPO (rhEPO) increases hemoglobin concentration and exercise capacity in humans. Small doses of rhEPO increase hemoglobin concentration and endurance performance.[106,107] Human athletes have used higher than recommended doses of rhEPO to further improve aerobic capacity. However, rhEPO can increase the resting hematocrit to values greater than 55%, increasing blood viscosity, hypercoagulability, and higher risk for heart attacks or stroke. This practice has also entered equine sports, with veterinarians and racing commission personnel reporting rhEPO being misused in racehorses to improve oxygen-carrying capacity.[108,109] Horses injected with rhEPO can develop several problems. Although horses can tolerate hematocrits of 50% to 60% during exercise, it is unclear what would happen to the cardiovascular system if the resting hematocrit were 70% to 80%. An increased hematocrit coupled with splenic mobilization may produce hyperviscous blood that could lead to sudden death during or after exercise.[109] It can be worse if blood hyperviscosity is coupled with lasix-induced fluid losses. A well-documented problem from rhEPO administration in horses is its immunogenicity, in which some animals develop anti-rhEPO antibodies that also block equine EPO, inducing aplastic anemia and often death.[110]

Studies on splenectomized and intact horses showed that low rhEPO doses increased the resting hematocrit level, red blood cell volume, maximal oxygen uptake, blood viscosity, and selected hemodynamic variables during incremental exercise performed on a treadmill.[111,112] In splenectomized horses, low rhEPO doses 3 times a week for 3 weeks increased the resting hematocrit from 37% to 46%.[112] This 13% hematocrit increase was associated with a 19% increase in $V_{O_{2max}}$ and increased blood viscosity.[112] In intact horses, rhEPO (50 IU/kg, 3 times a week for

3 weeks) increased red blood cell volume, $\dot{V}O_{2max}$ and velocity at $\dot{V}O_{2max}$.[111] Horses in that study developed antibodies to rhEPO (McKeever, unpublished data, 2006).

The Heart and Blood Vessels

The heart and blood vessels release paracrine and endocrine factors that control cardiovascular function. Although there are several mechanisms worthy of discussion, hormones that are major players during exercise are atrial natriuretic peptide (ANP) and endothelins (ETs).[3]

ANP is produced by the heart to regulate blood flow and blood pressure. ANP secretory granules are stored within the walls of the atria and released during atrial stretching.[3] Receptors for ANP are present in the posterior pituitary, kidneys, vascular smooth muscle, adrenal cortex, heart, and lungs. ANP causes rapid vasodilation and natriuresis.[3] ANP inhibits vasopressin, renin, and ALDO secretion, and interferes with ALDO actions in the renal tubules.[3] In the horse, ANP may be involved in accommodating exercise-related shifts of blood volume.[3] Evidence for this claim is provided by studies reporting that plasma ANP increases linearly with work intensity, from 5 to 10 pg/mL at rest to more than 60 pg/mL at speeds eliciting $\dot{V}O_{2max}$ and associated with HR.[3,113,114] ANP increased at steady-state submaximal exercise, from ~10 pg/mL at rest to 40 pg/mL at 40 minutes and remained increased through 60 minutes of exertion.[3,115] Nyman and colleagues[114] found that hyperhydrated horses had higher ANP concentrations during exercise than control and hypohydrated horses.[114] No difference was found between arterial and mixed venous ANP concentrations, suggesting that ANP is either not metabolized by the lungs or is secreted at a rate matching pulmonary metabolism.[24] It has been proposed that ANP remains increased after exercise as a response to increased blood volume rather than as a response to vasopressin or catecholamines.[39]

ET

The ETs are peptide hormones released by endothelial cells to control cardiovascular function. There are 3 isoforms (ET-1, ET-2, and ET-3), all with 21 amino acids. The half-life of ET-1 is very short (a few minutes), which is consistent with its role in controlling vascular tone. Factors affecting the release and metabolism of ET include increased blood flow, vasopressin, angiotensin, shear stress, and thrombin. ET-2 and ET-3 have limited vascular effects, and ET-1 has the most pronounced effect on vascular tone. ET-1 is involved in the pathogenesis of hypertension, in particular pulmonary hypertension. ET-1 and ET-2 (to a minor degree) are potent vasoconstrictors that increase systemic and pulmonary arterial blood pressures, and can alter cardiac output and blood flow distribution. ET-1 is likely to be involved in blood pressure regulation and redistribution during exercise. ET-3 seems to modulate vasopressin release. Resting ET-1 concentrations are similar in domestic animals and humans. Studies of ET-1 in horses have focused on its role in respiratory disease[116] or aging.[37] ET-1 concentration was increased in blood and bronchiolar alveolar lavage fluid in resting horses with respiratory disease.[117] No changes in plasma ET-1 concentrations were found in horses running at incremental exercise or increased work; however, ET-1 concentrations increased after the exercise, suggesting a cardiovascular adaptation after exercise.[37]

ET-1 concentrations are increased in humans with diseases such as chronic obstructive pulmonary disease and pulmonary hypertension. Benamou and colleagues[116] found that postexercise ET-1 concentrations were increased in plasma and bronchoalveolar lavage fluid of horses with recurrent airway obstruction. ET-1 may serve as a modulator for the acute response or slower phase of hypoxic pulmonary hypertension response to exercise. It remains unclear whether ET-1 and pulmonary hypertension are involved in the pathogenesis of exercise-induced pulmonary hemorrhage.

The Gonads and Reproductive Hormones

Reproductive hormones are essential for the health of mares and stallions. However, exercise performance is not affected per se by these hormones. Nevertheless, some studies have evaluated the effect of exercise on the reproductive cycle of women, and the interaction of prolactin, LH, FSH, estrogen and β-endorphin.[5] Work addressing the effect of exercise on reproductive hormones, in maiden and pregnant mares, in particular endurance and pleasure mares ridden while in foal, is needed.

ENDOCRINE MEDIATION OF SHORT-TERM CONTROL OF CARDIOVASCULAR FUNCTION

The cardiovascular response to exercise depends on a series of processes that ensure adequate blood flow to working muscles and obligate tissues along with the provision of adequate fluid volume for sweating and thermoregulation. Cardiovascular homeostasis during exercise is mediated by endocrine and neuroendocrine mechanisms. Anticipating exercise, humans and horses can withdraw parasympathetic control and enhance sympathetic activity to increase HR, cardiac contractility, stroke volume, and cardiac output. In horses HR can go from 30 to 40 beats per minute (bpm) at rest to ~120 bpm from parasympathetic withdrawal, whereas further increases result from sympathetic activity and catecholamine release.[3] This situation can increase cardiac output from 30 L/min at rest to 300 L/min at maximal exercise.[3] Adjustments of peripheral vascular resistance redistribute blood stored from compliant blood vessels to the arterial side, improving oxygen delivery. This situation is further enhanced by splenic contraction from sympathetic stimulation. From 6 to 12 L of blood can be delivered into central circulation at the onset of exercise, allowing equine athletes to reach maximal aerobic capacity (145–200 mL/kg/min), which is almost 3 times greater than that of human athletes.[3] This extra volume is rapidly accommodated through arterial vasodilation from increases in ANP.

Modulation of the blood pressure and flow response to exercise involves inputs from high- and low-pressure baroreceptors.[3,4] At the start of exercise, increased venous return stretches the atrium, eliciting a neuroendocrine response. Impulses are conducted via vagal afferent fibers and integrated into the central control of peripheral vascular tone. The endocrine response involves the release of ANP to induce vasodilation and inhibit vasopressin release.

Exercise and training produce cardiovascular adaptations that are mediated by neuroendocrine factors. Work from several species has shown that exercise expands plasma volume. Trained horses have greater blood volumes than untrained horses, with increases in plasma volume of 30% after 1 week of training.[38] Repeated exercise in humans alters sodium and water excretion by increasing ALDO concentrations.[21] Plasma ALDO concentration remained increased for almost 24 hours during the first days of training in horses.[38] It seems that ALDO mediates the retention of sodium and water by the kidneys and intestine in the hypervolemic response to training.

ENDOCRINE CONTROL OF METABOLISM DURING ACUTE EXERCISE

Exercise requires the transduction of stored energy into kinetic energy, and endocrine factors promote the mobilization and use of carbohydrates and free fatty acids to prevent central fatigue. At the onset of exercise catecholamines increase hepatic and muscular glycogenolysis, making more glucose available. Catecholamines stimulate hormone-sensitive lipase to mobilize free fatty acids, inhibit insulin, and stimulate glucagon release. Glucagon promotes gluconeogensis and inhibits glycogenesis, thus playing a key role in maintaining glycemia during exercise. Glucagon stimulates the breakdown of protein and release of amino acids to be used as fuel source by the liver. The effects of the catecholamines and glucagon can be augmented by cortisol. Cortisol stimulates gluconeogenesis, fatty acid mobilization, and protein breakdown. Amino acids not used to fuel exercise may be used for de novo protein synthesis and muscle repair.

REFERENCES

1. McKeever KH. The endocrine system and the challenge of exercise. Vet Clin North Am Equine Pract 2002;18:321–53.
2. Dickson WM. Endocrine glands. In: Swenson MJ, editor. Dukes physiology of domestic animals. Ithaca (NY): Cornell University Press; 1970. p. 1189–252.
3. McKeever KH, Hinchcliff KW. Neuroendocrine control of blood volume, blood pressure, and cardiovascular function in horses. Equine Vet J Suppl 1995;18:77–81.
4. Rowell LB. Human cardiovascular control. New York: Oxford University Press; 1993. p. 441–79.
5. Willmore JH, Costill DL. Hormonal regulation of exercise. In: Willmore JH, Costill DL, editors. Physiology of sport and exercise. Champaign (IL): Human Kinetics; 1994. p. 122–43.
6. Mehl ML, Schott HC, Sarkar DK, et al. Effects of exercise intensity on plasma β-endorphin concentrations in horses. Am J Vet Res 2000;61:969–73.
7. Yarasheski KE. Growth hormone effects on metabolism, body composition muscle mass, and strength. In: Holloszy JO, editor. Exercise and sport sciences reviews. Philadelphia: Williams and Wilkins; 1994. p. 285–312.
8. Horohov DW, Dimock AN, Gurinalda PD, et al. Effects of exercise on the immune response of young and old horses. Am J Vet Res 1999;60:643–7.
9. Malinowski K, Christensen RA, Konopka A, et al. Feed intake, body weight, body condition score, musculation, and immunocompetence in aged mares given equine somatotropin. J Anim Sci 1997;75:755–60.
10. McKeever KH, Malinowski K, Christensen RA, et al. Chronic equine somatotropin administration does not affect aerobic capacity or indices of exercise performance in geriatric horses. Vet J 1997;155:19–25.
11. Day TRJ, Potter GD, Morris EL. Physiologic and skeletal response to exogenous equine growth hormone in two-year-old horses in race training. Proc 15th Equine Nutr Physiol Soc Symp 1997. p. 53–8.
12. Gerard MP, Hodgson DR, Lambeth RR, et al. Effects of somatotropin and training on indices of exercise capacity in Standardbreds. Equine Vet J Suppl 2002;34:496–501.
13. Smith LA, Thompson DL, French DD, et al. Effects of recombinant equine somatotropin on wound healing, carbohydrate and lipid metabolism, and endogenous somatotropin responses to secretagogues in geldings. J Anim Sci 1999;77:1815–22.
14. Thornton JR. Hormonal responses to exercise and training. Vet Clin North Am Equine Pract 1985;2:477–96.
15. Alexander SL, Irvine CH, Ellis MJ, et al. The effect of acute exercise on the secretion of corticotropin-releasing factor, arginine vasopressin, and adrenocorticotropin as measured in pituitary venous blood from the horse. Endocrinology 1991;128: 65–72.

16. Marc M, Parvizi N, Ellendorff F, et al. Plasma cortisol and ACTH concentrations in the warmblood horse in response to a standardized treadmill exercise test as physiological markers for evaluation of training status. J Anim Sci 2000;78: 1936–46.
17. Nagata S, Takeda F, Kurosawa M, et al. Plasma adrenocorticotropin, cortisol and catecholamines response to various exercises. Equine Vet J Suppl 1999;30: 570–4.
18. Liburt NR, McKeever KH, Smarsh D, et al. The hypothalamic pituitary adrenal axis response to stimulation tests before and after exercise training in old vs. young Standardbred mares. Proceedings of the Havemeyer Foundation Geriatric Horse Workshop, Cummings School of Veterinary Medicine Tufts University. Cambridge (MA); October, 2010.
19. Liburt NR, Smarsh D, Avanatti R, et al. Response of the equine HPA axis to acute, exhaustive exercise before and after training in old vs. young Standardbred mares. Proceedings of the Havemeyer Foundation Geriatric Horse Workshop, Cummings School of Veterinary Medicine Tufts University. Cambridge (MA); October, 2010.
20. Malinowski K, Shock E, Roegner V, et al. Plasma beta-endorphin, cortisol, and immune responses to acute exercise are altered by age and exercise training in horses. Equine Vet J Suppl 2006;36:267–73.
21. Convertino VA. Blood volume: its adaptation to endurance training. Med Sci Sports Exerc 1991;23:1338–48.
22. Wade CE, Freund BJ. Hormonal control of blood volume during and following exercise. In: Gisolfi CV, Lamb DR, editors. Perspectives in exercise science and sports medicine volume 3: fluid homeostasis during exercise. Carmel (IN): Benchmark Press; 1990. p. 207–45.
23. McKeever KH, Hinchcliff KW. Neuroendocrine control of blood volume, blood pressure, and cardiovascular function in horses. Equine Vet J Suppl 1995;18: 77–81.
24. McKeever KH, Hinchcliff KW, Schmall LM, et al. Plasma renin activity, aldosterone, and vasopressin, during incremental exercise in horses. Am J Vet Res 1992;53:1290–3.
25. McKeever KH, Hinchcliff KW, Schmall LM, et al. Renal tubular function in horses during submaximal exercise. Am J Physiol 1991;261:R553–60.
26. Gonzalez O, Gonzalez F, Sanchez C, et al. Effect of exercise on erythrocyte beta-adrenergic receptors and plasma concentrations of catecholamines and thyroid hormones in Thoroughbred horses. Equine Vet J 1998;30:72–8.
27. Graves EA, Schott HC 2nd, Marteniuk JV, et al. Thyroid hormone responses to endurance exercise. Equine Vet J Suppl 2006;36:32–6.
28. Chiba S, Kanematsu S, Murakami K, et al. Serum parathyroid hormone and calcitonin levels in racehorses with fracture. J Vet Med Sci 2000;62:361–5.
29. Inzerillo AM, Zaidi M, Huang CL. Calcitonin: the other thyroid hormone. Thyroid 2002;12:791–8.
30. Aguilera-Tejero E, Garfia B, Estepa JC, et al. Effects of exercise and EDTA administration on blood ionized calcium and parathyroid hormone in horses. Am J Vet Res 1998;59:1605–7.
31. Aguilera-Tejero E, Estepa JC, Lopez I, et al. Plasma ionized calcium and parathyroid hormone concentrations in horses after endurance rides. J Am Vet Med Assoc 2001;219:488–90.
32. McKeever KH. Sympatholytic and sympathomimetics. Vet Clin North Am Equine Practice 1993;9:1–13.

33. Baragli P, Pacchini S, Gatta D, et al. Brief note about plasma catecholamines kinetics and submaximal exercise in untrained standardbreds. Ann Ist Super Sanita 2010;46(1):96–100.
34. McKeever KH. Fluid balance and renal function in exercising horses. Vet Clin North Am Equine Practice 1998;14:23–44.
35. McKeever KH, Geiser S, Kearns CF. Role of the renin-angiotensin aldosterone cascade in the pulmonary artery pressure response to exercise in horses. The Physiologist 2000;43:356.
36. Wade CE, Freund BJ. Hormonal control of blood volume during and following exercise. In: Gisolfi CV, Lamb DR, editors. Perspectives in exercise science and sports medicine, vol. 3: fluid homeostasis during exercise. Carmel (IN): Benchmark; 1990. p. 207–45.
37. McKeever KH, Antas LA, Kearns CF. Endothelin response during exercise in horses. Vet J 2002;164:41–9.
38. McKeever KH, Scali R, Geiser S, et al. Plasma aldosterone concentration and renal sodium excretion are altered during the first days of training. Equine Vet J Suppl 2002;34:524–31.
39. Kokkonen UM, Poso AR, Hyyppa S, et al. Exercise-induced changes in atrial peptides in relation to neuroendocrine responses and fluid balance in the horse. J Vet Med A Physiol Pathol Clin Med 2002;49:144–50.
40. Hyyppa S, Saastamoinen M, Poso AR. Restoration of water and electrolyte balance in horses after repeated exercise in hot and humid conditions. Equine Vet J Suppl 1996;22:108–12.
41. Farris JW, Hinchcliff KW, McKeever KH. Treadmill endurance of Standardbred horses with tryptophan or glucose. J Appl Physiol 1998;85:807–16.
42. Caloni F, Spotti M, Villa R, et al. Hydrocortisone levels in the urine and blood of horses treated with ACTH. Equine Vet J 1999;31:273–6.
43. Lassourd V, Gayrard V, Laroute V, et al. Cortisol disposition and production rate in horses during rest and exercise. Am J Physiol 1996;271:R25–33.
44. Toutain PL, Lassourd V, Popot MA, et al. Urinary cortisol excretion in the resting and exercising horse. Equine Vet J Suppl 1995;18:457–62.
45. Snow DH, Rose RJ. Hormonal changes associated with long distance exercise. Equine Vet J 1981;13:195–7.
46. Davie AJ, Evans DL, Hodgson DR, et al. Effects of muscle glycogen depletion on some metabolic and physiological responses to submaximal treadmill exercise. Can J Vet Res 1999;63:241–7.
47. De La Corte FD, Valberg SJ, Mickelson JR, et al. Blood glucose clearance after feeding and exercise in polysaccharide storage myopathy. Equine Vet J Suppl 1999;30:324–8.
48. Dybdal NO, Gribble D, Madigan JE, et al. Alterations in plasma corticosteroids, insulin and selected metabolites in horses used in endurance rides. Equine Vet J 1980;12:137–40.
49. Freestone JF, Wolfsheimer KJ, Kamerling SG, et al. Exercise induced hormonal and metabolic changes in Thoroughbred horses: effects of conditioning and acepromazine. Equine Vet J 1991;23:219–23.
50. Geor RJ, Hinchcliff KW, McCutcheon LJ, et al. Epinephrine inhibits exogenous glucose utilization in exercising horses. J Appl Physiol 2000;88: 1777–90.
51. Geor RJ, Hinchcliff KW, Sams RA. Beta-adrenergic blockade augments glucose utilization in horses during graded exercise. J Appl Physiol 2000;89: 1086–98.

52. Gordon ME, Betros CL, Manso HC, et al. Plasma leptin, ghrelin, and adiponectin concentrations in fit vs. unfit Standardbred mares. Vet J 2007;173:93–102.
53. Farris JW, Hinchcliff KW, McKeever KH, et al. Effect of tryptophan and of glucose on exercise capacity of horses. J Appl Physiol 1998;85:807–16.
54. Geor RJ, Larsen L, Waterfall HL, et al. Route of carbohydrate administration affects early post exercise muscle glycogen storage in horses. Equine Vet J Suppl 2006;36:590–5.
55. Pratt SE, Geor RJ, Spriet LL, et al. Time course of insulin sensitivity and skeletal muscle glycogen synthase activity after a single bout of exercise in horses. J Appl Physiol 2007;103(3):1063–9.
56. Lawrence LM, Williams J, Soderholm LV, et al. Effect of feeding state on the response of horses to repeated bouts of intense exercise. Equine Vet J 1995; 27:27–30.
57. Rodiek A, Bonvicin S, Stull C, et al. Glycaemic and endocrine responses to corn or alfalfa fed prior to exercise. In: Persson SG, Lindholm A, Jeffcott LB, editors. Equine exercise physiology 3. Davis (CA): ICEEP Press; 1991. p. 368–73.
58. Stull CL, Rodiek AV. Effects of post prandial interval and feed type on substrate availability during exercise. Equine Vet J Suppl 1995;18:363–6.
59. Williams CA, Kronfeld DS, Staniar WB, et al. Plasma glucose and insulin responses of Thoroughbred mares fed a meal high in starch and sugar or fat and fiber. J Anim Sci 2001;79:2196–201.
60. Carter RA, McCutcheon LJ, Valle E, et al. Effects of exercise training on adiposity, insulin sensitivity, and plasma hormone and lipid concentrations in overweight or obese, insulin-resistant horses. Am J Vet Res 2010;71(3):314–21.
61. Geor RJ, McCutcheon LJ, Hinchcliff KW, et al. Training-induced alterations in glucose metabolism during moderate-intensity exercise. Equine Vet J Suppl 2002;34:22–8.
62. Stewart-Hunt L, Geor RJ, McCutcheon LJ. Effects of short-term training on insulin sensitivity and skeletal muscle glucose metabolism in standardbred horses. Equine Vet J Suppl 2006;36:226–32.
63. Jablonska EM, Ziolkowska SM, Gill J, et al. Changes in some haematological and metabolic indices in young horses during the first year of jump-training. Equine Vet J 1991;23:309–11.
64. Farrell PA. Exercise effects on regulation of energy metabolism by pancreatic and gut hormones. In: Lamb DR, Gisolfi CV, editors. Perspectives in exercise science and sports medicine: energy metabolism in exercise and sport. Carmel (IN): Brown and Benchmark; 1992. p. 383–434.
65. Hall GM, Adrian TE, Bloom SR, et al. Changes in circulating gut hormones in the horse during long distance exercise. Equine Vet J 1982;14:209–12.
66. Ahren B, Rorsman P, Berggren PO. Galanin and the endocrine pancreas. FEBS Lett 1988;229:233–7.
67. Legakis IN, Mantzouridis T, Saramantis A, et al. Human galanin secretion is increased upon normal exercise test in middle-age individuals. Endocr Res 2000;26:357–64.
68. Furr M, Taylor L, Kronfeld D. The effects of exercise training on serum gastrin responses in the horse. Cornell Vet 1994;84:41–5.
69. Sandin A, Girma K, Sjöholm B, et al. Effects of differently composed feeds and physical stress on plasma gastrin concentration in horses. Acta Vet Scand 1998; 39:265–72.
70. Ferrari R, Ceconi C, Rodella A, et al. Temporal relations of the endocrine response to exercise. Cardioscience 1991;2:131–9.

71. Halaas JL, Gajiwala KS, Maffei M, et al. Weight-reducing effects of the plasma protein encoded by the obese gene. Science 1995;269:543–6.
72. Zhang Y, Proenca R, Maffei M, et al. Positional cloning of the mouse obese gene and its human homologue. Nature 1994;372:425–32.
73. Schwartz MW, Woods SC, Porte D Jr, et al. Central nervous system control of food intake. Nature 2000;404:661–71.
74. Saper CB, Chou TC, Elmquist JK. The need to feed: homeostatic and hedonic control of eating. Neuron 2002;36:199–211.
75. Giacobino JP. Uncoupling proteins, leptin, and obesity: an updated review. Ann N Y Acad Sci 2002;967:398–402.
76. Hamilton BS, Paglia D, Kwan AY, et al. Increased obese mRNA expression in omental fat cells from massively obese humans. Nat Med 1995;1:953–6.
77. Buff PR, Dodds AC, Morrison CD, et al. Leptin in horses: tissue localization and relationship between peripheral concentrations of leptin and body condition. J Anim Sci 2002;80:2942–8.
78. Kearns CF, McKeever KH, Roegner V, et al. Adiponectin and leptin are related to fat mass in horses. Vet J 2006;172:460–5.
79. Fitzgerald BP, McManus CJ. Photoperiodic versus metabolic signals as determinants of seasonal anestrus in the mare. Biol Reprod 2000;63: 335–40.
80. Frape DL. Dietary requirements and athletic performance of horses. Equine Vet J 1988;20:163–72.
81. McManus CJ, Fitzgerald BP. Effects of a single day of feed restriction on changes in serum leptin, gonadotropins, prolactin, and metabolites in aged and young mares. Domest Anim Endocrinol 2000;19:1–13.
82. Saad MF, Damani S, Gingerich RL, et al. Sexual dimorphism in plasma leptin concentration. J Clin Endocrinol Metab 1997;82:579–84.
83. Mulet T, Pico C, Oliver P, et al. Blood leptin homeostasis: sex-associated differences in circulating leptin levels in rats are independent of tissue leptin expression. Int J Biochem Cell Biol 2003;35:104–10.
84. Weltman A, Pritzlaff CJ, Wideman L, et al. Intensity of acute exercise does not affect serum leptin concentrations in young men. Med Sci Sports Exerc 2000; 32:1556–61.
85. Fisher JS, Van Pelt RE, Zinder O, et al. Acute exercise effect on postabsorptive serum leptin. J Appl Physiol 2001;91:680–6.
86. Leal-Cerro A, Garcia-Luna PP, Astorga R, et al. Serum leptin levels in male marathon athletes before and after the marathon run. J Clin Endocrinol Metab 1998; 83:2376–9.
87. Torjman MC, Zafeiridis A, Paolone AM, et al. Serum leptin during recovery following maximal incremental and prolonged exercise. Int J Sports Med 1999;20:444–50.
88. Halle M, Berg A, Garwers U, et al. Concurrent reductions of serum leptin and lipids during weight loss in obese men with type II diabetes. Am J Physiol 1999;277:E277–82.
89. Houmard JA, Cox JH, MacLean PS, et al. Effect of short-term exercise training on leptin and insulin action. Metabolism 2000;49:858–61.
90. Okazaki T, Himeno E, Nanri H, et al. Effects of mild aerobic exercise and a mild hypocaloric diet on plasma leptin in sedentary women. Clin Exp Pharmacol Physiol 1999;26:415–20.
91. Pasman WJ, Westerterp-Plantenga MS, Saris WH. The effect of exercise training on leptin levels in obese males. Am J Physiol 1998;274:E280–6.

92. Hickey MS, Houmard JA, Considine RV, et al. Gender-dependent effects of exercise training on serum leptin levels in humans. Am J Physiol 1997;272: E562–6.
93. Berg AH, Combs TP, Scherer PE. ACRP30/adiponectin: an adipokine regulating glucose and lipid metabolism. Trends Endocrinol Metab 2002;13:84–9.
94. Arita Y, Kihara S, Ouchi N, et al. Paradoxical decrease of an adipose-specific protein, adiponectin, in obesity. Biochem Biophys Res Commun 1999;257: 79–83.
95. Malinowski K, Betros CL, Flora L, et al. Effect of training on age-related changes in plasma insulin and glucose. Equine Vet J Suppl 2002;34:147–53.
96. Powell DM, Reedy SE, Sessions DR, et al. Effect of short-term exercise training on insulin sensitivity in obese and lean mares. Equine Vet J Suppl 2002;34:81–4.
97. Kojima M, Hosoda H, Date Y, et al. Ghrelin is a growth-hormone-releasing acylated peptide from stomach. Nature 1999;402:656–60.
98. Sugino T, Hasegawa Y, Kikkawa Y, et al. A transient ghrelin surge occurs just before feeding in a scheduled meal-fed sheep. Biochem Biophys Res Commun 2002;295:255–60.
99. Masuda Y, Tanaka T, Inomata N, et al. Ghrelin stimulates gastric acid secretion and motility in rats. Biochem Biophys Res Commun 2000;276:905–8.
100. Dall R, Kanaley J, Hansen TK, et al. Plasma ghrelin levels during exercise in healthy subjects and in growth hormone-deficient patients. Eur J Endocrinol 2002;147:65–70.
101. Otto B, Cuntz U, Fruehauf E, et al. Weight gain decreases elevated plasma ghrelin concentrations of patients with anorexia nervosa. Eur J Endocrinol 2001;145:669–73.
102. Ballinger A, McLoughlin L, Medbak S, et al. Cholecystokinin is a satiety hormone in humans at physiological post-prandial plasma concentrations. Clin Sci (Lond) 1995;89:375–81.
103. Matson CA, Reid DF, Ritter RC. Daily CCK injection enhances reduction of body weight by chronic intracerebroventricular leptin infusion. Am J Physiol Regul Integr Comp Physiol 2002;282:R1368–73.
104. Bagnasco M, Dube MG, Kalra PS, et al. Evidence for the existence of distinct central appetite, energy expenditure, and ghrelin stimulation pathways as revealed by hypothalamic site-specific leptin gene therapy. Endocrinology 2002; 143:4409–21.
105. Bodary PF, Pate RR, Wu PF, et al. Effects of acute exercise on plasma erythropoietin levels in trained runners. Med Sci Sports Exerc 1999;31:543–6.
106. Adamson JW, Vapnek D. Recombinant erythropoietin to improve athletic performance. N Engl J Med 1991;324:698–9.
107. Berglund B, Ekblom B. Effect of recombinant human erythropoietin treatment on blood pressure and some haematological parameters in healthy men. J Intern Med 1991;229:125–30.
108. Jaussaud P, Audran M, Gareau RL, et al. Kinetics and haematological effects of erythropoietin in horses. Vet Res 1994;25:1–7.
109. McKeever KH. Erythropoietin: a new form of blood doping in horses. In: Wade J, editor. Proceedings 11th International Conference of racing analysts and veterinarians. Newmarket (UK): R&W Press; 1996. p. 79–84.
110. Piercy RJ, Swardson CJ, Hinchcliff KW. Erythroid hypoplasia and anemia following administration of recombinant human erythropoietin to two horses. J Am Vet Med Assoc 1998;212:244–7.

111. McKeever KH, Agans JM, Geiser S, et al. Low dose exogenous erythropoietin elicits an ergogenic effect in Standardbred horses. Equine Vet J Suppl 2006; 36:233–8.
112. McKeever KH, McNally BA, Kirby KM, et al. Effect of erythropoietin on plasma and red cell volume, VO_{2max}, and hemodynamics in exercising horses. Med Sci Sports Exerc 1993;25:S25.
113. McKeever KH, Malinowski K. Endocrine response to exercise in young and old horses. Equine Vet J Suppl 1999;30:561–6.
114. Nyman S, Kokkonen UM, Dahlborn K. Changes in plasma atrial natriuretic peptide concentration in exercising horses in relation to hydration status and exercise intensity. Am J Vet Res 1998;59:489–94.
115. Kokkonen UM, Hackzell M, Rasanen LA. Plasma atrial natriuretic peptide in standardbred and Finnhorse trotters during and after exercise. Acta Physiol Scand 1995;154:51–8.
116. Benamou AE, Art T, Marlin DJ, et al. Effect of exercise on concentrations of immunoreactive endothelin in bronchoalveolar lavage fluid of normal horses and horses with chronic obstructive pulmonary disease. Equine Vet J Suppl 1999;30:92–5.
117. Benamou AE, Art T, Marlin DJ, et al. Variations in systemic and pulmonary endothelin-1 in horses with recurrent airway obstruction (heaves). Pulm Pharmacol Ther 1998;11:231–5.

Index

Note: Page numbers of article titles are in **boldface** type.

Vet Clin Equine 27 (2011) 219–231
doi:10.1016/S0749-0739(11)00012-5 vetequine.theclinics.com

N

O

P

Printed and bound by CPI Group (UK) Ltd, Croydon, CR0 4YY

03/10/2024

01040455-0006